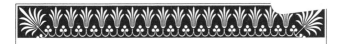

THE PRINCE
OF MEDICINE

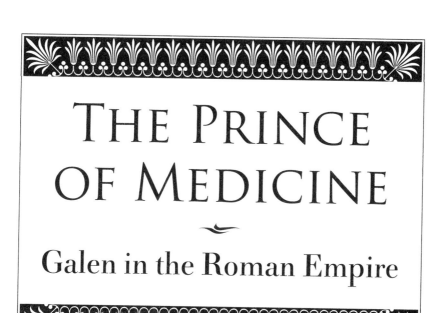

THE PRINCE
OF MEDICINE

Galen in the Roman Empire

Susan P. Mattern

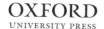

OXFORD
UNIVERSITY PRESS

OXFORD

UNIVERSITY PRESS

Oxford University Press is a department of the University of Oxford.
It furthers the University's objective of excellence in research, scholarship,
and education by publishing worldwide.

Oxford   New York

Auckland   Cape Town   Dar es Salaam   Hong Kong   Karachi
Kuala Lumpur   Madrid   Melbourne   Mexico City   Nairobi
New Delhi   Shanghai   Taipei   Toronto

With offices in

Argentina   Austria   Brazil   Chile   Czech Republic   France   Greece
Guatemala   Hungary   Italy   Japan   Poland   Portugal   Singapore
South Korea   Switzerland   Thailand   Turkey   Ukraine   Vietnam

Oxford is a registered trademark of Oxford University Press
in the UK and certain other countries.

Published in the United States of America by
Oxford University Press
198 Madison Avenue, New York, NY 10016

© Susan P. Mattern 2013

Library of Congress Cataloging-in-Publication Data
Mattern, Susan P., 1966–
The Prince of Medicine: Galen in the Roman Empire / Susan P. Mattern.
p. ; cm.
Galen in the Roman Empire
Includes bibliographical references and index.
ISBN 978–0–19–976767–0
I. Title.   II. Title: Galen in the Roman Empire.
DNLM: 1. Galen.   2. Physicians—Biography.   3. History of Medicine.   4. History,
Ancient.   5. Roman World. WZ   100
610.938 – dc23
2012035656

1 3 5 7 9 8 6 4 2
Printed in the United States of America
on acid-free paper

Acknowledgments

I thank Rob McQuilkin of Lippincott Massie McQuilkin for his exhaustive and most helpful efforts on the original proposal and manuscript of this book. Stefan Vranka, editor at Oxford University Press, and an anonymous reader for the Press also made invaluable suggestions. The cartography is the fine work of Wendy Giminski.

ABBREVIATIONS OF
GALEN'S WORKS

Abbreviations are followed by the full Latin title in Kühn or in the standard modern edition, the English title used in this book, and reference to the most reliable modern critical edition of the text, if this is not Kühn's edition. For all other works, the most recent edition is C. G. Kühn, *Claudii Galeni Opera Omnia*, 20 vols. (Leipzig: Cnobloch, 1821–33); reprinted in 22 vols. (Hildesheim: Olms, 1964–65). Modern English translations are also noted.

For the sake of simplicity I have referred to volume and page numbers in Kühn's edition throughout this book.

Adhort. Art. = *Adhortatio ad artes addiscendas*. Edition, with French translation: Véronique Boudon, *Galien*, Vol. 2, *Exhortation à l'étude de la médecine; Art medical* (Paris: Les Belles Lettres, 2000). English translation: P. N. Singer, *Galen: Selected Works* (Oxford and New York: Oxford University Press, 1997).

Adv. Jul. = *Adversus ea quae a Juliano in Hippocratis aphorismos enuntiata sunt* (*Against Julian's Criticisms of the Aphorisms of Hippocrates*). Edition: Ernst Wenkebach, Corpus Medicorum Graecorum 5.10.3 (Berlin: Akademie-Verlag, 1951).

Adv. Lyc. = *Adversus Lycum* (*Against Lycus*). Edition: Ernst Wenkebach, Corpus Medicorum Graecorum 5.10.3 (Berlin: Akademie-Verlag, 1951).

Aliment. Fac. = *De alimentorum facultatibus*. Edition: Konrad Koch et al., Corpus Medicorum Graecorum 5.4.2 (Leipzig: Teubner, 1923). Translations: O. W. Powell and John Wilkins, *On the Properties of Foodstuffs* (Cambridge and New York:

Cambridge University Press, 2003). Mark Grant, *Galen on Food and Diet* (London: Routledge, 2000).

An. Arter. Sang. = *An in arteriis natura sanguis contineatur* (*Whether the Arteries Naturally Contain Blood*). Translation: David J. Furley and J. S. Wilkie, *Galen on Respiration and the Arteries* (Princeton, NJ: Princeton University Press, 1984).

Anat. Admin. = *De anatomicis administrationibus* (*On Anatomical Procedures*). Edition of books surviving in Greek: Ivan Garofalo, *Galenus: Anatomicarum administrationum libri quae supersunt novem*, 2 vols. (Naples: Brill, 1986). Edition of books surviving in Arabic, with German translation: Max Simon, *Sieben Bücher Anatomie des Galen* (Leipzig: J. C. Hinrichs'sche Buchhandlung, 1906). Translation of books surviving in Greek: Charles Singer, *On Anatomical Procedures* (London: Oxford University Press for the Wellcome Historical Medical Museum, 1956). Translation of books surviving in Arabic: Malcolm Lyons and B. Towers, eds., and W. L. H. Duckworth, tran., *On Anatomical Procedures: The Later Books* (Cambridge: Cambridge University Press, 1962).

Anim. Affect. Dign., Anim. Peccat. Dign. = *De animi cuiuslibet affectuum et peccatorum dignotione et curatione* (*On Diagnosing and Curing the Affections and Errors of the Soul*). Edition: Wilko de Boer, Corpus Medicorum Graecorum 5.4.1.1 (Leipzig: Teubner, 1937). Translations: P. N. Singer, *Galen: Selected Works* (Oxford and New York: Oxford University Press, 1997); Paul W. Harkins and Walther Riese, *Galen on the Passions and Errors of the Soul* (Columbus: Ohio State University Press, 1963).

Anim. Mor. Corp. = *Quod animi mores corporis temperamenta sequantur* (*That the Soul Follows the Mixtures of the Body*). Edition: Johann Marquardt, Iwan von Müller, and Georg Helmreich, eds., *Claudii Galeni Pergameni Scripta Minora*, 3 vols. (Leipzig: Teubner, 1884–93), Vol. 2 (repr. Amsterdam: Hakkert, 1967). Translation: P. N. Singer, *Galen: Selected Works* (Oxford and New York: Oxford University Press, 1997).

Antid. = *De antidotis* (*On Antidotes*).

Ars Med. = *Ars medica* (*The Art of Medicine*). Edition, with French translation: Véronique Boudon, *Galien*, Vol. 2, *Exhortation à l'étude de la médecine; Art médical* (Paris: Les Belles Lettres, 2000). English translation: P. N. Singer, *Galen: Selected Works* (Oxford and New York: Oxford University Press, 1997).

Atra Bile = *De atra bile.* Edition: Wilko de Boer, Corpus Medicorum Graecorum 5.4.1.1 (Leipzig: Teubner, 1937). Translation: Mark Grant, *Galen on Food and Diet* (London: Routledge, 2000).

Bon. Hab. = *De bono habitu.* Translation: P. N. Singer, *Galen: Selected Works* (Oxford and New York: Oxford University Press, 1997).

Bon. Mal. Suc. = *De bonis malisque sucis* (*On Good and Bad Humors*). Edition: Konrad Koch et al., Corpus Medicorum Graecorum 5.4.2 (Leipzig: Teubner, 1923). Edition, with Italian translation: Anna Maria Ieraci Bio, *De bonis malisque sucis* (Naples: M. D'Auria, 1987).

Caus. morb. = *De causis morborum* (*On the Causes of Diseases*). Translation: Ian Johnston, *Galen on Diseases and Symptoms* (Cambridge and New York: Cambridge University Press, 2006).

Caus. Puls. = *De causis pulsuum* (*On the Causes of Pulses*).

Caus. Resp. = *De causis respirationis* (*On the Causes of Respiration*). Translation: David J. Furley and J. S. Wilkie, *Galen on Respiration and the Arteries* (Princeton, NJ: Princeton University Press, 1984).

Comp. Med. Gen. = *De compositione medicamentorum per genera* (*On the Composition of Drugs by Type*).

Comp. Med. Loc. = *De compositione medicamentorum secundum locos* (*On the Composition of Drugs by Part*).

Cris. = *De crisibus* (*On Crises*). Edition, with German translation: Bengt Alexanderson, *ΠΕΡΙ ΚΡΙΣΕΩΝ: Überlieferung und Text*, Studia Graeca et Latina Gothoburgensia 23 (Stockholm, 1967).

Cur. Ven. Sect. = *De curandi ratione per venae sectionem* (*On Treatment by Venesection*). Translation: Peter Brain, *Galen on Bloodletting* (Cambridge: Cambridge University Press, 1986).

Dieb. Decret. = *De diebus decretoriis* (*On Critical Days*).

Diff. Puls. = *De differentia pulsuum* (*On the Differences in Pulses*).

Diff. Resp. = *De difficultate respirationis*.

Dign. Insomn. = *De dignotione ex insomniis* (*On Diagnosis from Dreams*). Translation: Steven M. Oberhelman, "Galen, *On Diagnosis from Dreams*," *Journal of the History of Medicine and Allied Sciences* 38 (1983): 36–47.

Dign. puls. = *De dignoscendis pulsibus* (*On the Diagnosis of Pulses*).

Elem. Hipp. = *De elementis ex Hippocratis sententia* (*On the Elements According to Hippocrates*). Edition, with English translation: Phillip de Lacy, Corpus Medicorum Graecorum 5.1.2 (Berlin: Akademie-Verlag, 1996).

Exp. Med. = *De experientia medica* (*On Medical Experience*). Arabic. Edition, with English translation: R. Walzer, *Galen on Medical Experience* (London and New York: Oxford University Press for the Trustees of Sir Henry Wellcome, 1944). Translation reprinted in M. Frede and R. Walzer, *Three Treatises on the Nature of Science* (Indianapolis: Hackett, 1985).

Febr. Diff. = *De febrium differentiis* (*On the Differences in Fevers*).

Foet. Form. = *De foetuum formatione* (*On the Formation of the Fetus*). Translation: P. N. Singer, *Galen: Selected Works* (Oxford and New York: Oxford University Press, 1997).

Hipp. 1 Epid. = *In Hippocratis Epidemiarum librum primum commentarius*. Edition: Ernst Wenkebach and Franz Pfaff, Corpus Medicorum Graecorum 5.10.1 (Leipzig: Teubner, 1934).

Hipp. 1 Prorrh. = *In Hippocratis librum primum Prorrheticum commentarius*. Edition: Hermann Diels, Johannes Mewaldt, and Joseph Heeg, Corpus Medicorum Graecorum 5.9.2 (Leipzig: Teubner, 1915).

Hipp. 2 Epid. = *In Hippocratis Epidemiarum librum secundum commentarius*. Arabic. Edition, with German translation: Ernst Wenkebach and Franz Pfaff, Corpus Medicorum Graecorum 5.10.1 (Leipzig: Teubner, 1934).

Hipp. 3 Epid. = *In Hippocratis Epidemiarum librum tertium commentarius*. Edition: Ernst Wenkebach, Corpus Medicorum Graecorum 5.10.2.1 (Leipzig: Teubner, 1936).

Hipp. 6 Epid. = *In Hippocratis Epidemiarum librum sextum commentarius*. Edition, with German translation of parts surviving in Arabic: Ernst Wenkebach and Franz Pfaff, Corpus Medicorum Graecorum 5.10.2.2, 2d ed. (Berlin: Akademie-Verlag, 1956).

Hipp. Acut. Vict. = *In Hippocratis De victu acutorum commentarius*. Edition: Georg Helmreich, Corpus Medicorum Graecorum 5.9.1 (Leipzig: Teubner, 1914).

Hipp. Aph. = *In Hippocratis Aphorismos commentarius*.

Hipp. Artic. = *In Hippocratis librum De articulis commentarius*.

Hipp. Fract. = *In Hippocratis librum De fracturis commentarius*.

Hipp. Nat. Hom. = *In Hippocratis De natura hominis librum commentarius* (*On Hippocrates' The Nature of Man*). Edition: Johannes Mewaldt, Corpus Medicorum Graecorum 5.9.1 (Leipzig: Teubner, 1914).

Hipp. Off. = *In Hippocratis librum De officina medici commentarius*. Greek and Arabic. Edition of Arabic text, with English translation: Malcolm Lyons, Corpus Medicorum Graecorum, Supplementum Orientale 1 (Berlin: Akademie-Verlag, 1963).

Hipp. Prog. = *In Hippocratis Prognostica commentarius*. Edition: Hermann Diels, Johannes Mewaldt, and Joseph Heeg, Corpus Medicorum Graecorum 5.9.2 (Leipzig: Teubner, 1915).

Ind. = *De indolentia* (*Avoiding Distress*). Editions, with French translations: Véronique Boudon-Millot, "Un traité perdu de Galien miraculeusement retrouvé, le *Sur l'inutilité de se chagriner*: Texte grec et traduction française," in *La Science médicale antique: Nouveaux regards,* ed. V. Boudon-Millot, A. Guardasole, and C. Magdelaine (Paris: Beauchesne, 2007), 67–118; Véronique Boudon-Millot and Jacques Jouanna, *Galien*, Vol. 4, *Ne pas se chagriner* (Paris: Les Belles Lettres, 2010).

Instr. oder. = *De instrumento oderatus* (*On the Organ of Smelling*). Edition, with German translation: Jutta Kollesch, Corpus Medicorum Graecorum Supplementum 5 (Berlin: Akademie-Verlag, 1964).

Libr. Propr. = *De libris propiis* (*On My Own Books*). Edition, with French translation: Véronique Boudon-Millot, *Galien*, Vol. 1, *Introduction générale; Sur l'ordre de ses propres livres; Sur ses propres livres; Que l'excellent médecin est aussi philosophe* (Paris: Les Belles Lettres, 2007). English translation: P. N. Singer, *Galen: Selected Works* (Oxford and New York: Oxford University Press, 1997). Note: Singer's translation was made before the discovery of a new manuscript of this treatise, with a long passage that did not survive in the single manuscript previously known.

Loc. Affect. = *De locis affectis* (*On the Affected Parts*). Translation: Rudolph E. Siegel, *Galen on the Affected Parts* (Basel: S. Karger, 1976).

Meth. Med. = *De methodo medendi* (*On the Method of Healing*). Edition, with English translation: Ian Johnston and G. H. R. Horsley, *Galen: Method of Medicine*, 3 vols. (Cambridge, MA: Harvard University Press, 2011).

Meth. Med. Glauc. = *De methodo medendi ad Glauconem* (*On the Method of Healing to Glaucon*).

Mor. = *De moribus* (*On Characters*). Arabic. Edition: Paul Kraus, *Bulletin of the Faculty of Arts of the University of Egypt* 5.1 (1939): 1–51. English translation: J. N. Mattock, "A Translation of the Arabic Epitome of Galen's Book Περί ἠθῶν," in *Islamic Philosophy and the Classical Tradition*, ed. S. M. Stern, Albert Hourani, and Vivian Brown. Festschrift Richard Walzer (Columbia: University of South Carolina Press, 1972).

Morb. Diff. = *De morborum differentiis* (*On the Differences in Diseases*). Translation: Ian Johnston, *Galen on Diseases and Symptoms* (Cambridge and New York: Cambridge University Press, 2006).

Morb. Temp. = *De morborum temporibus.*

Motu Musc. = *De motu musculorum*. Edition, with Italian translation: Pietro Rosa (Pisa: Serra, 2009).

Musc. Dissect. = *De musculorum dissectione ad tirones* (*On the Anatomy of the Muscles*). Edition, with French translation: Ivan Garofalo and Armelle Debru, *Galien*, Vol. 7, *Les Os pour les debutants; L'Anatomie des muscles* (Paris: Les Belles Lettres, 2005). English translation: Charles Mayo Goss, "On the Anatomy of Muscles for Beginners," *Anatomical Record* 145 (1963): 477–501.

Nat. Fac. = *De naturalibus facultatibus* (*On the Natural Faculties*). Edition: Johann Marquardt, Iwan von Müller, and Georg Helmreich, eds., *Claudii Galeni Pergameni Scripta Minora*, 3 vols. (Leipzig: Teubner, 1884–93), Vol. 3 (repr. Amsterdam: Hakkert, 1967). Edition, with English translation: Arthur John Brock, *On the Natural Faculties* (London: Heinemann and Cambridge, MA: Harvard University Press, 1916).

Nerv. Dissect. = *De nervorum dissectione* (*On the Anatomy of the Nerves*). Edition of Greek, with French translation: Ivan Garofalo and Armelle Debru, *Galien*, Vol. 8, *L'Anatomie des nerfs; L'Anatomie des veines et des artères* (Paris: Les Belles Lettres, 2008). English translation of Greek version: Charles Mayo Goss, "On the Anatomy of the Nerves," *American Journal of Anatomy* 18 (1966): 327–36. Edition of Arabic version, with German translation: Ahmad M. Al-Dubayan, *Über die Anatomie der Nerven* (Berlin: Klaus Schwarz Verlag, 2000).

Nomin. Med. = *De nominibus medicis*. Arabic. Edition, with German translation: Max Meyerhof and Joseph Schacht, "Galen über die medizinischen Namen," *Abhandlungen der preussischen Akademie der Wissenschaften* 3 (1931).

Opt. Doct. = *De optima doctrina*. Edition: Johann Marquardt, Iwan von Müller, and Georg Helmreich, eds., *Claudii Galeni Pergameni Scripta Minora*, 3 vols. (Leipzig: Teubner, 1884–93), Vol. 1 (repr. Amsterdam: Hakkert, 1967).

Opt. Med. Cogn. = *De optimo medico cognoscendo* (*On the Examinations by which the Best Physicians are Recognized*). Arabic. Edition, with English translation: Albert Z. Iskandar, Corpus Medicorum Graecorum, Supplementum Orientale 4 (Berlin: Akademie-Verlag, 1988).

Opt. Med. Philosoph. = *Quod optimus medicus sit quoque philosophus* (*That the Best Physician is Also a Philosopher*). Edition, with French translation: Véronique Boudon-Millot, *Galien*, Vol. 1, *Introduction générale; Sur l'ordre de ses propres livres; Sur ses propres livres; Que l'excellent médecin est aussi philosophe* (Paris: Les Belles Lettres, 2007). Edition of Arabic version, with German translation: Peter Bachmann, *Galens Abhandlung darüber, dass der vorzügliche Arzt Philosoph sein muss* (Göttingen: Vanderhoeck & Ruprecht, 1966). English translation: P. N. Singer, *Galen: Selected Works* (Oxford and New York: Oxford University Press, 1997).

Ord. Libr. Propr. = *De ordine librorum suorum ad Eugenianum* (*On the Order of My Own Books*). Edition: Véronique Boudon-Millot, *Galien*, Vol. 1, *Introduction générale; Sur l'ordre de ses propres livres; Sur ses propres livres; Que l'excellent médecin est aussi philosophe* (Paris: Les Belles Lettres, 2007).

Oss. Tir. = *De ossibus ad tirones* (*On the Bones for Beginners*). Edition, with French translation: Ivan Garofalo and Armelle Debru, *Galien*, Vol. 7, *Les Os pour les debutants; L'Anatomie des muscles* (Paris: Les Belles Lettres, 2005).

Part. Med. = *De partibus artis medicativae*. Arabic and Latin. Edition, with English translation: Malcolm Lyons, Corpus Medicorum Graecorum, Supplementum Orientale 2 (Berlin: Akademie-Verlag, 1969).

Plac. Hipp. Plat. = *De placitis Hippocratis et Platonis* (*On the Doctrines of Hippocrates and Plato*). Edition, with English translation: Phillip de Lacy, Corpus Medicorum Graecorum 5.4.1.2, 2 vols., 3d ed. (Berlin: Akademie-Verlag, 1984).

Plac. Propr. = *De placitis propriis* (*On My Own Opinions*). Edition, with French translation, of the Greek text: Véronique Boudon-Millot and A. Pietrobelli, "Galien ressuscité: Édition *princeps* du texte grecque du *De propriis placitis*," *Revue des Études Grecques* 118 (2005): 168–213. Edition of the Latin translation from Arabic, with English translation: Vivian Nutton, Corpus Medicorum Graecorum 5.3.2 (Berlin: Akademie-Verlag, 1999). Note: No Greek manuscript of this treatise was known until recently; Nutton's edition pre-dates the discovery of the Greek text.

Plat. Tim. = *In Platonis Timaeum commentarii fragmenta*. Edition: H. O. Schröder, Corpus Medicorum Graecorum Supplementum 1 (Leipzig: Teubner, 1934).

Plen. = *De plenitudine* (*On Plenitude*). Edition, with German translation: Chrostoph Otte, *De plenitudine*, Serta Graeca: Beiträge zur Erforschung griechischer Texte 9 (Weisbaden: Reichert, 2001).

Praecog. = *De praecognitione* (*On Prognosis*). Edition, with English translation: Vivian Nutton, Corpus Medicorum Graecorum 5.8.1 (Berlin: Akademie-Verlag, 1979).

Praes. Puls. = *De praesagitione ex pulsibus* (*On Prognosis from Pulses*).

Puls. Tir. = *De pulsibus ad tirones* (*On the Pulse for Beginners*). Translation: P. N. Singer, *Galen: Selected Works* (Oxford and New York: Oxford University Press, 1997).

Purg. Med. Fac. = *De purgantium medicamentorum facultate.*

San. Tuend. = *De sanitate tuenda* (*On Healthfulness*). Edition: Konrad Koch et al., Corpus Medicorum Graecorum 5.4.2 (Leipzig: Teubner, 1923). Translation: Robert Montraville Green, *A Translation of Galen's Hygiene* (Springfield, IL: Thomas, 1951).

Sect. Intro. = *De sectis, ad eos qui introducuntur* (*On the Sects for Beginners*). Edition: Johann Marquardt, Iwan von Müller, and Georg Helmreich, eds., *Claudii Galeni Pergameni Scripta Minora*, 3 vols. (Leipzig: Teubner, 1884–93), Vol. 3 (repr. Amsterdam: Hakkert, 1967). Translation: M. Frede and R. Walzer, *Three Treatises on the Nature of Science* (Indianapolis: Hakkert, 1985).

Sem. = *De semine.* Edition, with English translation: Phillip de Lacy, Corpus Medicorum Graecorum 5.3.1 (Berlin: Akademie-Verlag, 1992).

Simp. Med. = *De simplicium medicamentorum temperamentis et facultatibus* (*On the Mixtures and Powers of Simple Drugs*).

Subfig. Emp. = *Subfiguratio empirica* (*Outline of Empiricism*). Edition: Karl Deichgräber, *Die griechische Empirikerschule: Sammlung der Fragmente und Darstellung der Lehre* (Berlin and Zurich: Weidmannsche Verlagsbuchhandlung, 1965). Translation: M. Frede and R. Walzer, *Three Treatises on the Nature of Science* (Indianapolis: Hakkert, 1985).

Sympt. Caus. = *De symptomatum causis* (*On the Causes of Symptoms*). Translation: Ian Johnston, *Galen on Diseases and Symptoms* (Cambridge and New York: Cambridge University Press, 2006).

Sympt. Diff. = *De symptomatum differentiis* (*On the Differences in Symptoms*). Translation: Ian Johnston, *Galen on Diseases and Symptoms* (Cambridge and New York: Cambridge University Press, 2006).

Syn. Puls. = *Synopsis librorum de pulsibus* (*Synopsis of the Books on Pulses*).

Temp. = *De temperamentis* (*On Mixtures*). Edition: Georg Helmreich, *Galeni De temperamentis libri III* (Leipzig: Teubner, 1904). Translation: P. N. Singer, *Galen: Selected Works* (Oxford and New York: Oxford University Press, 1997).

Ther. Pis. = *De theriaca ad Pisonem* (*On Theriac to Piso*).

Thras. Med. Gymn. = *Ad Thrasybulum utrum medicinae sit an gymnastices hygenie* (*To Thrasybulus on Whether Health belongs to Medicine or Gymnastics*). Edition: Johann Marquardt, Iwan von Müller, and Georg Helmreich, eds., *Claudii Galeni Pergameni Scripta Minora*, 3 vols. (Leipzig: Teubner, 1884–93), Vol. 3 (repr. Amsterdam: Hakkert, 1967). Translation: P. N. Singer, *Galen: Selected Works* (Oxford and New York: Oxford University Press, 1997).

Trem. Palp. = *De tremore, palpitatione, convulsione et rigore.*

Typ. = *De typis* (*On Types [of Fevers]*).

Usu Part. = *De usu partium* (*On the Usefulness of the Parts*). Edition: Georg Helmreich, *Galeni De usu partium libri XVII*, 2 vols. (Leipzig: Teubner, 1907–9) (repr. Amsterdam: Hakkert, 1968). Translation: Margaret Tallmadge May, *Galen: On the Usefulness of the Parts of the Body*, 2 vols. (Ithaca, NY: Cornell University Press, 1968).

Usu Puls. = *De usu pulsuum.* Translation: David J. Furley and J. S. Wilkie, *Galen on Respiration and the Arteries* (Princeton, NJ: Princeton University Press, 1984).

Usu Resp. = *De usu respirationis* (*On the Usefulness of Respiration*). Translation: David J. Furley and J. S. Wilkie, *Galen on Respiration and the Arteries* (Princeton, NJ: Princeton University Press, 1984).

Uter. Dissect. = *De uteri dissectione* (*On the Anatomy of the Uterus*). Edition, with German translation: Diethard Nickel, Corpus Medicorum Graecorum 5.2.1 (Berlin: Akademie-Verlag, 1971). English translation: Charles Mayo Goss, "On the Anatomy of the Uterus," *Anatomical Record* 144 (1962): 77–84.

Ven. Art. Dissect. = *De venarum arteriarumque dissectione* (*On the Anatomy of the Veins and Arteries*). Edition, with French translation: Ivan Garofalo and Armelle Debru, *Galien*, Vol. 8, *L'Anatomie des nerfs; L'anatomie des veines et des artères* (Paris: Les Belles Lettres, 2008). English translation: Charles Mayo Goss, "On the Anatomy of Veins and Arteries," *Anatomical Record* 141 (1961): 355–66.

Ven. Sect. Eras. = *De venae sectione adversus Erasistratum* (*On Venesection Against Erasistratus*). Translation: Peter Brain, *Galen on Bloodletting* (Cambridge: Cambridge University Press, 1986).

Ven. Sect. Eras. Rom. = *De venae sectione adversus Erasistrateos Romae degentes* (*On Venesection against the Erasistrateans at Rome*). Translation: Peter Brain, *Galen on Bloodletting* (Cambridge: Cambridge University Press, 1986).

CHRONOLOGICAL CHART

Emperors	Galen's Life
Trajan, 98–117	
Hadrian, 117–138	129, around the fall equinox in September: Galen is born.
Antoninus Pius, 138–161	143/144: Galen begins education with tutors in philosophy.
	145/146: Nicon's dream. Galen begins to study medicine with Satyrus and others.
	146, fall: Galen's serious illness begins.
	148: Nicon's death.
	150?: Galen leaves Pergamum to study with Pelops in Smyrna; travels to other cities seeking out the students of Quintus and Numisianus.
	151–153, fall: Galen arrives in Alexandria.
	156/157: Galen's serious illness cured by dream from Asclepius.
	157: Galen returns to Pergamum.
	157, fall, through summer 161: Galen is physician to the gladiators at Pergamum.

Emperors	Galen's Life
Marcus Aurelius, 161–180	161: Galen departs Pergamum.
Lucius Verus, 161–169	161/162?: Journeys to Lycia, Syria Palestina, and Cyprus.
	162, spring/summer: Galen arrives in Rome.
	162/163: Showdown with Martianus over the plethoric young woman. Winter: Cure of Eudemus; showdown with Martianus over Eudemus.
	164, summer: Wrestling injury.
	166, summer?: Galen leaves Rome for Pergamum.
	168: Galen summoned to Aquileia.
	168–169, winter: Galen treats victims of "the great plague" at Aquileia.
	169: Galen appointed personal physician to emperor's heir Commodus; begins receiving imperial salary?
	169–176: Galen professedly retires from public life. Appointed official maker of theriac for Marcus. Cure of Commodus. Publication of *On the Usefulness of the Parts.*
	176: Cure of Marcus Aurelius.
Commodus, 177–192	192, late winter/early spring: Great fire at Rome.
Pertinax, 193	
Didius Julianus, 193	
Septimius Severus, 193–211	
Caracalla, 197–217	
Geta, 209–211	
	216/217: Galen's death.
Macrinus, 217–218	
Elagabalus, 218–222	

Note: All dates are C.E.

MAPS

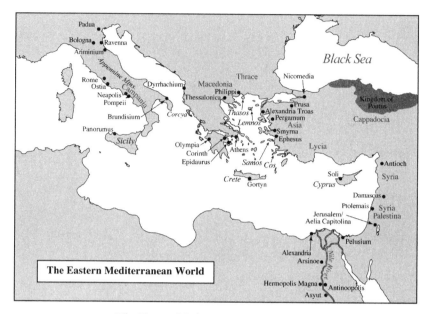

MAP 1: The Eastern Mediterranean. By Wendy Giminski.

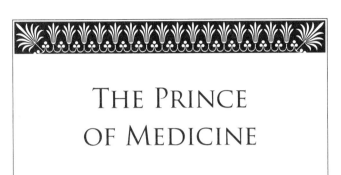

THE PRINCE
OF MEDICINE

THE RANCID CHEESE

 ne day when Galen was debating with his household slaves about what to do with a rancid cheese, a patient appeared at his door. It was an old man, arthritic with "chalkstones" (Galen's word) in his joints. Unable to walk, he was being carried in a litter. Galen had what seemed to him the brilliant idea of mixing some of the cheese with cooked, pickled pig's leg, blending it in a mortar and applying it to the affected joints. The plaster caused the patient's skin to rupture ("spontaneously, without cutting") and the chalkstones oozed away through the wound, over a period of several days. Both Galen and the patient found this outcome highly satisfactory; there was some difficulty when the supply of rancid cheese ran out, but the patient managed to procure another one and remained an enthusiastic user of, and evangelist for, the cure Galen had invented on the spur of the moment.

We can hazard a modern explanation of happened in the case of this patient. He probably suffered from gout; in advanced cases, uric acid crystals form deposits in the joints and over time can cause severe debility. Large accretions of crystals in the hands and feet are sometimes called "chalkstones" today. These can rupture spontaneously, and this is most likely what happened with Galen's patient; there is no obvious reason why the rancid cheese plaster would have helped.[1] It is inevitable that, reading Galen's anecdotes from so long ago, we will refocus them through the lens of our own, very different ideas and experience, and in some places I have helped the reader to do this. But we should not lose sight of the fact that the story is a clue to Galen's own perspective, in some ways so different from our own, in others startlingly familiar, and it is this—the experience of medicine in antiquity—that I hope most of all to convey to the reader.

I offer the story, then, not to suggest that Galen had some preternatural healing ability that transcended the limits of his understanding. There can be no comparison between the state of medical knowledge in antiquity and that following the "paradigm shifts" of the Renaissance and modern periods—for example, the discovery of the blood's circulation, germ theory, or genetics. No paradigm shift occurred with Galen, who practiced what Thomas Kuhn, the inventor of that term, would describe as "normal science."[2] I have not belabored Galen's errors about physiology, disease, the humors, and so forth, as our understanding of medicine has fundamentally changed in the last five centuries in ways that would make a catalog of his mistakes both overwhelming and unnecessary. I have pointed out intellectual contributions still relevant today—Galen's anatomy, although based on that of animals, was the foundation of Renaissance anatomy, for example; and he was a keen observer of human nature with unnervingly accurate insights into psychological disorders. But this is not mainly a work of intellectual history.

Rather, the story of the elderly man with chalkstones, which appears in one of Galen's works on pharmacology, his treatise *On the Mixtures and Powers*

---

1   The story is *Simp. Med.* 10.2.9 (12.270–271K). Thanks to Thomas C. Garland, MD, for help interpreting this passage.

2   I do not mean here to endorse every aspect of Thomas S. Kuhn's *The Structure of Scientific Revolutions*, first published in 1962 (Kuhn 2012), although much of Galen's work fits his description of "normal science." Kuhn's central concept of paradigm shift is relevant to medicine, as well as to physics, the discipline he originally described. A revolution in medical knowledge paralleled the nineteenth-century shift away from Aristotelian ideas of the four elements and qualities in physics, on which ideas Galenic medicine had partly depended.

of Simple Drugs, illustrates the everyday practice of medicine by one of the most skilled experts of his time. This is what makes it historically significant: the patient arriving at Galen's door even in the middle of a dispute with his domestic servants; Galen's immediate, focused, apparently unmediated attention as he examines the patient, mixes the plaster, places it on the affected part; his characterization of the patient as old (this is one of very few patients so described); his lack of comment on the patient's social status, which is probably, given the circumstances, humble. A richer patient would have sent for Galen, and Galen would have appeared at his house, even in the middle of the night, if it was urgent.

Galen practiced medicine in the Roman Empire for more than fifty years. In his own lifetime, as I shall describe, he achieved so much prestige through his reputation as a healer, his social standing, his prolific writing, and his ruthless demolition of his enemies in every debate and showdown, that he became virtually the last word on medicine. His works, for this reason preserved in scattered European locations and in Arabic translations, and collected in the massive editions of the Renaissance, represented the culmination of what was then known of medical science, the premodern "paradigm." Until the twentieth century, he was the most influential figure in western medicine and perhaps in western culture generally. The most modern edition of his corpus runs to twenty-two volumes, including about 150 titles, and is one-eighth of all the classical Greek literature that survives.

Today, we are most accustomed to seeing Galen as an disembodied corpus of texts—a set of ideas about the body that became first canonical, then obsolete; a stultifying influence from which western medicine struggled, heroically and successfully, to escape. We fail to appreciate the extent to which Galen's works are grounded in his life and in his practice, in what he observed, experienced, dared, performed, and accomplished. The Galen of this biography is a tireless interrogator of nature, an attentive inquisitor of patients and reader of diagnostic clues, a ruthless critic of ideas unsupported by experience, skeptical of nearly all received medical knowledge, and an aggressive and competitive public figure. When Vesalius used dissection to disprove many of Galen's assertions about anatomy and then mercilessly skewered the followers of his remote predecessor for their mistakes, he was imitating the very methods that Galen had delighted in hundreds of years before.

One day, if humanity is lucky, our own state of medical knowledge will seem as quaint as that of Galen and his contemporaries. In modern medicine there is no shortage of mystery, of inefficacy, of ignorance. How then do we understand its place in our culture and in history? Galen's life can offer us this perspective. This is the story of a brilliant and driven, privileged and highly educated, but otherwise normal person practicing normal science on normal people. My main emphasis is not on Galen's ideas, but on his life.

I close this preface with a note on Galen's personality; for ever since antiquity, one cannot write biography without consideration of the moral example set by one's subject, nor disregard the historian's traditional obligation of assigning praise and blame. Galen's defects of character will be very obvious even to the casual reader of this book. In the modern, western world he might be diagnosed with a personality disorder, once megalomania, today narcissism. He also epitomizes the much-maligned "type A" personality. All of this, however, was typical of his time, place, and social stratum, and Galen was not more competitive, hostile, or self-aggrandizing than his peers. For these reasons I have chosen to call attention to qualities that the reader might more easily overlook, qualities that did distinguish him from his peers and contributed to his success and long-standing influence; among these are not only insatiable drive, intellectual curiosity, and self-discipline but also unusual powers of observation and a profound understanding of human nature.

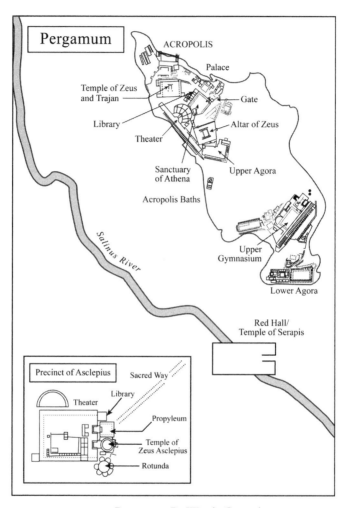

MAP 2: Pergamum. By Wendy Giminski.

Chapter One

PERGAMUM

ven when he had not seen it for years, Galen always called Pergamum home. It was the jewel in the Greek Middle East's crown of cities, sprawling over the plain near the river Caicus 16 miles from the Aegean Sea, in what is now western Turkey. Over its maze of streets and markets loomed the rock spur of the acropolis on which it was founded. In Hellenistic times the entire city was settled on its steep slopes, within the crowning perimeter wall built by its kings, in the decades after the death of Alexander the Great. In Galen's time this remained the old part of the city, home to its most prominent families, perhaps including his own—a crowded, dense settlement of steep, narrow, stepped streets and level after level of terracing.

On the acropolis's height the Attalids, Pergamum's ruling dynasty, constructed the most magnificent building complex of any Hellenistic city. The royal palace rose step by step in a sequence of terraced plateaus, flanked by buildings and monuments famous throughout the Greek world. Among these was the Great Altar of Zeus, one hundred feet long, covered (as was the wall that enclosed it) in a sculpted frieze depicting the mythical battle of gods and giants. Reconstructed in the Pergamon Museum in Berlin, this frieze is perhaps the most spectacular artistic work to survive from antiquity. Another renowned monument stood further up the slope, in a plaza dedicated to Athena: a bronze group of sculptures commemorating King Attalus I's victory over the migrant Celts of neighboring Galatia, in the 230s B.C.E. The bronzes have disappeared, but two survive in marble copies, and today the "Dying Gaul" is famous for the pathos it evokes and for its image of the shaggy-haired, mustachioed "barbarian." Above Athena's precinct stood Pergamum's famous library, second in size and renown only to that of Alexandria in Egypt. (Rumor told that together the libraries of Pergamum contained 200,000 scrolls, considered an astounding number at that time; and that in Roman times they were all transported to Alexandria, a gift from Mark Antony to Queen Cleopatra.)[1] And into the hill's precipitous western slope was set a stone theater, with seating for 10,000, where spectacles were played out against a heart-stopping backdrop view of western Turkey's austere, arid landscape. The acropolis of Pergamum is a most eloquent monument to the egotism, manic militarism, and cultural pretensions of the Hellenistic world's dynastic families.

The city boasted all of the usual Greek amenities, on a magnificent scale reflecting centuries of patronage by its kings and, later, the ambitions of its aristocracy to emulate and impress the Roman emperors. The social epicenter of every Greek city was its marketplace, or *agora*. The cultural epicenter was its gymnasium, a public space for the nude exercises, especially wrestling, that defined the lifestyle of Greek men of elite status.

Within the Hellenistic walls, Pergamum had at least two monumental *agorai*, three gymnasia, and four major bathing complexes (and, like all cities and towns, a host of minor ones). Besides the theater on the acropolis, Pergamum had theaters attached to its Upper Gymnasium and to the precinct of Asclepius, and a Roman-style freestanding theater on the plain, in the newer part of the town, that could seat 30,000. Nearby was an amphitheater, the city's largest public building and one of the few of its kind in the Roman East. Today Pergamum's buildings testify to the urban culture that dominated the Middle East of Galen's time.[2]

---

1   Plutarch, *Life of Antony* 58.
2   On the archaeology of Pergamum, see Halfmann (2004); Radt (1999); and the collection of essays in Koester (1998). On the gymnasium in Greco-Roman culture, see especially the articles of van Nijf (2003), (2000), and (1999).

Galen's world and experience was that of a Greek in the Roman Empire. To understand his life is impossible without understanding the ancient intertwining between Greek culture and Roman imperialism, a topic illustrated very conveniently by the history of his city. I offer, then, a brief political and cultural history of Pergamum by way of orienting the reader to Galen's world; and also, as a way of introducing Galen himself. His city—its monuments, its great and eccentric kings, its foundation legends, and its culture heroes—was a large part of Galen's identity. He was proud of his origin and identified as a Pergamene until the end of his life.[3]

Pergamum had been a Greek city probably since the eighth century B.C.E., but its early history is lost in myth. The Pergamenes traced their ancestry to Telephus, bastard child of Heracles and an Arcadian princess, abandoned to drift across the Aegean in a chest. The city became important late in the fourth century B.C.E., in the wake of Alexander the Great's death, when his generals, the so-called Diadochi, fought for control over his empire. What is now western Turkey, including Pergamum, changed hands several times in the early decades of this ferocious struggle. In the course of affairs an opportunistic man of ordinary background, named Philetaerus, acquired control over the city and its large treasury, which he proceeded to make into the capital of a new, emergent kingdom.

In the reign of Attalus I, whose victory over the Galatians was commemorated in the famous bronze statue group, and largely through his own actions, the tentacles of Roman imperialism reached Asia. Threatened by the Macedonian King Philip V, who was seeking to expand his territory into Asia, Attalus appealed to Rome for help. Pergamum proved a loyal ally in Rome's subsequent conflicts with the kingdoms of Macedonia and Syria, and Attalus's successor, Eumenes II, was rewarded with a large swath of territory wrested from Syria, comprising the most fertile and populous region of Asia Minor. From a petty principality Pergamum overnight became a large kingdom. It was this Eumenes who planned and paid for the spectacular building program on the acropolis—the Altar of Zeus with its famous frieze, the

---

3   Galen's lifelong references to his birthplace as "among us" or "our Asia" have often been noticed: e.g., Swain (1996, 377–78); Nutton (1995a, 365–66).

precinct and temple of Athena, the Upper Agora, the theater, the library, and a new fortification wall of which large sections survive today. Like his predecessors he fought constantly with the Celts and with rival kings and chiefs, celebrated his militaristic achievements loudly and visibly, and died exhausted.

The last of the Pergamene kings was the notoriously unstable, misanthropic, and bloodthirsty Attalus III, about whom historians tell us little other than that he murdered most of his family and sent homegrown poisons to his friends for his own amusement. Galen, however, mentions with praise his pharmacological discoveries and his complex antidote, even complaining that Attalus did not leave enough written records. (Attalus's antidote, however, was not as famous as that of Rome's great enemy, the ill-fated Mithradates VI "Eupator"—see below.)[4]

Attalus III died without heirs at age thirty-six, after ruling less than five years, and left his kingdom in his will to the Roman people. The Romans had not expected this legacy; they usually avoided annexing new lands that they were ill-equipped to garrison and preferred to rule hegemonically through local kings. But Pergamum was a wealthy kingdom and, although they gave away some of its territory to local allies, most of Attalus's former realm became the Roman province of Asia. From most of the province Rome collected a hefty tax, which every five years was auctioned to corporations of wealthy Roman citizens and sold to the highest bidder. The tax collectors did their job ruthlessly, keeping any profits over whatever they had promised to pay the treasury. To communities unable to pay the tax, wealthy Romans lent money at exorbitant rates of interest—Marcus Junius Brutus's loan to the city of Salamis on Cyprus, at 50 percent interest, was not considered exceptionally usurious—and they found other ingenious ways to exploit the

---

4   On the history of Pergamum, see Halfmann (2004); Radt (1999); Allen (1983); Magie (1950). Evans (2012) appeared too late to be incorporated into this study. On the aggressive and hypermilitaristic character of Hellenistic kingdoms, see Eckstein (2006). On Attalus III's pharmacology: Galen, *Simp. Med.* 10.1 (12.251K); *Comp. Med. Gen.* 1.13 (13.416K), 1.14 (13.419K), and 1.17 (13.446K). Galen calls him "our king Attalus" and "our Attalus, ruler of the Pergamenes." On Attalus's theriac: *Antid.* 1.1 (14.2K).

province economically.[5] As for Pergamum itself, Attalus had specifically left the city free, and there were many similarly "free" cities in Asia and in the Greek East. By his bequest he probably intended Pergamum to be subject to its own magistrates and laws and relieved of taxation, but it is not clear what privileges the Romans actually recognized.

This was the situation in the early first century B.C.E., when the Near East was roiled by the spectacular career of King Mithradates VI "Eupator" of Pontus. Mithradates was one of Rome's great enemies, along with Hannibal of Carthage and Cleopatra VII of Egypt—cruel, unscrupulous, shrewd, arrogant, and manically energetic; demonized as evil incarnate, lionized as that rare phenomenon, a truly worthy adversary. Rumor made him superhuman in size and strength and portraits display him as a young Heracles and Alexander the Great, with fanged lion's head helmet. Rumor also credited him with extraordinary intelligence and erudition: reportedly he could speak all twenty-two languages of his kingdom. His prowess in pharmacology was legendary, his recipe for theriac—an antidote of profound complexity—is cited not only in Galen but in several other ancient sources, and he remained famous for this through modern times. ("Mithridate" mixed according to ancient prescriptions was a highly prized drug in the Renaissance and is the subject of a poem by A. E. Housman.) Galen adds what is also repeated in other sources, that after his defeat and exile by the Roman general Pompey, Mithradates tried twice to commit suicide by poisoning himself, but the antidote to which he had accustomed his body was so effective that he had to beg one of his officers to run him through with a sword instead (*Antid.* 1.1, 14.3–4K).

Mithradates ruled the kingdom of Pontus, the southeastern coast of the Black Sea. By the age of thirty-one he had already vastly extended his territory and set his sights on much more, perhaps all of Alexander's former

---

5   On the province of Asia and Roman rule, see Dmitriev (2005, especially part 3, "General Overview"); Mitchell (1993); Sherwin-White (1977); A. H. M. Jones (1971); Magie (1950). An excellent discussion of Roman foreign policy in the later Republic is Morstein-Marx (1995). On the corporations of the late Republic and their activities, Badian's classic monograph (1983) is still instructive; see more recently Nicolet (2000, part 4).

empire. Again and again he sparred with the Romans over the control of the neighboring kingdoms of Bithynia and Cappadocia, until finally in 89 B.C.E. the Romans declared war on Mithradates through their proxy, the king of Bithynia. The Pontic king promptly defeated him with a small contingent of infantry and his famous scythed chariots. Mithradates then swept southeastward to the Roman province with the bulk of his army, said to have numbered 150,000, proclaiming himself the liberator of the Greeks. Three generals sent from Rome with much smaller forces were routed or fled. Most cities received him with enthusiasm, though some remained loyal to the Romans and stood siege. Pergamum was in the former category and surrendered immediately.

Mithradates appointed "satraps" to rule the former territory of the Romans. And then, notoriously, he proclaimed a genocidal slaughter of all Romans and Italians in Asia, male and female, adults, children, and slaves. Ancient sources tell us, but with no basis for accuracy, that 80,000 or 150,000 were murdered on the fatal day. Among the most enthusiastic participants were the cities of Pergamum and Ephesus, both of whom hunted down and massacred their Roman populations even as they took refuge in the sacred precincts of the gods.

The Roman general Sulla defeated Mithradates a few years later. The Romans reimposed taxes and tax collectors with a vengeance, with the additional burden of a colossal indemnity payment. Mithradates himself survived to plague the Romans for twenty-five years and two more major military campaigns, until finally driven into exile and suicide by Pompey the Great in 63 B.C.E.[6]

Pergamum suffered in the decades after the massacre of its Roman residents. Its "free" status was revoked; building languished; the festival in honor of its mythical ancestor Heracles ceased because no one was able to pay for it. But gradually the city's fortunes picked up. In the brief dictatorship of Julius Caesar, it regained its "freedom." Caesar also reduced the amount of

---

6   On Mithradates Eupator, see the excellent new biography of Mayor (2010); also Sherwin-White (1977, 70–75). On Pergamum in the revolt and under Roman rule, see also Halfmann (2004, 25–34); Radt (1999, 27–48).

tribute that Asia owed to Rome and put an end to the practice of collecting it through corporations of publicans, shifting the burden onto local aristocrats. The economy slowly recovered from years of merciless exploitation.

In the relatively peaceful imperial period, freed from the burden of warfare and the aggressions of its neighbors, Pergamum and the Greek East's other cities flourished. The resources that they had once poured into war now fueled cultural rivalry—each city wanted the best theaters and gymnasia, the most splendid festivals, and the most renowned orators and philosophers. Aristocrats who had once competed for military commands now bankrupted themselves in their efforts to win the gratitude and respect of their fellow-citizens, paying for games and festivals, handouts, and gargantuan public buildings. In the second century C.E., Pergamum reached its apogee; its temple of Asclepius, the god of medicine, was renowned the world over; its population, as Galen claimed, was 120,000; it boasted famous orators and culture heroes.[7]

The nobility defined itself by its participation in Greek urban culture. They held the civic offices that supervised and paid for the city's festivals and its elite gymnasia; their names were inscribed on its public buildings, as donors; they competed in the games as athletes, poets, and even as doctors (medical competitions are attested in at least one city of Asia Minor—see chapter 3). In their leisure time they wrestled in the gymnasia and took massages at the baths. They debated each other in the *agorai*, temple precincts, and other open spaces. They proudly styled themselves Pergamene citizens, *bouleutai* (members of the local senate), officeholders, and members of the gymnasium. They thought of themselves, above all, as Greeks.[8]

Rome ruled through the social ties between its ruling class and the elite classes of cities like Pergamum. Those ties were very complicated. Many of Pergamum's aristocratic citizens held Roman citizenship too, including,

---

7   On euergetism, see recently Zuiderhoek (2009) and the classic studies of MacMullen (1980a) and Veyne (1976). On the population of Pergamum: *Anim. Affect. Dign.* 9 (5.49K).

8   On the participation of the ruling class in competitive athletics, see the articles of van Nijf, cited in n. 2 above. On athletics in Greco-Roman culture at this time, see also König (2005), including a chapter on Galen; and Newby (2005), focusing on visual evidence.

probably, Galen's father and Galen himself. There is some doubt about this—Galen never mentions his citizen status—but two inscriptions from Pergamum from about the right time, honoring an Aelius Nicon, an architect, may refer to his father.[9] Citizens usually took their Roman names from the emperor who granted them citizenship: Aelius was one of the names of Emperor Hadrian, who ruled from 117 to 135.

Galen mentions in passing a youthful connection with another prominent Roman citizen:

> I was still living in my homeland at that time, studying under Satyrus; he was then spending his fourth year in Pergamum with Costunius Rufinus, who was constructing the new temple of Zeus Asclepius for us.
>
> (*Anat. Admin.* 1.2, 2.224–225K)

Other sources tell us that the proper name of this benefactor was L(ucius) Cuspius Pactumeius Rufinus (it was probably distorted by copying error in Galen's text), a Pergamene appointed to the Roman senate by Emperor Hadrian. Galen goes on to mention Satyrus's teacher Quintus, another Roman citizen and very famous doctor who taught and practiced at Rome—that is, Galen's teacher Satyrus had studied in Rome.

The entanglements between the Pergamene aristocracy and the Roman ruling class can also be read in the archaeological record; for Pergamene culture increasingly linked it to Rome. The Upper Gymnasium, on the acropolis, had baths adjoining, which were put together in such a way that the complex resembled the great imperial baths at Rome; although in which direction the influence extended, we do not know. Rufinus's new temple of Zeus Asclepius was a miniature replica of the renovated Pantheon, Hadrian's

---

9   See Schlange-Schöningen (2003, III.3) on Galen's possible Roman citizenship and 46–51 on the inscriptions. On the inscriptions, see Habicht (1969, no. 104). It is also possible that another architect named Julius Nicodemus or Nicon, also a Roman citizen, attested on two Pergamene inscriptions, was Galen's father. Modern scholars have tended to favor Aelius Nicon, but no compelling evidence argues for either one, and Nicon was a common name.

latest architectural triumph in Rome, complete with a domed roof. At the same time, on the crown of the acropolis, an elegant and highly visible temple dedicated jointly to Zeus Philios ("Friendly" Zeus) and the deified Emperor Trajan was also under construction. (The temple was completed in Hadrian's reign, and contained cult statues of both emperors, so that in Galen's time it was probably called the "Temple of Hadrian.") Pergamum already had, in common with many Greek cities, a temple of Augustus and Rome and associated games; in fact, it proudly advertised that it had been granted the first imperial temple and cult, in 29 B.C.E. The Roman emperors were worshipped as gods, like the Hellenistic kings before them, and not only after they were dead and officially "deified." Their festivals, their temples, their statues—mostly funded not by the emperors themselves, but by eager members of Pergamum's local nobility—were only the most blatant advertisements of Pergamum's place in the Roman Empire.[10]

It is therefore not surprising then that Galen made the journey to Rome, twice, and lived there most of his life. But his attitude to Roman culture was ambivalent at best. He proudly portrays himself as Greek. If he had a Roman name, he never used it; no reference to himself as "Aelius" survives. He never quotes a Latin author and, although he lived in Rome for many decades, we have no real evidence that he knew Latin at all. He did not need to; every educated person at Rome, and most of their slaves, spoke Greek. He considered his connection to the emperor Marcus Aurelius his highest accomplishment; but he otherwise remained aloof from Roman culture and vested all his political loyalty in his home city.

Greek culture in some ways reached its height of aggressive self-consciousness in the Roman Empire and especially in Galen's time. In the second century the movement that scholars today call the "Second Sophistic"—and it is called this also in one ancient source—reached its height. The "sophists"

---

10   On the Pergamene elite, see White (1998). On second-century renovations of the Asclepius precinct, see Hoffmann (1998). On the image of the emperor and provincial loyalty, see Ando (2000, especially chapters 7 and 9).

were professional orators, but much more than that—they were entertainers, educators, public benefactors, culture heroes, and ambassadors. They could capture audiences of thousands with their virtuoso performances, often in the city's huge public theaters. Disdaining prepared topics, they made a display of soliciting random topics from the audience and then declaiming on them. Certain themes were traditional, mostly from the classical and Hellenistic Greek past; for example, "Demosthenes denounces himself after the battle of Chaeronea." They affected the classical Athenian dialect, which had not been spoken in many centuries but which survived in the works now considered the foundations of Greek culture. The most famous sophists commanded enormous fees and prizes. They and their students came from the highest classes of the Hellenized East, and they embodied Hellenism itself.[11]

Sophists competed with each other for prestige and students; cities competed for famous sophists. Polemo, perhaps the most illustrious sophist who ever lived, was won over to the city of Smyrna (modern Izmir, about 66 miles by road from Pergamum in Galen's day) by the deluge of honors they voted him, opened a school there, and was commonly believed to be a native of the city although he was actually born in Laodicea on the Lycus, some 150 miles to the southeast.[12]

The sophists' complex relationship to Rome and to the empire, like Galen's, illustrates the paradox of Greek culture: Hellenism's high prestige among its conquerors. The sophists' disdain for the Romans mixed awkwardly with subservience and assimilation. Polemo's family included consuls in the Roman senate; many sophists held office by imperial appointment; some were "friends" or regular advisors to emperors. Sophists often served as ambassadors from their cities to the emperor, pleading a cause—disaster relief, or

---

11   On sophists and the Second Sophistic, a large literature exists; especially relevant here and for what follows are Whitmarsh (2001); Schmitz (1997); Swain (1996); Bowersock (1969).

12   A brilliant online tool for calculating distances, travel times, transport costs, and many other logistical factors in the Roman Empire is now available in *Orbis: The Stanford Geospatial Network Model of the Roman World*, created by Walter Scheidel and Elijah Meeks (http://orbis.stanford.edu).

a new gymnasium, or asking for judgment in one of the continual disputes with other cities over some minute signifier of primacy. Every self-respecting sophist had met at least one emperor and had a story to tell about the experience. Polemo was famous for having thrown the Emperor Antoninus Pius out of his house in Smyrna in the middle of the night. Of Dio Chrysostomus of Prusa, a sophist of the early second century C.E. from what is now Bursa in northwestern Turkey, a biographer writes that the Emperor Trajan let him ride next to him in his chariot during a triumphal procession and often said "I don't understand what you are saying, but I love you as myself." Here as often, the emperor is the butt of the story; sophists affected an arrogance that no one else could get away with. To the empire's proudly Hellenic population the sophists represented the antiquity, sophistication, and superiority of Greek culture; but for all their posturing, they were not in conflict with the Roman ruling class nor even distinct from it. They held positions of power in the imperial bureaucracy, they often held Roman citizenship and came from the same families as Roman senators, and they educated the sons of Roman aristocrats.[13]

I mention the sophists because in many ways Galen was one of them. Erudition, competitiveness, Hellenism; public displays of skill; rivalries, political power, and an intimate but complicated relationship with Roman authority—the sophists were the most visible exemplars of these qualities, but the latter were typical of the Greek urban aristocracy generally and of Galen in particular. Like the sophists, Galen was an expert on classical Athenian language: for most of his writing he used a more straightforward, pedestrian style suitable for its technical subject, but he was perfectly capable of high Sophistic style, which he adopted for florid polemical passages. His longest work, now lost, was a two-part dictionary of Attic words. Like the sophists he was an educator; like them he staged dramatic public speeches, debates, and performances; like them he mingled with the Roman aristocracy and was proud of his association with the emperor. Like most of them, he came from

---

13   Trajan's comment to Dio: Philostratus, *Vitae Sophistarum* 7. On the status of sophists vis-à-vis imperial power, see references in n. 11.

a Greek city in Asia Minor. Galen is a very accurate mirror or microcosm of Greek elite society in his time.[14]

Women were a shadowy presence in Greek public life. Hellenic aristocratic culture prized modesty above all things in women; and its ideals relegated them to the domestic sphere, to the *thalamoi* or "chambers," the more private areas of the house. When women appeared outside in the Greek East, they were heavily draped and veiled. Besides the production of new citizens, religion was their primary duty to the city—the celebration of cults, some of them very ancient. Pergamene women held some civic offices and even, like their male counterparts, occasionally appeared on coins. Many were wealthy and could be honored as public benefactors. But they did all of these things much less frequently than men, and with important differences in how the inscriptions that honored them described their accomplishments.[15]

For the most part, life was lived in the open air. Even within houses, life centered around courtyards and, in larger houses, colonnaded interior gardens. Not enough of residential Pergamum has been excavated to describe it specifically; but it was probably like other cities of the Roman Mediterranean. Commercial and private life mixed promiscuously. Among the houses, on every block and street corner one found workshops, bakeries, bars, and brothels. Artisans clustered in certain areas of the city, well known to the patrons who needed to find them—shoemakers, glassmakers, barbers, butchers; on the outskirts the more noxious professions, potters, fullers (who used human urine to prepare cloth), and blacksmiths. Some merchants occupied stalls in the city's spacious, monumental fora; others hawked their wares in the streets.

---

14 On Galen and the sophists, the articles of von Staden (1997) and (1995) are especially important. See also chapters on Galen in Swain (1996) and Bowersock (1969). On Galen's style, see Johnston and Horsley (2011, 1: xciv–cvi).

15 On the veiling and seclusion of women, see Llewelyn-Jones (2003). See also however Nevett (2002, 81–100), arguing that Greek houses became more integrated as women became less secluded and their domestic roles changed in the Roman period. On women in Greek civic life in the Hellenistic and Roman periods, the most important work is van Bremen (1996). The appendices catalog civic titles for women (see especially Appendix 2, 334–35 on Pergamum). The classic article of MacMullen (1980b) is still well worth reading.

Office buildings and schools did not exist. Professionals worked at home; later, in Rome, Galen's clinic was in his house. Schoolteachers taught their pupils outside, wherever they could find shelter, for example under the porticoes that lined some streets. Libraries and temples lacked indoor space—one read outside, where the light was better. Temple buildings functioned mainly as repositories for the items dedicated to the god and as imposing frames and shelters for the cult statue. The action—debates and speeches, spectacles, processions, sacrifices, contests, and festivities—occurred in the space around, the open temple precinct and nearby theaters. All Greco-Roman theaters and amphitheaters were open air, though some had awnings that could be unfurled in hot weather. Likewise the gymnasium was mostly open space—a large inner courtyard for wrestling and other sports, and an attached theater.[16]

The main activity that occurred indoors was bathing. Baths were the only structures with heat, and at Pergamum they were likely a welcome refuge from the cold in winter, when average low temperatures dip to the thirties Fahrenheit, and snow is not unheard of. Today baths are often recognized by their hypocaust floors, raised on brick pillars, beneath which steam from the boilers circulated. These floors were dangerously hot; at Rome one master's slaves attacked him in the baths and then threw him on the floor to test whether he was really dead. Stoking the boilers and cleaning up after the patrons was the unhappy duty of public slaves.[17]

Today, tourists and archaeologists know the ancient city as a scattered collection of bleached stone: some of it reasonably intact, some of it rebuilt as poignant ruins, most of it foundations and rubble, requiring a great effort to imagine the original structure. It is even more difficult, confronted only with these remains, to capture the squalor of the ancient city, in which sanitation was rudimentary, animals were herded through the streets and also butchered there, settlement was much denser than modern Westerners are used to, and

---

16   On Pergamene residences, see Wulf-Rheidt (1998). On urban life in the Roman Empire, see MacMullen (1974, chapter 3). On urban architecture, two surveys are especially important: Gros (1996–2001) and MacDonald (1982).

17   On baths in the Roman era, see Yegül (2010) and Fagan (1999). On the master attacked by slaves: Pliny the Younger, *Letters* 3.14.

plague and famine were frequent events. Average life expectancy at birth in the Roman Empire was probably about twenty-five or thirty. Because most people died of infectious disease, that figure varied with ecological conditions and was lower in the cities and somewhat higher in the countryside, though it was probably not higher than about thirty-five anywhere. (It may be helpful to note for comparison that in Bangladesh today, average life expectancy at birth is close to seventy.)[18] The city best attested in ancient literature is Rome, bigger and fouler than any other in the empire; I will describe it in its own place. Pergamum was a miniature version, although probably safer from malaria and some other diseases because of its elevated situation.

Baths were undrained, the water often visibly filthy:

> Someone recently asked us why we piss cold in the [hot water of the] baths, but outside [we piss] hot, not understanding that the piss itself is lukewarm …
>
> (*Simp. Med.* 3.8, 11.554K)

Baths were also common sites of violence, theft, and illicit sex. Fainting at the baths was common, especially if the wood from the boilers gave off too much smoke. Houses lacked indoor plumbing and many people emptied their refuse into the streets rather than use the few public latrines. At the gymnasium, wrestling injuries—such as a crushed larynx, fractured ribs, or dislocated shoulder—were common (Galen will suffer a dislocation himself, in chapter 5). Galen does however praise the fountains of Pergamum; their water, some of it brought 43 miles from Soma by aqueduct, is not "smelly or toxic or muddy or hard," as it is in many locations in which, Galen explains, he has given patients boiled water.[19]

---

18   For up-to-date discussions of life expectancy and well-being in the Roman Empire, see Scheidel (2010a).

19   On public health and mortality in Rome and other cities, see further discussion in chapter 4. Especially important studies are Scheidel (2001b); Scobie (1986). On Bangladesh, see Central Intelligence Agency, "The World Factbook, Country Comparison: Life Expectancy at Birth," https://www.cia.gov/library/publications/the-world-factbook/rankorder/2102rank.html

Some of Galen's most vivid experiences of famine and epidemic date to his childhood and young adulthood in Pergamum. While an adolescent student of the physician Satyrus, he and his teachers witnessed an epidemic outbreak of what he calls "anthrax" (the disease was perhaps the most common, cutaneous form of what is now called anthrax, transmitted by infected livestock; this has a fatality rate of about 20 percent if untreated): "of many patients parts were stripped of skin, and of some also of the very flesh" (*Anat. Admin.* 1.2, 2.224–25K). In a famous passage, he describes the effects on the peasantry of a famine that raged for years in many parts of the empire. The good grain and other produce went to the cities, as was customary. Peasants, forced to eat green twigs, bulbs, and grasses, began to suffer from a huge variety of noxious symptoms, especially ulcerative skin disease, dysentery, and fever; their sweat smelled foul; when doctors let their blood it oozed thick and dark, and the wounds refused to heal (*Bon. Mal. Suc.* 1, 6.749K). In another passage, Galen writes that during food shortages the peasants in his homeland consume the acorns they normally feed to pigs; first they slaughter the pigs, then eat the acorns (*Aliment. Fac.* 2.21, 6.620K). In a bad year farmers neglect to remove the darnel, a toxic weed, from the wheat that they send to the city, and consumers become sick with headaches and ulcerated skin (*Aliment. Fac.* 1.37, 6.553K).

In Galen's view, food flows from the countryside to the city as from (he believed) the intestines to the liver—along roads, which are like veins (*Hipp. Nat. Hom.* 2.6, 15.145K). The city was parasitic on the countryside and had power over it—not only economic power as the sole consumer market for the land around it, but the power to extort its produce if necessary, as taxes, rent, or by requisition. Cities were not, however, immune from food shortages, which are well-attested and occurred frequently. Most cities had an

---

(accessed December 17, 2011). On fainting in the baths, see Galen, *Usu Resp.* 4 (4.494K), *Hipp. Aph.* 2.41 (17B.540K). On illicit sex, the study of Ward (1992) is especially interesting. On wrestling injuries, see Galen, *Anat. Admin.* 7.13 (2.632–33K), 11.1 (85 Simon); *Loc. Affect.* 4.8 (8.262K), 4.11 (8.287–88K); *Meth. Med.* 5.8 (10.339–40K); *Hipp. Artic.* 1.22 (18A.347–51K); *Opt. Med. Cogn.* 11 (118 Iskandar). On Galen's injury: *Hipp. Artic.* 1.61 (18A.401–4K). Galen on the fountains of Pergamum: *Hipp. 6 Epid.* 4.10 (17B.159K).

official especially in charge of the grain supply; when it failed, mob violence often resulted. A fourth-century grammarian recalls rioting during a food shortage, and he himself was in danger of being stoned by the crowd when he defended the local magistrates from accusations of corruption; this was in his hometown of Antioch (modern Antakya, then in the Roman province of Syria, today a part of Turkey). The pagan saint Apollonius of Tyana is supposed to have rescued a magistrate from being burnt alive at Aspendus in southern Asia Minor, where a hungry mob besieged him as he clung to a statue of the emperor. At Prusa, a mob beset the property of the philosopher and wealthy citizen Dio Chrysostomus, intending to burn it, because they suspected he was hoarding grain. In his speech on this episode he refers to "stones and fire" as the habitual weapons of the city's populace—here as elsewhere, lynching is represented as the normal behavior of an urban population under stress, not a ghastly aberrant act. A stone-wielding mob set on another sophist of Dio's generation, Lollianus, who at the time was the official in charge of the food supply in Athens, during a riot in the baker's district.[20]

Lynchings did not only happen during famine, as we know from familiar passages of the New Testament and other sources. In Ephesus, a mob incited by the guild of silversmiths kidnapped two associates of the apostle Paul and dragged them to the theater, where a menacing crowd shouted "Great is Artemis of the Ephesians" in unison for two full hours. In the gospel of John, an adulteress narrowly escapes death by stoning. In Apuleius's novel *The Golden Ass*, a mob condemns a woman to death by stoning as a witch, and a widow is nearly lynched at her husband's funeral by a crowd that suspects her of murder. All of these are routine episodes mentioned in passing or invented to flesh out a story with plausible detail, and many of them are set in Asia Minor (both Prusa and Ephesus are within 100 linear miles of Pergamum). Emperor Trajan considered the province of Bithynia to the north—Prusa

---

20   On famine, see especially the work of Garnsey (1999) and (1988); and the recent collection of articles in Alston and van Nijf (2008), especially the contribution of Erdkamp for discussion of Dio Chrysostomus. Libanius on stoning: *Orations* 1.205–9. Apollonius of Tyana: Philostratus, *Life of Apollonius* 1.15. Dio's speech: *Orations* 46. Lollianus: Philostratus, *Lives of the Sophists* 23.

was one of its cities—so volatile that he banned all trade organizations and would not even allow a fire brigade.[21]

Despite its occasional horrors, Galen considered city life normal. To him, the countryside was an alien environment and peasants were almost another species. Urbanites were not cut off from the country—they traveled through it, slowly, on foot; they owned property there, since real property was the mainstay of most wealthy citizens' income; they managed those properties and visited them and dealt with their tenants. In middle age, Galen's father took up residence in the countryside as a gentleman-farmer and taught himself, among other things, to distinguish the seeds of different kinds of grain and weeds; weeds, as he thought based on experiments of his own design, resulted from spontaneous changes in the cultivated plant (*Aliment. Fac.* 1.37, 6.552–53K). Galen often refers to the peasants in the environs of his home city and of other areas—especially in his works on food, where he is interested in local diet, and on drugs, where he remarks on indigenous herbal remedies and on the challenges of treating patients with only locally grown ingredients, far from the marketplaces of the city. Sometimes he speaks admiringly of the simplicity and self-sufficiency of peasant life; but he also portrays the countryside as a world of isolation and hardship where people live more like animals. Peasants eat food indigestible to city folk; they suffer sickle wounds and snakebite; they often self-treat or their problems go untreated; their bodies are harder than those of city-dwellers (*Simp. Med.* 10.2.22, 12.299K) and require adjusted remedies for that reason. While Galen's urbane fellow-citizens work out in the gymnasium, backbreaking labor is the peasant's exercise.[22]

The Greek culture with which Galen identified was urban culture. In some of the rural hinterlands of Asia Minor, Greek was not even spoken; about two dozen native languages are attested, including Luwian, the ancient language of the Hittites still spoken by the bandit tribes of the Cilician highlands to the south. Galen never mentions meeting a peasant who did not

---

21   Ephesus: Acts 19. Adulteress: John 8. Apuleius: *The Golden Ass* 1.10, 2.27. Fire brigade: Pliny the Younger, *Letters* 10.34, 117.

22   On peasants, see Mattern (2008a, 53–55, 116); and see further below, chapter 4.

speak Greek or speaking through an interpreter; but he barely mentions Latin either, though he lived in Rome for decades, and we do not really know what language or languages the peasants he encountered spoke.[23] (For more on Galen's encounters with peasants, see chapter 4.)

To the east of the city of Pergamum, far outside the Hellenistic walls and on the outskirts of the Roman development, stood the temple of Asclepius, the Greek god of medicine. It was founded around 200 B.C.E., in the time of king Eumenes II. In 88 B.C.E., on the day of Mithradates' genocidal edict, the city's Roman population took refuge in Asclepius's sacred precinct. The Pergamenes tracked them down and slaughtered them where they stood. As a result, after the Roman reconquest, the temple temporarily lost its status as asylum—a devastating blow, since temples were their own jurisdiction, their power coextensive with the territory sacred to them. The temple regained its status in 44 B.C.E., the same year that Pergamum was once again declared a "free" city, and in the next centuries Asclepius became Pergamum's most important god and his temple was renowned everywhere.[24]

The Roman Emperor Hadrian visited Pergamum in 123 C.E. He typically traveled with a corps of architects and engineers and was renowned for his love of Greek culture, his skill at architecture, and his generous support of large-scale building projects in the Greek world. His visit inspired a massive remodeling of the temple precinct that swept away its accumulated clutter of small buildings and replaced them with a spacious complex of grand and opulent design. A covered colonnade enclosed an area almost twice that of an American football field (100 meters by 93 meters) on three sides. The builders leveled the precinct, cutting into rock to the north and supporting the long southern portico with elaborate subterranean vaulting. On the eastern side stood a porticoed, monumental gateway and the new temple of Zeus Asclepius, a miniature replica of Hadrian's most famous project, the renovated Pantheon at Rome. Its domed roof and circular, niched interior

---

23   On the languages of Asia Minor, see Mitchell (1993, 1:172–76).
24   On the temple and the rebellion of Mithradates, see Hoffmann (1998, 42). On the restoration of rights, see Magie (1950, 1: 417).

were the height of modern innovation at the time and were reduplicated faithfully at Pergamum. The complex also included a theater; a library; two sets of latrines; a large, round structure with semicircular niches usually called the Rotunda, which was probably not constructed until about 200 C.E.; and in the center a number of old Hellenistic cult buildings including the main temple of Asclepius, several sacred wells and fountains, and an incubation complex where pilgrims slept and where Asclepius spoke to them, and healed them, in dreams. A colonnaded "Sacred Way" (the last hundred feet or so survive) led from the city to the temple precinct.[25]

In the Greco-Roman world, healing was the main business of medicine. On inscriptions thanking gods for favors, healing is the benefit most often mentioned, by a wide margin. Most gods could heal, but Asclepius was the healing god par excellence, and his temples stood all over the Mediterranean world:

> We never find any country, or any city, without places where recovery is sought through divine medicine, some named after Asclepius, others after Apollo.
>
> (*Opt. Med. Cogn.* 1, tr. Iskandar)

Some were small and local, while others—like the temple at Pergamum—attracted pilgrims from far and wide. By Galen's time Pergamum was so closely tied to Asclepius that the latter was often called "the god of Pergamum" and Galen calls him his "ancestral god" (*Libr. Propr.* 2, 19.18–19K; *San. Tuend.* 1.8, 6.41K). Those who were healed dedicated offerings, often simple terracotta models of the part healed: feet, ears, breasts, and genitalia festooned the temple precinct. Wealthier patrons sometimes dedicated plaques with scenes of healing, or more expensive treasures. Each object commemorated a story of healing, and the stories also circulated as testimony to Asclepius's power. At some sanctuaries the priests collected and published the temple's stories

---

25   On Hadrianic renovations of the Asclepieion, see Petsalis-Diomidis (2010, 151–220); Hoffmann (1998).

on stone inscriptions for pilgrims to admire. The most famous and complete of these collections is at Epidaurus in Greece and dates to the fourth century B.C.E., but there are examples from the Roman period, including one inscription from Pergamum in which the god cured the dedicator by prescribing a diet of onions and white pepper.[26]

The cult of Asclepius was not hostile to rational medicine, or vice-versa. Asclepius was the god of doctors. Legend told how he learned the art of medicine from the centaur Chiron. Many doctors visited his shrine and made dedications to him, including medical instruments. Medical families often named their offspring Asclepiades or "son of Asclepius" and the Hippocratic Oath invokes him. The god's prescriptions, as communicated in dreams, were baths, vomiting, purging, plasters—the same things that doctors prescribed. But Asclepius's cures could have extreme or counterintuitive twists, and the legends that surrounded his cures attracted the exaggerated, unlikely elements typical of oral history:

> Nicomachus of Smyrna's whole body grew so disproportionately [huge], that he finally was unable to move; but Asclepius cured him.
>
> (*Morb. Diff.* 9, 6.869K)

The god healed Galen himself when he contracted a dangerous illness as a teenager (see chapter 2); as a result of which Galen "proclaimed myself a servant of the ancestral god" (*Libr. Propr.* 2, 19.18–19K). Galen occasionally expresses frustration at patients' greater willingness to consult or obey the god rather than their doctors, but he never criticizes the god's cures or doubts their efficacy.[27]

---

26   On healing in pagan religion, see Cruse (2004, chapter 5); Nutton (2004, chapter 18); MacMullen (1981, 49–51). On the cult of Asclepius, see the classic work of Edelstein and Edelstein (1945). For archaeological evidence, see further the studies of Hausmann (1948) and van Straten (1981). On the inscriptions from Epidaurus, see LiDonnici (1995). On the Pergamene inscription, see Müller (1987); cf. Christopher Jones (1998, 66).

27   On patients' willingness to obey Asclepius: *Hipp. 6 Epid.* 4.8 (17B.137K); *Opt. Med. Cogn.* 3 (43 Iskandar).

The temple at Pergamum is well-known today through the diaries of Aelius Aristides, a sophist and older contemporary of Galen who spent a lot of time there. Aristides lived most of his life in Smyrna and identified with that city. He visited Rome at age twenty-six and met the emperor. The journey was a nightmarish one during which he became very ill and never fully recovered. He spent the rest of his life seeking cures at temples of Asclepius, surrounded by his entourage of doctors along with his friends and servants. Dreams were the normal method by which gods communicated with humans, and Asclepius instructed Aristides in dreams, which the latter recorded—in an immense work of some 300,000 lines now lost to us, compiled over the years, but also in the six *Sacred Tales* that survive among his orations. Most of the time Aristides did not dream about the god directly—he dreamt about declaiming, or about his nurse or his foster father, his friends, the temple personnel; or about the emperors or the governor or the king of Parthia. His dreams are quite ordinary, but he interprets elements of them as divine instruction—for example, the excavation of a drainage ditch signifies vomiting (*Sacred Tales* 1.46, 50).[28]

Aristides recounts a long history of ailments, most notably a monstrous tumor on his thigh, and a plague that killed much of his household at Smyrna (*Sacred Tales* 2.4). This was the same plague Galen faced in 166 C.E. (see chapter 6), probably smallpox; Aristides was narrowly spared when, as he believed, his foster son died in his place. During one of his extended stays at Pergamum, the god advised him to cover himself with mud and bathe in the Sacred Well. It was a very cold day, but Aristides obeyed Asclepius's commands, as always. He also bathed in a linen tunic in freezing weather, ran naked around the temple complex in icy winds, went barefoot throughout the whole winter, and slept in the open air everywhere in the temple precinct. Very frequently Aristides' entourage of friends and doctors would object to

---

28 On Aelius Aristides, Asclepius, and dreams, see Petsalis-Diomidis (2010); Harris (2009, 118–22); the recent collection of articles in Harris and Holmes (2008), especially the contributions of Holmes, Downie, and Petsalis-Diomidis (chapters 5, 6, and 7); Christopher Jones (1998); Perkins (1995, chapter 7); Behr (1968). On his journey to Rome, see Mitchell (1993, 1: 165–67). An English translation of Aristides' orations, including the *Sacred Tales*, is available in Behr (1981).

the god's advice; but Asclepius was always right. Aristides' devotion to the god was profound. He kept up a running dialogue with him, through dreams, all his life; he joined the community of initiates at Pergamum; he considered the god his savior multiple times over; he believed the god had the power to predict and remit death.

Pergamum, the city founded on pilfered treasure, the city of Attalus and of Asclepius, the city that had turned on its Roman inhabitants and slaughtered them by the thousands on one dark day in 88 B.C.E., and had then become the light of Roman Asia, beloved of Hadrian, adorned with every architectural glory—Pergamum was Galen's city.

We do not know how long his family had lived there, but it seems that they were prominent citizens. Galen's father and grandfather were architects. In the Greek world that placed high value on skill and intellectual accomplishment, work of this type was no disgrace but, depending on the profession, could be very prestigious. Like sophists, architects could command huge fees or gifts from their clients; but as a point of pride Galen's ancestors, like Galen himself, probably declined to be paid by the piece or by the day. Galen writes that he never charged a patient a fee and even donated medicine and servants to those who could not afford them. I will say more about Galen's clientele in chapter 7, but I note here that in his surviving works Galen scrupulously portrays himself as a man of independent means, living off the landed property he inherited from his father. Galen owned property in Pergamum—which he kept, with its staff of slaves, long after he had ceased to live there—and a house in Rome and a country home in Campania, in southern Italy. He owned a large contingent of slaves, including domestic servants, professional assistants, and stenographers. He mentions all of these things in passing, without comment, as a matter of course. There is no doubt that Galen's prowess and renown as a physician brought material advantage. He mentions with pride a huge gift of 400 *aurei*—gold coins—that he accepted from his enormously wealthy and powerful friend, the senator and ex-consul Flavius Boethus, for curing his wife; although this is the only time Galen describes receiving money for a cure, it was probably not the only time it happened. But Galen would have been horrified if people thought he practiced medicine to amass money. He was a gentleman, a Greek, a leading citizen of Pergamum. His lifestyle came to him by birthright; but his skill and reputation, by hard work, exhaustive study, experiment, experience, and proven superiority over his rivals. Galen's sense of professionalism was highly developed, and its various aspects will be explored in the chapters that follow. But it did not include working for money.[29]

Galen no doubt inherited these values from his father, whom he idolized. A late antique encyclopedia, the Suda, tells us that his father's name was Nicon and that he was an architect. Galen confirms the detail about his father's profession in his treatise *Avoiding Distress*, a work long thought lost but rediscovered, along with new manuscripts of several other Galenic treatises, in 2007 at a monastery in Thessaloniki. Among other things Galen reports that his father and his father's father were architects, and that his great-grandfather was also a professional, a geometer—most likely an engineer, but possibly a land surveyor. The Suda's information on the name of Galen's father probably traces to one of Galen's lost works. If it is correct, he may be attested in Pergamene inscriptions honoring an Aelius Nicon, a Roman citizen, as I have mentioned. The Nicon of the inscriptions is a small-scale public benefactor and a man of great erudition, composer of a poetic diatribe on geometry and a hymn to the Greek sun-god Helios; it is quite plausible, but by no means certain, that he was Galen's father.[30]

Galen tells us very little about his childhood. We know, calculating from later events, that he was born in 129, and, perhaps more tenuously, from a

---

29   On professionalism: for further discussion and references, see Mattern (2008a, 21–27). On fees and donations, see Meyerhof (1929, 84). The relevant fragment, surviving only in Arabic, is from Galen's lost work *How to Profit from One's Enemies*. On Galen's social status and property, see Schlange-Schöningen (2003, III.1–2). On gold coins: *Praecog.* 8 (14.647K).

30   On Nicon, see Habicht (1969, no. 140); Schlange-Schöningen (2003, 40–60). The *editio princeps* of *Avoiding Distress* (*Peri Alupias* or *De Indolentia*) is Boudon-Millot (2007b). It is more accessible, also with French translation, in the Budé edition of Boudon-Millot and Jouanna (2010). We will soon have a new English translation by Vivian Nutton, whose English version of the work's title I adopt here. On father and grandfather: *Ind.* 59.

chance comment, that he was born around the time of the autumn equinox in September.[31] None of his autobiographical anecdotes takes place before his mid-teens. We do not know whether he had siblings or pets or a nurse or favorite caretaker, or how he remembered his childhood years, if he did at all. This may be related to Galen's reticence on the subject of "private" or family life in general. That is, while he talks about his postsecondary education, his friends, his classmates, and his father, Galen never mentions a wife or concubine, a child, a male or female lover, or a sibling. It is possible that he had all of these and never found them worthy of mention. It is also possible that he had none of them. Siblings, in particular, may have died very young in a population with horrific child mortality; and aristocratic families often sought to limit the number of heirs. (Galen writes as though he were the only heir to his father's estate.) One patient he describes, Theagenes the Cynic, when he died was mourned only by a crowd of friends:

> No one inside was wailing. For Theagenes had neither servant nor boy nor wife, but only his philosopher friends were around him, who behave properly in the care of the dead, not being inclined to mourn.
>
> (*Meth. Med.* 13.15, 10.915K)

For Galen, Theagenes lived an ideal; and his own life, what he lets us see of it, is defined by his intensely competitive, masculine relationships with friends and rivals and not by domestic attachments. Our image of Galen is a very public one in that sense. The sole woman in his family whom he mentions is his mother, in one notorious passage:

> My mother was very irascible, so that she sometimes would bite her maidservants, and she constantly screamed at my father and fought with him, like Xanthippe with Socrates. When I compared the good

---

31   On the year of Galen's birth, see most recently Boudon-Millot (2007a, xi–xviii). On the month: *Comp. Med. Gen.* 3.2 (13.599K); Galen was entering his twenty-ninth year when he was first appointed physician to the gladiators, by a priest who probably took office at the equinox.

actions of my father with the disgraceful passions of my mother it occurred to me to embrace and love the former, and to avoid and hate the latter.

(*Anim. Affect. Dign.* 8, 5.40–41K)

It would, of course, be irresponsible, based on this passage alone, to speculate about the long-term effects of growing up in a troubled household with a violent and irascible mother. We should remember that Galen's mother was probably not his primary caretaker; most likely, he was raised by domestic servants. The minor significance of women in his later works (and perhaps in his life) is not necessarily the result of bad mothering; it is comparable to what we see in other Greek autobiographical writers, such as Aelius Aristides and Libanius, especially if we consider that Galen offers us only anecdotes in medical treatises and no extended narrative of his life.

Still, the contrast with Galen's father is very obvious. Galen mentions the latter many times and always with the deepest reverence, emphasizing his moral qualities and the values that he transmitted to Galen.

I had a father who attained the height of geometry, architecture, logic, mathematics, and astronomy; and those who knew him praised him for his justice, goodness, and moderation beyond all the philosophers.

(*Bon. Mal. Suc.* 1, 6.755K)

My father accustomed me to disdain reputation and honor, and to value truth alone.... If a cow, a horse or a domestic servant died, it was not enough to make me grieve, when I remembered what my father advised, not to grieve for the loss of material goods as long as what remained was adequate for the care of the body.... If means beyond this existed, he said they ought to be used for good works.

(*Anim. Affect. Dign.* 8, 5.43–44K)

I had the great good fortune to have the least irascible, most just, best and most philanthropic of fathers …

(*Anim. Affect. Dign.* 8, 5.40K)

> He was drawn into political business by his fellow-citizens, since he
> seemed to them to be the only one who was just and above material
> wealth, and approachable and mild.
>
> *(Anim. Affect. Dign.* 8, 5.41K)

Here Galen's father embodies the sober reserve that Greek and Roman
philosophers alike espoused as their ethical ideal. A gentleman did not
indulge in lavish displays of emotion, did not hit slaves in anger, was neither acquisitive of luxuries nor aggrieved at material losses, did not pursue
romantic passions (a subject Galen barely mentions in all his works), and
scorned fame.

And yet for all his insistence on these values, the vices they were meant to
suppress—competitiveness, rancor, anger with occasional explosive violence,
and especially the pursuit of prestige at all costs—were very characteristic
of Galen's class. The tension between philosophy and reality is obvious in
some passages:

> I have never struck any of my servants with my hand, which was also
> my father's practice, and he reproved many of his friends, seeing their
> bruises from hitting servants in the teeth, saying that they deserved to
> have convulsions and die from the inflammation that resulted.
>
> *(Anim. Affect. Dign.* 4, 5.17K)

Widely held values about emotional restraint did not prevent some of Galen's
contemporaries, including his own mother as I have mentioned, from brutal-
izing their domestic servants. Most disingenuous is Galen's oft-professed lack
of concern for honor and reputation. Nothing, as we shall see in the following
chapters, drove him more. It drove his father too:

> not a few of my fellow-students answered me, "you have the advan-
> tage of an excellent nature and an astounding education because of the
> ambition (*philotimia*, love of honor) of your father, and you are at the

stage of life when it is possible to learn, and you have wealth with which to obtain leisure for studies. And we do not have these things."

(*Meth. Med.* 8.3, 10.560–61K)

Philotimia, the defining quality of the Greek urban aristocracy, is ambivalently praised, critiqued, and dissected in the ethical treatises of the philosophers who nearly invariably came from its ranks, including Galen himself. It was *philotimia* that built the architectural wonders of the East and adorned them so splendidly; and that fueled the incessant litigation, rancor, *stasis* or internal unrest, even low-level insurrection endemic in the East at all times, as the wealthy competed for rank and honor and drew their friends, families, and dependents into the struggle. *Philotimia* was even arguably the basis of Roman rule; Roman emperors and senators participated in the drama as arbiters or allies, heard cases, resolved round after round of disputation, suppressed violence when necessary and feasible, and occasionally rescued the colossal wreckage of failed, hugely expensive architectural projects with their engineers and expertise.[32]

As I have mentioned, Galen acknowledges, hints, or boasts in several places that he lived off the assets he inherited from his father, which gave him leisure to devote all his time to his intellectual and professional life, to disdain fees, and to be magnanimous in the tradition of his class. But he also attributes to his father his most important asset of all, his education. *Philotimia* drove Galen's father to desire for his offspring all the cultural capital— *paideia*, education—that alone, along with landed wealth, could ensure his success in the exclusive and intensely competitive society into which he was born. Nicon homeschooled Galen rigorously in geometry, mathematics, and arithmetic, just as he had been educated by his own father and grandfather. Nicon also was deeply versed in grammar and taught Galen proper Greek. For the rest of his life Galen claimed expertise in geometry, mathematics,

---

32 On the Hellenic or Hellenized ruling class of the Roman East, especially important are Zuiderhoek (2009), Quass (1993), and Halfmann (1979).

and logic, and brought all of these to bear on medicine in both valuable and infelicitous ways. Later, he claimed that no physician could be competent without a background in these disciplines; and one of his longest works, *On Demonstration* in fifteen books (now lost), expounded on the principles of geometric proof, which he considered far superior to the kinds of proof offered by most philosophers.[33]

Galen's education in philosophy, the specialty that his father first chose for him, began quite young. As Galen explains, when he was about fourteen, Nicon became more active in city politics and had less leisure to supervise Galen's education himself; but he interviewed and handpicked his son's philosophical teachers with care. Galen studied with a Stoic, a Platonist, a Peripatetic, and an Epicurean; and attributes to his father's advice one of the defining features of his own intellectual life:

> "These commands," I said, "of my father I hold to and preserve to this day, never professing myself an adherent of any sect, making rigorous investigation of them with all diligence … "
>
> (*Anim. Affect. Dign.* 8, 5.43K)

Had Galen uncritically adopted the ideology of the Empiricists, his first medical teachers—who forswore anatomy, among other things—his life and Western medical history would have taken a very different course. But Galen went to his grave insisting that he was neither Dogmatist, nor Empiricist, nor Methodist—the three main "sects" we today identify in Greco-Roman medicine, based largely on a simplified reading of Galen's works, our main source. I shall discuss them further in the next chapter.

---

33   On homeschooling: *Libr. Propr.* 14 (19.39–40K); *Anim. Affect. Dign.* 8 (5.41–43K). On proper Greek: *Diff. Puls.* 2.5 (8.587K); *Ord. Libr. Propr.* 4 (19.59K). Note: For *De Libris Propriis*, I refer to the chapter divisions in the edition of Boudon-Millot (2007a), which includes material not known or printed in earlier editions. *On Demonstration: Libr. Propr.* 14 (19.39–41K); *Ord. Libr. Propr.* 1 (19.52–53K). For Galen on the relationship of philosophy and medicine, see Mattern (2008a, 23–27) for further references; and also the edition, with commentary, of *That the Best Physician is Also a Philosopher* (*Opt. Med. Philosoph.*) in Boudon-Millot (2007a).

From what Galen tells us of his father, combined with the barest scraps available from other sources and a moderate amount of speculation, a brief biography of the latter can be sketched. Nicon may have been a Roman citizen; if so, he was probably the first one in his family. He was a professional architect like his own father and was trained in mathematics, geometry, logic, and architecture by his father and grandfather. He also laid claim to the linguistic erudition in Greek that partly defined his class. He owned a house in the city with some domestic staff and land in the countryside. His marriage was troubled and Galen was perhaps his only surviving child. He invested heavily in his legacy, schooling Galen himself in the disciplines traditional to his family and supervising his later education closely. He deeply impressed on his offspring the values of temperance, self-control, and magnanimity. In Galen's mid-teens, perhaps under pressure from his peers who felt he was shirking his fair share of the expense involved, he became more active in city politics, probably holding office. A few years later—psychologically and financially depleted?—he retired to the countryside and the life of a gentleman-farmer. When Galen was nineteen he died, probably still in middle age. At the time his son had not yet left Pergamum, and he could never have foreseen the remarkable career in store for him.

Chapter Two

LEARNING MEDICINE

hen Galen was an adolescent of fourteen, his father—busy with civic responsibilities and no longer able to dedicate himself full-time to his son's education—handed him over to teachers of philosophy, whom he interviewed with care. So Galen tells us in a passage from his treatise *On Diagnosing and Curing the Affections of the Soul*, written much later, in the 190s (see chapter 7). Galen's teachers represented most of the major philosophical sects, and all had impeccable credentials and illustrious intellectual pedigrees. One was a Stoic in the tradition of the great Chrysippus of Stoli; Chrysippus's works remained influential in Galen's later life and form much of the subject-matter of one of his most important philosophical works, *On the Doctrines of Hippocrates and Plato*, written years later in Rome. Another of his early teachers was a Platonist student of Gaius, with whom Galen studied only "for a short time" (Gaius, whose name indicates Roman citizen status, is mentioned in several other sources and was famous in the second century, though his works are lost today). Galen also mentions a Peripatetic (Aristotelian) student of Aspasius; Aspasius's works would later be cited by the late antique philosophers Porphyry and Boethius, and part of his commentary on Aristotle's *Nicomachean Ethics* survives today. The Peripatetic, anonymous in this passage, is possibly Eudemus, one of Galen's first patients in the city of Rome (see chapter 4). Finally, Galen mentions an Epicurean about whose background he is more reticent, but this teacher came from Athens, still considered the epicenter of philosophical education. Galen identifies the other three tutors as Pergamene citizens, probably with some pride and nostalgic reference to Platonic ideas of civic pedagogy, though the Peripatetic had just returned from a long journey abroad. Galen does not name his teachers—perhaps because their reputations were modest and these names would not have been impressive on their own; he identifies *their* teachers (except in the case of the Epicurean) and their intellectual affiliation. Intellectual influence, transmitted mostly orally, and pedigree was a matter of some importance (see below). Galen here stakes a claim to intellectual independence or philosophical "eclecticism" from his earliest youth.[1]

Galen continued to seek education from philosophers throughout his life and considered himself a philosopher, as well as a physician. He long argued that all truly educated doctors were philosophers and that Hippocrates had been a philosopher; he wrote philosophical treatises on logic and ethics and a brief work *That the Best Physician is Also a Philosopher*; he boasts of his reputation as a philosopher, which is attested independently of his works. Galen was what the Greeks called a *pepaideumenos*, a cultured man, proud of his broad education, of his mastery of mathematics, geometry, Greek grammar, and especially philosophy, queen of the academic disciplines.[2]

---

1   On Galen's early philosophical education, see Schlange-Schöningen (2003), 68–71. Nicon's distractions: Most translators of *Anim. Affect. Dig.* 8.3 (5.41K) have read Galen's clause "because he had no leisure, having been drawn by his fellow citizens into civic business" as referring to Galen's father; but Schlange-Schöningen (2003, 69) interprets this clause as applying to Galen's teacher, the student of Gaius, and explaining why Galen studied with him only briefly; Gaius's student, as he imagines, must have been a non-Pergamene called home. But Galen implies in the next sentence that the Platonist was a Pergamene like his next teacher the Peripatetic; and the encomium to his subject's character ("because they [the citizens] considered him alone to be just, possessing superior wealth, and approachable and mild") resembles Galen's other statements about his father (see chapter 1); Galen says nothing similar about anyone else. On Galen's Stoic teacher, see also *Libr. Propr.* 14 (19.43K).

2   On Galen's continued philosophical education, see *Foet. Form.* 6 (4.695–96K, 4.700K); *Anim. Affect. Dign.* 1 (4.767K). His philosophical acquaintances in Rome included Boethus's friends Eudemus the Peripatetic, his first patient in the city, and Alexander of Damascus, the Peripatetic with whom he enacts a funny showdown in *Praecog.* 5 (14.628K; see also *Anat. Admin.*

Only a very small number of those calling themselves *iatroi*, doctors, acquired this type of education, as well as Galen's astounding erudition in the whole medical tradition up to his time. Some epitaphs commemorate doctors as young as seventeen, suggesting a traditional apprenticeship (perhaps similar to those common in rural China today) and not an exhaustive, liberal intellectual education. In Italy and especially in the city of Rome, many doctors were slaves or freedmen, trained in the households of the rich. But medicine also had a place among the Greek world's prestigious and esoteric disciplines, and Galen was not the only one who thought so. At Rome he would exploit medicine's cachet among the ruling class, as I shall describe.[3]

Like most people, Galen believed that the gods spoke in dreams and he followed their commands. (He also believed that dreams could be the soul's reflections on humoral imbalances in the body, thus useful for medical diagnosis; and that the soul could prophesy in dreams.) When Galen was sixteen, dreams convinced his father to alter the path of his only son's education: "Exhorted by distinct dreams, he had me study medicine together with philosophy." Galen offers no details and does not identify which god, if any, spoke to his father, but his readers might have assumed the dreams came from Pergamum's most famous divine resident, Asclepius.[4]

1.1, 2.217–18K and chapter 5 below); a Platonist named Antisthenes, addressee of some anatomical treatises (*Libr. Propr.* 1, 19.12K; *Ven. Art. Dissect.* 7, 2.804K); and Glaucon, the addressee of *On the Method of Healing to Glaucon.* Galen also has great respect for Boethus himself as an Aristotelian (*Libr. Propr.* 1, 19.13K). Friends like these may be whom he has in mind when he writes of investigating the soul "together with my teachers and the greatest philosophers" (*Anim. Affect. Dign.* 1, 4.767K). On Galen's reputation, see Nutton (1984b). For Galen on medicine and philosophy, see Mattern (2008a, 23–27, with further references).

3   On China's rural doctors, see Zaminska (2007, 2008). On apprenticeship and other "low" forms of medical training in the Roman Empire, see recently Nutton (2004, chapter 17; and 1995c). For the epitaphs of teenage doctors, see Gummerus (1932, nos. 53, 169, 309). On slaves and freedmen, see Mattern (2008a, 22, with note 73 for references). Especially important are Korpela (1987) and Kudlien (1986).

4   For Galen on dreams, see Kudlien (1981). Following the commands of dreams: *Cur. Ven. Sect.* 23 (11.314–15K); *Libr. Propr.* 2 (19.18–19K); *Usu Part.* 10.12 (3.812, 814K). On the medical interpretation of dreams, see the fragment *Dign. Insomn.* (6.832–35K) and Oberhelman (1983, 37–38). An excellently scholarly study of dreaming in antiquity, including sections on Galen, is now available

Galen was now to take up the study of medicine; but not, as he emphasizes, to the exclusion of philosophy: "We came to cultivate the study of medicine, and throughout our whole life we applied ourselves to both disciplines [medicine and philosophy] in deeds more than in words" (*Meth. Med.* 9.4, 10.609K). Thus, a few years later at Smyrna, we find him studying with the physician Pelops and also the Platonist philosopher Albinus. Like Galen's Platonist teacher at Pergamum, Albinus was a student of Gaius, and the publisher of what became Gaius's main written legacy, his lectures on Plato.[5] In retrospect, Galen emphasizes the diligence with which he attacked his studies while others, as he writes, spent more time socializing with the rich and powerful and cultivating their favor:

> When I began to study medicine I repudiated all pleasure.... I spent all my time in the study of medical practice, deliberating and reflecting on medicine. Generally, I have gone without sleep at night in order to examine the treasures left to us by the Ancients.
>
> (*Opt. Med. Cogn.* 9, 100–102 tr. Iskandar)

> It is no wonder that, while others wandered around the whole city performing salutations, and dined with the rich and powerful and escorted them about, and we on the other hand labored diligently the entire time, we first learned all the things that were creditably discovered by the ancients; then through deeds we both tested and practiced them.
>
> (*Meth. Med.* 9.4, 10.609K)

We know the names of some of his medical teachers at Pergamum: the most important, the one with whose intellectual legacy Galen later identified most, is Satyrus, a pupil of the illustrious Quintus who had practiced in Rome in the decades preceding Galen's birth. Satyrus had been living at Pergamum

---

in Harris (2009). Nicon's dreams: *Ord. Libr. Propr.* 4 (19.59K); see also *Meth. Med.* 9.4 (10.609K) and *Praecog.* 2 (14.608K) for similar language, and see Schlange-Schöningen (2003, 71–73).

5   On Galen's early medical education in Pergamum, see Schlange-Schöningen (2003, 73–76); Boudon-Millot (2007a, xxvii–xxxii). Pelops and Albinus: *Libr. Propr.* 2 (19.16K).

for three years with Rufinus, the native Pergamene, Roman senator, and ex-consul who was apparently funding and overseeing the construction of the spectacular new Temple of Zeus Asclepius (see chapter 1). Satyrus had possibly met Rufinus in Rome while studying with Quintus, and returned to Pergamum with Rufinus as part of his entourage.[6]

Satyrus appears in Aelius Aristides' account of his relationship with Asclepius, the *Sacred Tales*: "The doctor Satyrus was in Pergamum at that time, a sophist of no humble birth, as it was said" (3.8). The date of the story may be around 147 C.E., while Galen was Satyrus's student; it may have been in his teacher's company that Galen met Aristides, whom he describes as an example of a strong soul joined with a weak body—"I have seen only a few of these. One was Aristides, a resident of Mysia" (*Plat. Tim.*, 33 Schröder). Satyrus advised his patient to leave off the harsh regimen of venesection commanded by Asclepius and use a simple plaster to treat his abdominal complaint. Aristides tried the remedy, but it only made his condition worse; the dream prescriptions of Asclepius were, of course, effective.[7]

Besides Satyrus, Galen mentions other physicians from whom he acquired his early education at Pergamum, in passing. These include "Aeschrion the Empiric, that old man most experienced in drugs, my fellow-citizen [of Pergamum] and teacher" (*Simp. Med.* 11.1.34, 12.356–57K), whose cure for rabies Galen describes with approval. The main ingredient was the ashes of crawfish. The crustaceans were collected on a single day in summer, between the rising of the dog star Sirius and the transition of the sun into the sign of Leo (that is, between July 22 and August 20 or thereabout), in the eighteenth day of the moon's cycle, and cooked alive in a pan of red bronze. Galen also mentions a teacher called Stratonicus, "a student of Sabinus the Hippocratic" (*Atra Bile* 4, 5.119K): he once cured a long-standing abscess in the leg by extracting thick, black blood from the patient's elbow over a number of days. Thus, Galen seems to have studied

6   Schlange-Schöningen (2003, 75) assumes that Satyrus was Rufinus's "house doctor," but I think the relationship is likely to have been more complicated than one of simple dependency. It may, for example, have resembled Galen's relationship with Boethus (chapter 5).

7   For the date of Aristides' story, see the annotation of Behr (1981, ad loc).

with several physicians at Pergamum, and it is likely that he does not tell us all of their names. It is unclear whether the "Empiricist teacher" Galen debates in his treatise *On Plenitude* (9, 7.558K) is Aeschrion or not, or possibly identical with another Empiricist teacher, Epicurus, whom Galen mentions only once, in an obscure passage. Galen also describes an argument in which he humiliated yet another teacher—a Pneumatist (the sect was founded by Athenaeus of Attaleia, and named for the role of the vaporous *pneuma* in its natural theory)—without transmitting his name; he was eighteen years old when the episode occurred and probably still living at Pergamum. It is tempting to identify this Pneumatist with Aeficianus, a student of Pelops, whom Galen mentions in *On the Order of My Own Books* as a Stoic-influenced interpreter of Hippocrates and in another passage identifies as one of his teachers. Pneumatist doctrine was heavily tinged with Stoicism, and Galen mentions Aeficianus in connection with Satyrus, suggesting that he learned from them at about the same time.[8]

Much of Galen's medical training was intellectual—he clearly heard Satyrus and others expound on Hippocrates, for example, and I will discuss the intellectual heritage of medicine further below. But from the very beginning, his training also or mainly involved practical demonstration and clinical experience. With Satyrus, Galen observed the horrific effects of an epidemic whose victims "were stripped of skin, and of some also of the very flesh" (*Anat. Admin.* 1.2, 2.224–25K). Galen calls the epidemic "anthrax," and as I mentioned in chapter 1, this was possibly the disease known today as cutaneous anthrax, caused by the *Bacillus anthracis*; although the symptoms he describes are much more extreme than what would be seen today, in an era when the infection is treated with antibiotics. Satyrus would demonstrate anatomy on the patients, instructing them to move in ways that

---

8   Epicurus: *Hipp. 6 Epid.* 7 (412 Wenkebach and Pfaff); see von Staden (2004, 214). Debate with Pneumatist: *Elem. Hipp.* 1.6 (1.462–65K); see Temkin (1973, 20–22) for an English translation. Aeficianus's Stoicism: *Ord. Libr. Propr.* (3, 19.58K). Aeficianus as Galen's teacher: *Hipp. 3 Epid.* 1.40 (17A.575K); as Pelops's student, ibid.; and see further references in von Staden (2004, 213). Tenuous evidence in the Arabic tradition connects Aeficianus with Corinth, and Galen may have met him there rather than in Pergamum; see Grmek and Gourevitch (1994, 1514, 1520–21).

showed the action of the muscles, even displacing muscles to better expose arteries and nerves:

> As we practiced anatomy on one or another of the exposed parts, those of us who had observed Satyrus [previously, demonstrating on animal subjects?] recognized them [the parts] right away and made detailed distinctions, instructing the patients to make certain movements, which we knew to be controlled by certain muscles. We saw that some students, because, like the blind, they did not recognize the exposed parts, were forced to try each of two [experiments], or they raised and moved many parts of the naked muscles, and the patients were unnecessarily distressed.
>
> (*Anat. Admin.* 1.2, 2.225K)

> Sometimes putrefying diseases strip the whole of this region of the surrounding skin, so that the naked veins are seen clearly. This happened frequently over all parts of the body especially at the time when the epidemic of anthrax happened in Asia.
>
> (*Ven. Art. Dissect.* 7, 2.803K)

These experiments on live, suffering patients disfigured by a hideous necrotizing disease were Galen's earliest exposure to human anatomy and must have been unforgettable, although he tells the story without a hint at any emotion other than pride in his own training and disdain for the inferior skills of other students. The story occurs in a complicated passage explaining the importance of observing human anatomy by any available method, in a world in which the dissection of human corpses was taboo and rarely practiced.

The story implies that Galen had observed animal dissections under Satyrus, and animal dissection was certainly part of his early training. His teachers had demonstrated, for example, the muscles responsible for the motion of the lungs. Although he tells no explicit stories about youthful experiences with animal dissection, by the time he left Pergamum (around age nineteen or twenty) he had written his first anatomical treatise, *On the Anatomy of the Uterus*, composed for a midwife; the treatise survives. Galen was certainly a virtuoso anatomist by the time he returned to Pergamum from Alexandria in 157 and humiliated his rivals for the position of physician to the gladiators (see chapter 3).[9]

Clinical practice was a part of Galen's medical training from the beginning—many of Galen's anecdotes illustrate this point. Thus, his story about Stratonicus extracting black blood from a patient day after day, mentioned above, probably derives from his own observation. In an argument with "my Empiric teacher" about the indications for bloodletting, Galen cites several cases treated by the teacher himself, cases Galen had observed: "those whom I saw phlebotomized by you" (*Plen.* 9, 7.560K). Some of these early experiences remained with Galen throughout his life. One case, that of an emaciated and apparently incurable 40-year-old man with digestive problems, Galen recalls many years later in the seventh book of *On the Method of Healing* (7.8, 10.504–6K): "together with my teachers I first saw a patient, a man of mature age, who had been troubled for many months, but none of them could identify his condition, nor could I." Here Galen attends the patient together with several other doctors, all called his "teachers." The physicians consult together on the management of the illness ("And the doctors considered whether the man ought to bathe, some in favor, others opposed, and the opinion won out of those who thought he should bathe"); and Galen, though a student, has a voice ("we all decided that the weakness of the belly had been cured, but that the stomach had been chilled").

Similarly, Galen describes a boy suffering from epilepsy whom he observed "in my youth, together with the best physicians of my homeland, who had come together to consider his treatment" (*Loc. Affect.* 3.11, 8.94K). This happened later, while he was at Smyrna (by "homeland" here Galen means the province of Asia). It was Galen's first case of epilepsy; the boy was suffering horribly, having seizures every day. Among the physicians called to

---

9   Teachers demonstrate muscles for respiration: *Anat. Admin.* 8.2 (2.660K). *Anatomy of the Uterus*: *Libr. Propr.* 2 (19.16K); the treatise is 2.887–908K.

the consultation was Pelops, Galen's teacher; Galen recalls Pelops's diagnosis, and the treatment prescribed, although this treatise was written about fifty years later.

With Galen's medical training, then, began his clinical experience, although he mostly played the role of observer. Thus, of an early encounter with a patient with amnesia, he writes that "I was still young, and had neither observed any of my teachers treating this condition, nor had I read about the treatment in the [works of] any of the ancients" (*Loc. Affect.* 3.5, 8.147K).[10]

Galen's youthful stories not only show him observing and participating in treating patients but also vigorously debating his teachers in what seem like dramatic, even tumultuous scenes that foreshadow his conflicts and performances in Rome. Galen's detailed catalog of cases, recalled perfectly from the physician's own practice, stumped his "Empiric teacher": "after these things, however, he was silent ... he hesitated a long time about what he should answer." His confrontation with the Pneumatist is decidedly dramatic—under the assault of Galen's aggressive, Socratic-style questioning about ambiguities in his classification of the elements, the teacher is at first flummoxed ("he hesitated a long time"), then agitated ("now becoming angry and disturbed"), and finally cannot suppress a hostile outburst:

> Looking at the other students, he said: "This man, raised on dialectics and therefore full of mange (for thus he himself called it), turns everything upside down and twists it around and mixes it up, and confuses it by playing the sophist with us, so that he may demonstrate his logical skills."
>
> (*Elem. Hipp.* 1.6, 1.462–65K)

This all happened, as the last quotation makes clear, in front of the other students, which was probably also the case in Galen's debate with the Empiricist. Furthermore, we have seen Galen and his teachers consulting and debating at

---

10   For similar statements referring to cases observed with his teachers among his other clinical experiences, see *Loc. Affect.* 3.3 (8.143K), 3.4 (8.145–46K).

the patient's bedside. Medical education was not the monotonous transmission of knowledge from authority to pupil; it was a passionate dialogue in which everyone participated.

It was probably also at Pergamum "as a lad" (*meirakion*—a word Galen uses for males in their late teens and early twenties) that Galen began to acquire his lifelong expertise in pharmacology; not only from his physician-teachers (Satyrus and Aeschrion are both cited in his compendia on drugs, as is Pelops, his next teacher)[11] but also he paid an exorbitant sum to an unnamed expert who taught him to prepare certain exotic drugs "so that what I prepared was indistinguishable from the genuine item" (*Simp. Med.* 9.3.8, 12.216K). Galen lists among the drugs he learned to produce those made from *diphryges* (a metallic mining by-product, possibly a pyrite), also signets of Lemnian earth and "Indian lycium" (catechu). Later in life he traveled widely around the eastern Mediterranean to obtain a lifetime supply of these ingredients: "for this reason I was zealous to travel to Lemnos and Cyprus and Palestinian Syria to acquire for myself a large enough quantity of each of these drugs for my whole life" (ibid., and see chapter 4 on these journeys). Did Galen learn, from the teacher who demanded such a high price ("a huge fee," *misthos megas*), to counterfeit the genuine drugs or did he learn local secret recipes and methods for preparing the rare ingredients he later went to such effort to obtain? His comment above—that his own products looked exactly like the "genuine items" (*alethina*)—suggests that he had hired an expert pharmaceutical counterfeiter to teach him the tricks of the trade, and that perhaps this knowledge inspired him to acquire quantities of the true materials.[12]

Like his philosophical education, Galen's medical education was eclectic: one or more of his early teachers was an Empiricist; one was a Pneumatist; and one, Satyrus, was not (at least, not strictly) aligned with either of these traditions, although he may have shared the Empiricist leanings of Quintus

---

11   Satyrus on pharmacology: *Antid.* 1.14 (14.69K); Schlange-Schöningen (2003, 83). Aeschrion: see p. 40 above. Pelops: *Simp. Med.* 11.1.34 (12.359K).

12   Galen goes on, in the same passage just quoted, to recount how he acquired some "Indian lycium" from a camel caravan after convincing himself that it was the genuine, imported-from-India article.

(see below). Throughout his life Galen vigorously proclaimed his independence from any sect. This intellectual independence he attributed to the influence and advice of his father, who warned him not to align himself with any tradition but to choose the best ideas from each (*Anim. Affect. Dign.* 8, 5.42, 43K). "I consider," he writes, making his point sharply, "those who name themselves Hippocrateans or Praxagoreans or after any man at all to be slaves" (*Libr. Propr.* 1, 19.13K), that is, intellectually servile. There was a certain virtuosity to his position. "Whenever I chose to advocate a single sect, it was difficult for anyone to convict me of hesitation in improvised speech; for I learned them not from handbooks [*hypomnemata*], as some do, but from the most prominent teachers of each sect" (*Loc. Affect.* 3.3, 8.143–44K).

From the early Hellenistic period, medicine had encompassed vigorously competing intellectual traditions. Galen identifies three sects, or *haireseis* (from the Greek word for clinging or adherence), in his treatise *On the Sects for Beginners* and refers to them often in other works, notably *Outline of Empiricism* and *On the Method of Healing* (the title of the latter mocks the detested Methodists—Galen meant *The [True] "Method" of Healing*). The Empiricists defined themselves according to their epistemology, or theory of how knowledge is obtained: this, as Galen writes, they considered so important that they disdained the more usual appellation deriving from a founding figure. Their founder was in fact Philinus of Cos, renegade student of the renowned anatomist Herophilus. Philinus broke from his master and founded his own school in Alexandria on radical principles.[13]

Empeiria is "experience" in Greek, the sole source of medical knowledge in Empiricist doctrine. This experience could be an observation, usually of a cure (because of their methods, much surviving Empiricist writing—all fragments, as no complete work survives—concerns therapy and especially drugs). The cure might occur randomly, by accident; or the physician might make an educated guess and deliberate experiment; or, as Galen writes, he might be

---

13   For an excellent brief discussion of the medical sects, see von Staden (1982, 76–100, 199–206). The fundamental study of Empiricism and collection of the fragments is Deichgräber (1965). Empiricists not named for a founding-figure: *Subfig. Emp.* 1 (42 Deichgräber).

advised by a dream (*Sect. Intro.* 2, 1.3K). Empiric methods of discovery could thus have a tinge of mysticism. Galen, although he mentions without comment dream cures of Asclepius and the dream instructions given to his father about his own education, even criticizes Empiricists because "they refer nearly all the compound drugs [they devise] to dreams and fortune and chance" (*Comp. Med. Gen.* 1.1, 13.366K). One might speculate that Aeschrion's aforementioned magical cure for rabies, using crawfish gathered by moonlight on a single day in summer, was inspired by a dream.

For a conclusion to be valid (*x* drug cures *y* condition), the observation had to be made repeatedly. Lest medical knowledge be limited to what each individual physician might observe in a lifetime, it was permissible to use conclusions based on the observations of other physicians, as recorded in books or transmitted orally—these reports Galen calls history (*historia*). History, in turn, must be evaluated according to specific criteria, especially the trustworthiness of the source, the number of sources attesting to a specific cure, and the degree of consensus among sources. It was also allowable to use simple reasoning based on similarity (a condition similar to *y* might also be treatable by *x*). But most forms of deductive reasoning, especially theorizing about the cause of disease, the Empiricists rejected as irrelevant or impractical. According to Galen they also rejected anatomical dissection; close observation of wounds in living persons was, they believed, an adequate method of studying anatomy, a position Galen excoriates.[14]

But some of his earliest training was in Empiricist methods. Not only did Galen study with two or more Empiricist teachers at Pergamum, but Satyrus himself, his main and most respected teacher, was the product of an Empiricist-leaning tradition. In particular, Galen attributes to Satyrus's teacher Quintus—about whom more below—an Empiricist interpretation of Hippocrates, of which he is critical: "Quintus interpreted these books and also the *Aphorisms* badly ... for Quintus says that this is known only by experience, without reasoning about the cause" (*Hipp. 1 Epid. Proem.*, 17A.6K).

---

14   Empiricists reject dissection and Galen's disapproval: *Sect. Intro.* 5 (1.11K); *Anat. Admin.* 2.3 (2.288–90K); *Comp. Med. Gen.* 3.2 (13.607, 609K).

Galen considered Satyrus the most faithful transmitter of Quintus's views on Hippocrates, suggesting that Satyrus, too, had Empiricist leanings.[15]

Galen's early exposure to Empiricism permanently influenced his vision of medicine as above all grounded in practice. Throughout his life, Galen would continually refer to "deeds among the patients" as the most conclusive form of medical proof and heap scorn on those who clung to theories contradicted by the observable facts or accepted the doctrines they read in written sources without testing them against experience.[16] Late in life, in his treatise *On the Affected Parts*, he writes:

> I myself, if truth be told, whenever I hear Empiricist doctors talking about [how knowledge is acquired, and particularly how it is not necessary to know the mechanism by which something is effective if it demonstrably works], I consider their arguments highly persuasive, and I find the counterarguments raised by the Dogmatists not especially genuine; but just as in all other things, for my whole life, I have always refrained from unconsidered approval, also in these matters I strove for a long time in clinical practice [literally, "among the patients"] to discover whether I needed in addition some logical demonstration of remedies, or whether what I had learned from my own experience and from that with my teachers was enough.
>
> (*Loc. Affect.* 3.3, 8.141–43K)

He adds, "I have no hatred for the Empiricists, on whose arguments I was raised, nor against any of the Dogmatists" (ibid. 8.144K). And in another late passage, from the second half of *On the Method of Healing* (9.4, 10.609K): "If

---

15   On Quintus's Empiricist views, see also *Hipp. 1 Epid.* 1.1 (17A.24K), 2.7 (17A.99K); *Hipp. 3 Epid.* 1.4 (17B.502K); and Grmek and Gourevitch (1994, 1509–10). Satyrus as transmitter of Quintus's views: *Ord. Libr. Propr.* 3 (19.57K).

16   For example: *Hipp. 6 Epid.* 3.29 (17B.95K), here relying on the experience of midwives regarding the alteration of the breasts during lactation "for these women state the phenomena truly, rather than those who bumble blindly around it because of dogma." On testing the writings of the ancients, ibid. 2.28 (17A.951K); on those who practice "sophistic" medicine uninformed by experience with patients, ibid. 2.10 (17A.806K); *Diff. Resp.* 1.12 (7.792K); and many other references.

everyone who undertook to teach and write something would first demonstrate these things with deeds, altogether few false things would be said."

Galen credited his skill with the pulse (a field in which, as he writes, Empiricist contributions had been very extensive) and understanding of the "critical days" of fever, among other things, to exhaustive and repeated observation and experience; that is, experience was not only helpful in therapeutics. Galen credits midwives and athletic trainers with valuable knowledge gained purely from their experiences with injury and regimen. Like modern physicians, he refers often to what he has seen personally in proving a point, for example: "all those that we have seen, suffering from *phrenitis* in this way, died on the seventh day; a few, rarely, survived longer" (*Hipp. 3 Epid.* 3.75, 17A.760K).[17]

The Empiricists did not differ from what Galen calls "Rationalist" or "Dogmatist" physicians in the symptoms they observed or the remedies they prescribed; Galen insists that they all used the same therapies. Empiricists, like Dogmatists, took account of age, location, season, occupation, and regimen in their prescriptions, but apparently without theorizing a cause explaining the relevance of these factors. Empiric method emphasized acute observation—of the patient, the symptoms, the effects of remedies, the body and its wounds, or as Galen writes, the phenomena, the "the things that are evident"—above all else.[18]

Galen's early Empiricist training may explain the prominent role of case histories in his writings, although they are also attested in other ancient medical authors and especially in the Hippocratic Corpus, the canon of Greek medicine's earliest texts associated with its half-legendary founder, Hippocrates of Cos, and already about five hundred years old by Galen's time. The seven books of Hippocratic *Epidemics* were composed mostly or entirely of case histories. When Galen argues with his Empiricist teacher about the indications

---

17   Empiricists and the pulse: *Dign. Puls.* 1.1 (8.771–73K); Deichgräber (1965, 132–39). "Critical days": *Dieb. Decret.* 1.3 (9.780K). Midwives: *Hipp. 6 Epid.* 3.29 (17B.95K). Athletic trainers: *Meth. Med.* 6.3 (10.407K), 7.6 (10.490K).

18   Empiricists and Dogmatists use the same remedies: *Sect. Intro.* 4 (1.7–8K). Age, location, etc.: *Exp. Med.* 6 (92 Walzer).

for bloodletting or explains how he confirmed the efficacy of snake venom as a cure for elephantiasis in his treatise *Outline of Empiricism*, he recalls cases from his own experience or that of his teacher, or even stories whose origin may lie in folklore; it is possible that this reflects an Empiricist tradition of using case narratives as evidence, though it is not attested elsewhere.[19] Several of Galen's stories recount his first use or discovery of a treatment that proved efficacious with further testing, reflecting Empiricist ideas of knowledge, although he may use forms of reasoning not allowed in strict Empiricist doctrine in deciding which remedy to try. For example, at the end of the story of how he miraculously cured a patient with "chalkstones" using rancid cheese— the story with which this book begins—Galen writes that "this, which was known from our own ingenuity (*epinoia*), was confirmed by experience." He introduces another story with a complex epistemological statement reflecting his debt to Empiricism and particularly the value he ascribed to repeated testing of a remedy:

> But I shall tell you about a patient of this type on whom I first dared, led by reason, to disregard the *diatritos* [a Methodist remedy] and to aim at strength[ening the patient]. Afterward, seeing others similarly [afflicted], I was encouraged to treat them in the same way as [I had treated] him. For when the first trial has affirmed those things that were [originally] discovered by indication (*endeixis*, a type of logical inference forbidden in Empiricist doctrine), it renders people more confident in using it a second time.
>
> (*Meth. Med.* 10.3, 10.671K)

Thus the modern case history traces its intellectual roots to antiquity, where it served many of the same functions: encoding the knowledge gained by clinical experience.[20]

---

19   On case narrative and Empiricism, see Mattern (2008a, 31–33).
20   On the case history in modern medicine, a large scholarship exists; Hunter (1991) is especially relevant. See Mattern (2008a, 27–28) for more references.

Galen contrasts the Empiricists with two other schools of medical thought, the Dogmatists or Rationalists, and the Methodists. The designation "Rationalist" or "Dogmatist" was relevant mainly in opposition to Empiricists, as it signified all sects that used long-traditional theories of causation and deductive reasoning; these were, then, very nonspecific words that encompassed several important and conflicting traditions, some of which also referred to themselves—or each other—as *haireseis*.

Galen, citing his father's admonitions, did not consider himself an adherent of any sect. Had he completely rejected Empiricist views, however, Galen should have qualified as a "Rationalist" of some sort—certainly he makes ample use of deductive reasoning and accepts most Rationalist theories of the nature of the body and the etiology of disease. It may be his continued sympathy for some Empiricist principles, or possibly his intensely critical attitude toward the writings of virtually all his predecessors—except Hippocrates, who played a foundational and complex role in his thought—that qualified Galen as a free agent in his own mind.

As I have mentioned, Galen also distinguished a third sect, called the Methodists. Galen detested Methodists with an unwavering hostility that did not diminish at any point in his life. Methodists rejected Empiric epistemology because they postulated a theory of disease, based on Democritus's "atomist" theory of physics: bodies are made of atoms and pores, and all diseases either result from compaction (where the atoms are pressed too tightly together) or flux (where the atoms are too dispersed) or some combination of those two things. Methodists differed from the other schools in the radical reductionism of their theory, which led them to reject (as Galen claims) anatomy and the study of most other medical traditions. The art of medicine, they believed, could be mastered in six months.

The Methodist school was founded in the first century B.C.E. by the shadowy Themison and made famous in the reign of Nero by the charismatic Thessalus of Tralles, who authored a famous letter to the emperor (quoted by Galen) denouncing the worthlessness of all previous medical writers, and called himself "champion physician" on his monumental tombstone that graced the Appian Way.[21] Methodism maintained a glamorous appeal also in Galen's day and may have been the dominant doctrine of the time, at least in aristocratic circles. Many of Galen's stories describe triumphs over rival Methodist physicians, including some of the most renowned doctors of his era. The royal lady Annia Faustina travels with an entourage of Methodists with which she confronts Galen during his treatment of the prince Commodus. One of the most illustrious physicians of the second century C.E. after Galen himself, Soranus of Ephesus, was a Methodist; the latter is the author of the *Gynecology*, one of the few surviving medical treatises of the second century C.E. besides Galen's own work; of treatises *On Acute and Chronic Diseases*, of which a fifth-century Latin translation by Caelius Aurelianus also survives; and of many lost works.[22]

Galen heaps invective on the sect and the figure he treats as its founder, deriding Thessalus as an uneducated, low-class quack, son of a weaver and trainer of household slaves and craftsmen; contemporary Methodist rivals of Galen are incompetent, "amethodic," or "the Thessalian ass."[23] He particularly mocks the *diatritos*, the Methodist three-day unit of therapy (especially, a three-day fast at the onset of fever) that was apparently much in vogue in his day. But the extreme quality of his polemic only underlines that the Methodists were worthy rivals, over whom Galen's intellectual legacy triumphed presumably with some difficulty.

The tripartite division of medicine into the Empiricist, Dogmatist, and Methodist traditions was not Galen's invention but is attested earlier in the Latin medical writer Celsus. It is, however, in some ways an oversimplification of a complex intellectual heritage, as the discussion of Dogmatism above suggests. Within Empiricism and Methodism also there were separate

---

21   Galen, *Meth. Med.* 1.2 (10.8K); Pliny, *Naturalis Historia* 29.9.

22   For a recent, sympathetic history of Methodism, see Nutton (2004, chapter 13); see also von Staden (1982, 83–85). Fragments are collected and discussed in Tecusan (2004). Annia Faustina: *Praecog.* 12 (14.663–64K). Galen mentions Soranus several times, and one of his most entertaining stories recounts his own humiliation of Attalus, a student of Soranus: *Meth. Med.* 13.15 (10.910K).

23   Mattern (2008a, 73).

and competing traditions; and Galen often identifies rival physicians not as Empiricists, Dogmatists, or Methodists but as followers of a specific tradition identified by its founding figure. Among these are notably Asclepiadeans or followers of Asclepiades, who in adopting atomist physics was a founding influence on the Methodist sect but did not count as Methodist himself; and Erasistrateans or followers of Erasistratus, who argued that the arteries contained air (*pneuma*) rather than blood and eschewed venesection, positions Galen criticizes.[24]

Empiricists declined to buy into speculative assumptions about disease and the body; but as I have mentioned, Galen insists that they used the same remedies as Rationalists and considered most of the same factors as relevant. But Methodist theories of disease as the constriction or flux of atoms departed radically from what was by then a long tradition. The earliest Greek medical texts, the treatises of the Hippocratic Corpus, share (although it is not always explicit) a humoral idea of the body and its relationship to the world. The humors, essential bodily fluids, literally "juices," were thus an ancient concept by Galen's time. The Hippocratic treatise *The Nature of Man* is the most coherent and explicit description of a humoral doctrine (it is not, however, in all ways consistent with the ideas of other Hippocratic authors, who mostly postulated two or three essential humors). *The Nature of Man* is sweeping and schematic in its view, identifying no less, or more, than four humors. The new humor—the one lacking in other Hippocratic texts, the one probably added to make up the canonical number four—was black bile. The other humors were blood, phlegm, and yellow bile, and all together they were the essential components of man, whose health depended on their proper balance. Linked to the four humors were the four elemental qualities of hot, cold, wet, and dry; the four seasons, each matched to a pair of qualities and a corresponding humor; and four stages in human life.

---

24   Celsus: *proem.* 10, 57, and see von Staden (1982, 83–84). On "Asclepiadeans," e.g., *Nat. Fac.* 1.12–17 (2.28–67K); *Usu Part.* 1.21 (3.74K), 5.5 (3.364K), 7.4 (1.363K); *Purg. Med. Fac.* 2 (11.328K). On Erasistrateans, *Nat. Fac.* passim; *Anat. Admin.* 7.4 (2.597–98K); *Usu Part.* 5.5 (3.364K); *Purg. Med. Fac.* 2 (11.328K); *An Arter. Sang.* (4.703–36K); and *Ven. Sect. Eras.*

Galen had a special affinity for this treatise, of which he believed Hippocrates himself was the genuine author, despite that Aristotle clearly attributed it to Polybus, Hippocrates' son-in-law. Galen wrote two commentaries on it in the course of his life: the first called *On the Elements According to Hippocrates*, and a second, written much later, which comes down to us simply as *On Hippocrates' The Nature of Man*. Galen would take the Hippocratic treatise's schema further by linking (in some respects, loosely) the four humors to the four elements of fire, earth, air, and water, in the theory of physics first expounded by the mystic philosopher Empedocles in the fifth century B.C.E. Galen also seems to have originated the idea of what he called the "mixtures," or temperaments, in which each humor, except phlegm, affected the state and character of the *psyche* or soul. Galen also wrote a separate treatise *On Mixtures*, here emphasizing "mixtures" not so much of humors as of the elemental qualities of hot, cold, wet, and dry, and their manifestations in body and soul. In his view there were nine possible temperaments: one dominated by each of the four elemental qualities; one dominated by each of the four possible combinations of two qualities; and an ideal temperament in which all were equally balanced. Still, the theory of the equivalence of four canonical temperaments with four humors—the phlegmatic, sanguine, choleric, and melancholic temperaments—that became popular in medieval Europe is not found in Galen's work but is a later development.[25]

Although he avoided adherence to any sect, Galen was proud of his intellectual descent from Quintus, the pre-eminent physician practicing in Rome under Hadrian; "the best doctor of his time." Quintus, who was of Galen's father's generation, died shortly before Galen began his medical education; but Galen sought out Quintus's students and learned from as many of them as possible, sparing no effort or expense. He only disdained, as he writes, to seek out Lycus, whom, as he claimed later, he considered a mediocre physician. Quintus's Roman first name reflects a grant of citizenship, either to himself or to one of his ancestors; he was an ethnic Greek, for Galen apparently

---

25   On the origin and development of the four-humor theory and the idea of temperament, see recently Jouanna (2010, 1–21). Polybus: Aristotle, *Historia animalium* 3.3.

calls him a fellow Pergamene. Galen may have seen himself as following, eventually, in his illustrious predecessor's footsteps, rising to prominence in Pergamum and then moving to Rome.[26]

Quintus was especially renowned as an anatomist: he is called "the most anatomical man" by the hostile audience at one of Galen's demonstrations (*Libr. Propr.* 2, 19.22K), and Galen mentions him several times in his treatise *On Anatomical Procedures* (where, for example, his distinguished predecessor dissects the scrotum of a living goat). Quintus's teacher had been Marinus, the author of the most comprehensive work on anatomy known to Galen or available in his student years, before the appearance, in the 170s, of a work of comparable length (nineteen books) by the despised Lycus, and before the composition of Galen's own great treatises *On the Usefulness of the Parts* and *On Anatomical Procedures*. Marinus's exhaustive work ran to twenty books, and Galen eventually published a summary of it in four (both the original and Galen's summary are now lost, but Galen describes the contents of his summary at length in *On My Own Books*, chapter 4; here Galen writes, not to be accused of ignorance of his rival's work that, he also summarized the inferior treatise of Lycus, but in only two books). Galen credited Marinus with reviving the art of anatomy in his era and clearly considered his work fundamental, but he also found it full of errors, which he would demonstrate before audiences in live anatomical dissections in Rome. His surviving criticisms of Marinus, however, are mixed with respectful praise of his predecessor.[27]

---

26   Quintus's pre-eminence: *Anat. Admin.* 14.1 (230 Simon); *Praecog.* 1 (14.602K). Quintus's death: *Anat. Admin.* 1.2 (2.225K). "Quintus, who practiced in Rome in the time of our fathers," *Hipp. 6 Epid.* 4.10 (17B.151K). Sparing no effort: *Anat. Admin.* 4.10 (2.469–70K). Lycus: *Anat. Admin.* 4.10 (2.469K), 14.1 (232 Simon). Fellow Pergamene: *Hipp. 6 Epid.* 4.9 (17B 151K). In most readings of this passage, Galen calls Quintus a "fellow countryman," but one manuscript variant casts doubt on the word, which is the only evidence for Quintus's Pergamene citizenship. See Grmek and Gourevitch (1994, 1505 n. 45). It was common for Galen and other Greeks to call Roman citizens by their first names only: ibid., 1505.

27   Scrotum of goat: *Anat. Admin.* 12.7 (155 Simon). Errors: *Anat. Admin.* 1.3 (2.234K), 2.1 (2.280–81K), 4.10 (2.469–70KK), 14.1 (233 Simon); and see Grmek and Gourevitch (1994, 1497–1501) on Galen's many references to Marinus on individual points of anatomy, emphasizing that Galen usually combines praise of his predecessor with censure of his errors. Marinus revived anatomy: *Plac. Hipp. Plat.* 8.1 (5.651K); *Hipp. Nat. Hom.* 2.6 (15.136K); and see Grmek and Gourevitch (1994, 1493–94). Twenty volumes: *Libr. Propr.* 3 (19.25K). Summary: ibid. 4 (19.25–31K).

(Later, in the Renaissance, Galen's own works will play roughly the same role in the anatomical career of his remote intellectual descendant Vesalius as Marinus's played in Galen's; see the Epilogue.)

But Quintus, like Galen himself and all the other physicians with whom he studied, was not only an anatomical expert; he taught Hippocratic textual criticism, pharmacology, and presumably other subjects, and also practiced medicine. Galen's anecdotes about Quintus suggest a vigorous, rough-and-ready man whose patients complained that he stank of wine and who was forced to flee a conspiracy of his rivals to charge him with murdering his patients.[28]

Quintus left only an exiguous written legacy. Galen learned of his views on Hippocrates through his pupils: "We first heard Satyrus's exposition of Quintus, and later I read some of those of Lycus" (*Ord. Libr. Propr.* 3, 19.58K). On anatomy—the subject for which he was most renowned—Quintus composed no written works at all. Galen considered Satyrus's memory of Quintus's anatomical knowledge to be the most reliable; and Satyrus also left written works on anatomy.[29]

Quintus's most famous pupil Numisianus, whose instruction Galen sought (see below), also left few written works: he composed prolifically, but his son Heraclianus was jealous of his legacy and did not allow the works to circulate. One story even told that the son burned his father's books on his deathbed. Galen wanted to see Numisianus's books and tried to persuade Heraclianus to show them to him, when he was in Alexandria, but without success. Numisianus's student Pelops, also Galen's teacher, kept Numisianus's works a secret—Galen accuses him of wishing to take credit for some of Numisianus's ideas. Pelops's own works, apparently, were mostly

---

Lycus: ibid. 4 (19.25K); and Galen describes his summary of Lycus's work in a passage restored to the text based on the new *Vlatadon* manuscript (Boudon-Millot (2007a, 153–54).

28   Wine smell: *Hipp. 6 Epid.* 4.9 (17B.151K). Murder: *Praecog.* 1 (14.601K); *Opt. Med. Cogn.* 3 (52 Iskandar). On this episode, see Schlange-Schöningen (2003, 77).

29   Quintus wrote nothing on anatomy: *Anat. Admin.* 14.1 (231 Simon); *Hipp. Nat. Hom.* 2.6 (15.136K). Satyrus's memory best: *Anat. Admin.* 14.1 (231 Simon). Satyrus's works on anatomy: *Hipp. Nat. Hom.* 2.6 (15.136K).

lost in a fire, though some books he composed for his students were still in circulation.[30]

Galen never describes himself and his teachers as "followers of Quintus" or "Quinteans," nor does he identify a specific and unifying set of doctrines that would distinguish them from competing "schools" or *haireseis*. Furthermore, Galen shows no dogmatic loyalty to his predecessors, proclaiming his advances over their mistakes and errors many times.[31] But his intellectual genealogy is important to him: he takes great pains to identify himself as a second- and third-generation student of the great Quintus, the most famous anatomist in recent history. And not only this, he suggests that medical knowledge and discoveries particular to Quintus, Numisianus, and Pelops were transmitted personally from teacher to student and not available to others; Galen inherited a body of knowledge that was, in some ways, secret. His claim to adhere to no sect must be qualified in this sense.

A massive written medical literature had accumulated by Galen's time, and there can be no doubt that Galen considered mastery of these texts fundamental to professional competence. Besides the Hippocratic Corpus (on which see more below) he recommends the works of many of the "ancients;" one list mentions Diocles, Pleistonicus, Phylotimus, Praxagoras, Dieuches, Herophilus, Erasistratus, and Asclepiades. Some of these authors are lost entirely; others survive in fragments (especially Diocles of Carystus, who wrote in the fourth century B.C.E.; Erasistratus and Herophilus of Alexandria, in the early third century B.C.E.; and Asclepiades of Bithynia, in the first century B.C.E.), largely in quotations from Galen's works. But Galen believed that every educated physician should master them. Galen himself continually flaunted his knowledge of his predecessors' work; huge percentages of some treatises are given over to blow-by-blow analysis (most often, criticism) of the arguments of previous medical writers. After the fire of 192 that destroyed

---

30 All of this is described in *Anat. Admin.* 14.1 (230–33 Simon).

31 Mistakes: e.g., regarding the motion of the lungs, *Anat. Admin.* 8.2 (2.657–58 and 660K); Pelops's theory that all blood vessels originate with the brain, *Plac. Hipp. Plat.* 6.3 (5.527K); Pelops was also wrong about crab meat being a cure for rabies, *Simp. Med.* 11.1.34 (12.359K); Galen's discovery of the "phonetic nerves," unknown to his teachers, *Loc. Affect.* 1.6 (8.53K).

his most valuable possessions, the loss he mourned most was not that of his own works, but of the precious manuscripts of ancient writers, to which he had added his own notes and comments. Clearly, medicine of the type that Galen learned and practiced was at least partly a textual discipline and medical education depended partly on a long and, by Galen's time, extensive and exhaustive written tradition.[32]

Most of the authors Galen names in his recommended curriculum wrote many centuries before him, illustrating that the modern obsession with currency—only the most recent work can be valuable—did not obtain in his time; in some ways the reverse was true, although a sense of medical progress is also evident in Galen, who especially perceives anatomical discoveries as building on predecessors (see chapter 5). But a unique role in medical education was played by the oldest body of works, the treatises attributed to Hippocrates. Hippocratic exegesis had a long history by Galen's time. Galen considers his own educators, "Quintus and his students," explicitly including his own teacher Satyrus, mediocre commentators on Hippocrates ("they did not understand the mind of Hippocrates accurately," *Ord. Libr. Propr.* 3, 19.57–58K). He goes on to direct explicit criticism against the despised Lycus, while recommending the Hippocratic commentaries of one of Quintus's other students, Numisianus, and Numisianus's student Pelops, who was also Galen's own teacher. Pelops, as Galen mentions elsewhere, wrote an introductory work on Hippocrates in at least three books. Stratonicus, one of Galen's teachers at Pergamum, had been the student of Sabinus the Hippocratean, whose Hippocratic commentaries were the most exhaustive known to Galen.[33]

Hippocrates and Hippocratic commentary clearly played a foundational role in Galen's medical education and in medical education generally. Almost all significant medical writers had, apparently, commented on Hippocrates, and Galen's own commentaries cite the interpretations of many predecessors dating at least as far back as Herophilus, Hippocrates' first known

---

32   List: *Opt. Med. Cogn.* 5 (68 Iskandar). On Diocles, see van der Eijk (2001). On Erasistratus, see Garofalo (1988). On Herophilus, see von Staden (1989). On Asclepiades, see Vallance (1990). Loss in fire: *Ind.* 13.

33   Pelops: *Musc. Dissect.* (18B.926K). For references on Stratonicus, see Nutton (2004, 212).

commentator, in the early third century B.C.E. Galen himself had hoped to publish commentaries on all genuine Hippocratic works before his death (*Ord. Libr. Propr.* 3, 19.57K).

Galen mentions Hippocrates more than 2,500 times in his surviving works.[34] To do justice to his relationship to the Hippocratic Corpus would require a volume in itself. Later, Renaissance scientists would criticize Galen as a mere transmitter of Hippocratic views, but this is not the case; his use of the Hippocratic Corpus is much more complex. Galen was like early Christian exegetes who expanded on biblical texts and altered their meaning with their interpretations. The genuine Hippocrates, in Galen's work, is laconic, often enigmatic, and virtually never wrong; but Galen did not consider all works transmitted in the Corpus to be genuine—nor are modern scholars able to identify which, if any, of the dozens of treatises it contains were written by Hippocrates.[35]

The latter is a shadowy figure, known to Plato as a famous physician of the previous century; his name attracted folktales, spurious documents, and late biographies written centuries after his death, but few reliable facts are transmitted about him. The founding father of Greek medicine was said to have lived on the island of Cos in the later fifth century B.C.E., and the works that survive under his name, the Hippocratic Corpus, are the earliest Greek medical writings; but ancient commentators recognized contradictions and inconsistencies within the corpus and had long postulated multiple authors and competing schools (the ancient theory that a rival tradition had arisen on the nearby island of Cnidus is still widely accepted today, on no real evidence). Some Hippocratic treatises were very influential in antiquity and even through the modern period, for example the treatise *On the Sacred Disease*, which demystified epileptic seizures, arguing that they were caused by a blockage of phlegm in the brain and not by divine disfavor. Also the treatise *Airs, Waters, Places*, on the relationship between climate, health, and

---

34   Jouanna (1999, 352).

35   On the influence and interpretation of the Hippocratic Corpus in antiquity, including a chapter on Galen, see Wesley Smith (1979); and for a brief account of Hippocratism in the Roman period, Nutton (2004, 206–9, 212–13, 219–21).

race; its descriptions of Scythians, Egyptians, and other peoples contrasted with Greeks resonated through centuries of imperialism and colonialism (notwithstanding that the Hippocratic author considered white northern Europeans as different from, and inferior to, his own people as Asians or Africans). The *Oath* is a statement of ethics that has served, off and on and with long hiatuses, as a touchstone of the medical profession's identity over centuries; modern versions (mostly unrelated to the original in content) are used today in many western countries, especially the United States. The canonical *Oath* began with a long section on the obligations of the apprentice to his master and to his master's family, and also included an abjuration of surgery, of sexual contact with the men and women of patients' households (both slave and free), of giving patients lethal drugs even if they ask for them, and famously, of providing women with drugs for abortion. Much of it was obsolete even in Galen's time.[36]

Galen disdained to name himself the follower of any sect or individual and did not call himself a "Hippocratean," as some other doctors did. But he considered knowledge of the Hippocratic Corpus a basic foundation of medical expertise. While he subjects virtually all other authorities in the long tradition of medical literature—including the iconic Plato and Aristotle, and all of his own teachers—to at least some criticism, and in some cases to hundreds of pages of outright polemic, Hippocrates is the exception, rarely if ever attacked in his work. In his treatise *That the Best Physician is Also a Philosopher*, Galen holds up (his version of) Hippocrates' life, education, and ethics as the ideal.

While Galen and other sources list Hippocrates as the first Dogmatist, Empiricists also claimed him as their founder, emphasizing different texts—and Galen learned some of this Empiricist Hippocrates from his early teachers, as I have mentioned. Only the Methodists treated Hippocrates like any

---

36 I oversimplify many subtle points. For a good introduction to Hippocratic medicine, see Jouanna (1999); on *Airs, Waters, Places* in the early modern period, see, for example, Wear (2008); on the *Oath*, four articles in a special edition of the *Journal of the History of Medicine and Allied Sciences* are most informative: von Staden (1996), with a translation of the original text; Galvão-Sobrinho (1996); Rütten (1996); and Dale C. Smith (1996).

other authority, accepting what was valuable but mercilessly attacking the errors they perceived as typical of an entrenched, outmoded approach to medicine. It is one of Galen's accusations against Lycus, the subpar student of Quintus, and Julian the Methodist and others of his sect, that they published critical interpretations of Hippocrates or, as Galen sees it, attacks on the ancient physician's views (both wrote commentaries on the Hippocratic *Aphorisms*, of which Galen published his own refutations). Not that this was inappropriate in theory; Hippocrates' accusers are just profoundly ignorant and wrong:

> No blame should attach to Lycus or to anyone who wishes to write against Hippocrates. Still more blameless are those who are able to demolish the accusations badly pronounced against him … and especially when the one who accuses has made bold first to learn the things said [by Hippocrates], and when the spokesman for the defense has been educated in the ancient dogma.
>
> (*Adv. Lyc.* 1, 18B.196K)

Lycus, of course, does not meet the criterion of a learned accuser, as Galen proceeds to demonstrate in the rest of his treatise.[37]

Thus, Galen has a complicated relationship to the written medical tradition. In the earliest, foundational work lies medical truth; the skilled physician knows and understands the Hippocratic Corpus thoroughly, has commented on it (as several or all of Galen's teachers had published commentaries), and can recall or quote any part of it at will, at the patient's bedside:

> I arrived and saw that the youth's face was of the type which Hippocrates once described in his *Prognostic* in the following terms:

---

37   On the Dogmatic and Empiricist Hippocrates, see Wesley Smith (1979, 177–214). On Asclepiades and the Methodists, ibid. 225–28. Lycus: *Ord. Libr. Propr.* 3 (19.57K); *Adv. Lyc.* (18A.196–245K, passim). Julian: *Adv. Jul.* (18A.246–299K, passim).

'sharp nose, concave eyes,' and the other things which, we know, are said by him after that ...

(*Meth. Med.* 10.3, 10.673–74K)

or in oral combat with a rival on the streets of Rome:

> On his way down to the Sandaliarion he [Martianus, a leading Erasistratean physician in Rome who is following Galen's treatment of the philosopher Eudemus] met me by chance, and straightaway, without greeting me as his custom was, he asked whether I was familiar with the second book of the *Prorrhetics* of Hippocrates, or whether I was entirely ignorant of that work; and hearing that I was familiar with it, and that it seemed to me that those doctors were correct who declared that it was not one of the genuine books of Hippocrates, "In any case you know therefore," he said, "the statement in it, 'I make no prophecy about these things?'"

(*Praecog.* 4, 14.620K)

Here Galen flaunts his status as expert on Hippocratic textual criticism, dismissing as spurious a work aggressively deployed by a rival in a high-profile case.

Thus, Galen studied and mastered the writings of his predecessors. Sometimes, he demonstrated his erudition in spectacular public displays—as when he produced all of the anatomical works then in circulation, amounting to an enormous pile of dozens of scrolls, claiming that he would prove the superiority of his own views over those of his predecessors in a live display of animal dissection. Galen also, in his turn, wrote didactic works for his own students—calling several of his treatises "for beginners" and recommending that these be read first.[38] But Galen intended these books to be used in conjunction with practical experience, not on their own. His anatomical treatises

---

38   Public demonstration: see *Libr. Propr.* 2 (19.20–23K) and chapter 5. On Galen's works for "beginners," see Boudon (1994, 1421–67); Oser-Grote (1997, 95–117).

were handbooks for live dissection. Galen remarked on the difficulty of recognizing parts that one has not repeatedly observed—those who rely only
on reading will have difficulty recognizing what they see the first time (*Anat.
Admin.* 1.2, 2.223–24K). Indeed, as he writes,

> of those who have seen the parts of the body shown by a teacher,
> none is able to remember accurately having seen them only once or twice,
> but it is necessary to see them many times.
>
> (*Comp. Med. Gen.* 3.2, 13.608K)

Galen labels anatomical treatises a late phenomenon, originally unnecessary—the ancient physicians, in his imagination, learned dissection even as
children and had no need for the works he calls "memoranda" or "notes" of
the kind first produced by Diocles in the mid-fourth century B.C.E.; he uses
the same word (*hypomnemata*) to characterize many of his own anatomical
works.[39] The written anatomical tradition is a concession to what he perceives
as the decline of medicine in later times. Not only anatomical treatises, but
written works in general are only supplementary to medical teaching:

> The best teaching is the teaching by live voice, and … from a book
> neither the helmsman nor the practitioner of any craft can be trained.
> These [books] are memoranda for those who are already learned, not a
> complete education for the ignorant.
>
> (*Aliment. Fac.* 1.1, 6.480K)

> The learning of methods only, without a variety of practices in them,
> is unable to produce well-trained students.
>
> (*Loc. Affect.* 2.10, 8.123K)

Galen's literary erudition has been much appreciated by modern scholars.
But much of Galen's medical education, as I have shown above, was also

---

39   *Anat. Admin.* 2.1, 2.280–83K; on *hypomnemata* and other terms in Galen, see von Staden
(1997b), especially 67–75.

practical: he saw and even treated patients together with his teachers and drew on these experiences throughout his lifetime; he watched animal dissections and performed them himself; he mixed drugs; he will, at Rome, use these same methods to train his own students. Far from deferring passively to his teachers' authority, he argued with them vigorously; his arrogance and, at times, open contempt must have been a trial to them. "I looked down on many of my teachers," as he writes, "even as an adolescent" (*Anim. Peccat. Dign.* 3, 5.70K).

The last years of Galen's adolescence at Pergamum were pivotal, as a story from *On Good and Bad Humors* indicates. His father was, at that time, no longer living in the city; perhaps exhausted and financially drained by the civic responsibilities he had taken on a few years earlier (and which had called him away from his personal instruction of his teenage son), he took up residence in the countryside as a gentleman-farmer. Galen remained in town to study. "I pursued my studies beyond all of my fellow students not only every day, but at night as well." Now free from direct parental supervision, in the "dog days" of the late summer, he and his friends indulged their love of fresh fruit (which Galen considered unhealthy, and which, available only in season, was in any case eaten much less commonly than cooked, dried, or pickled fruit). In fall, Galen became very ill. His symptoms, from what we can tell based on other stories that may refer to the same incident, included a piercing pain in the abdomen and the excretion of clear mucus, and possibly a burning fever with delirium causing him to pluck at straws and imaginary pieces of wool. The modern medical term for the latter symptom is carphology, and it is an ominous sign. His father, who had apparently never allowed Galen to eat fresh fruit, returned to the city and reproached him for succumbing to peer pressure and altering his long-standing dietary habits; no doubt alarmed by the dangerous condition of his beloved and only son, he supervised Galen's lifestyle personally for the next year. Then, when Galen was nineteen, he died.[40]

---

40   The story of Galen's illness: *Bon. Mal. Suc.* 1 (6.755–57K). On Galen's stance on fresh fruit, see also Nutton (1995b, 366–67). On this episode, see also Grmek and Gourevitch (1986). Carphology: *Loc. Affect.* 4.1 (8.226–27K). Mucus: *Loc. Affect.* 2.5 (8.81–82K).

Letting blood from a vein relieved Galen's symptoms, but not for long. Galen had never, from childhood, had an especially healthy constitution, as he tells us in his treatise *On Healthfulness* (5.1, 6.308–9K)—"in childhood and later as a pubescent boy and an adolescent I suffered from no few and no trivial diseases." In another passage he writes that in his youth he suffered four times from tertian fever, and once from the intense and burning fever called *kausos* (*Trem. Palp.* 7, 7.638K). As for the particular illness that struck him at eighteen, one modern study tentatively diagnoses amoebic dysentery; amoebic infections, if untreated, can persist for years and lead to abscesses in the liver, and are one of the world's leading causes of mortality today. Galen's condition recurred in the year following his father's death, when Galen, once more a free agent, indulged liberally in the fruits of late summer and suffered a relapse. His condition returned annually—but skipping some years—until Galen was twenty-seven, when it reached a critical point: "I arrived at danger, lest there might be an abscess in the part at which the liver adheres to the transverse septum." Galen was then at Alexandria; I shall take up the continuation of the story below.[41]

Galen makes no comment, here or elsewhere in his surviving work, on his father's death. But he writes of him always with love and reverence, and this event must have affected him deeply; a sense of loss could explain the vehemence with which he excoriates his youthful dietary mistakes in the story from *On Good and Bad Humors*. It may also have catalyzed his decision to leave Pergamum to pursue his education in the wider world. This happened some time shortly after his father's death; we do not know exactly when, but Galen was still an "adolescent," *meirakion*, when he studied under his next teacher, Pelops, at Smyrna.[42] Perhaps, having inherited his father's estate, Galen was freer to indulge an increasing thirst for knowledge and professional advancement. He seems to have known he was a special student and may have already formed the project in his mind of tracking down and

---

41   For the diagnosis of amoebic dysentery, see Grmek and Gourevitch (1986).
42   On Galen and Pelops, and his studies in Smyrna, see Schlange-Schöningen (2003, 85–90); Boudon-Millot (2007a), xxxii–xxxiv. *Meirakion*, *Atra bile* 3 (5.112K). "Pelops, my second teacher, after Satyrus," *Anat. Admin.* 1.1 (2.217K).

learning from all the students of the legendary Quintus. He perhaps hoped and believed that he would one day be the next Quintus.

Galen had already met Pelops. He had seen him debate medical episte-mology with an Empiricist named Philippus who argued that medicine can be known through experience alone. He had later written up their arguments in one of his first treatises—this work *On Medical Experience* survives today in Arabic translation, although the Greek has been lost. Together with *On the Anatomy of the Uterus*, mentioned above, and another lost treatise *On the Diagnosis of Eye Diseases*, it made up the juvenile written legacy he left behind him at Pergamum. The works circulated in his absence and he came across them again when he returned from his first sojourn in Rome, almost twenty years later. Galen also describes a debate between Pelops and his Pergamene teacher Satyrus, which he may have witnessed as Satyrus's student: the sub-ject was similar, for Satyrus argued skeptically that most people do not know what blood is (Galen's subject in this treatise is words and their meaning).[43]

In any case, sometime not long after his father's death in 148 C.E. Galen left Pergamum to study at Smyrna, principally, as he writes above, under Pelops, "my second teacher after Satyrus." He would not return until 157. Pelops was the foremost student of Numisianus, Quintus's most illustrious student; Galen will later seek out the latter as a teacher. I have mentioned above some of the details of Galen's studies with Pelops—Galen visited patients with him, and particularly remembered a consultation on an epilep-tic boy of thirteen; from Pelops he learned "the signs of the humors," anat-omy, pharmacology, Hippocratic exegesis, and probably many more subjects that he does not mention; he criticized Pelops's ideas that crab meat was a good cure for rabies, and that the source of all the blood vessels was the brain. Pelops wrote sparingly and was secretive about his books; he failed to copy them, he kept them in his house, and they mostly perished after his death. Among the lost treatises was an exhaustive work on anatomy of which Galen

---

43   *On Medical Experience*, see Walzer (1944); translation reprinted in Frede and Walzer (1985). Juvenile works: *Libr. Propr.* 2 (19.16K). Debate between Pelops and Satyrus: *Nomin. Med.* 99ʳ–100ᵛ (27–28 Meyerhof and Schacht).

thought very highly. Only "such writings as he used to hand over to his pupils ... when his pupils wished to return to their homes" survived and circulated (*Anat. Admin.* 14.1, 1:232 Simon, tr. Duckworth). We learn incidentally in this passage that Pelops had died by the time Galen wrote the first books of *On Anatomical Procedures,* in the early 170s.

While a student of Pelops, Galen himself produced one anatomical work, *On the Motion of the Chest and Lungs,* in three books

> doing a favor for fellow student who was about to depart on a journey to his homeland, so that he could practice according to it, to perform a certain anatomical demonstration.
>
> (*Libr. Propr.* 2, 19.17K)[44]

The book does not survive, but Galen's work on these muscles became one of his most important contributions to anatomy. This example, and also the story of Pelops's works, illustrate once again how texts were produced not for their own sake, but for social and practical reasons—as memoranda to students about to depart, who would no longer be able to benefit from the live instruction of their teachers; as guides to dissection, which might be performed as a public demonstration; as favors to friends.

We do not know how long Galen stayed with Pelops. It is certain that during this period he traveled to cities he does not mention and studied with individuals whose names he does not record. "I knew all the students of Quintus, and I was not deterred by the length of the journey by land or by sea" (*Anat. Admin.* 4.10, 2.469–70K); "all of whom I took great pains to meet, and whom I found to be inferior to Satyrus and Pelops" (*Anat. Admin.* 14.1, 232 Simon, tr. Duckworth). As I have mentioned, he never met Lycus of Macedonia, a decision he defends in retrospect; "he ... had no great reputation among the Greeks. Had that not been the case, I most certainly would not have omitted to go and see him also" (ibid., tr. Duckworth). Lycus would go on to publish a lengthy and well-received treatise on anatomy that appeared just

---

44 See also *Anat. Admin.* 1.1 (2.217K) for another reference to this work and to Pelops.

before Galen's own masterpiece on the subject, *On the Usefulness of the Parts* (see chapter 5), and Galen was obliged to dedicate considerable energies to demolishing that work and, perhaps, to explain why he never studied with the man who became Quintus's most influential student of anatomy. (Later Galen will meet one Antigenes in Rome, also a student of Quintus, whom he either thought, like Lycus, unworthy of learning from, or of whom he had not heard previously; *Praecog.* 3, 14.613K)

Galen tells us that he pursued Pelops's teacher, Quintus's brilliant student Numisianus, to several locations: "Next [after Smyrna], I was in Corinth on account of Numisianus, who was himself the most famous of the students of Quintus, and in Alexandria and some other places in which I learned that Numisianus, the famous student of Quintus, was living" (*Anat. Admin.* 1, 2.217–18K). An alternate version of this passage is preserved in Arabic translation: "places in which I learned that a famous student of Quintus or of Numisianus was living," which makes more sense—it seems unlikely that Galen pursued Numisianus around the Mediterranean without ever meeting him, as the first version of the passage implies, but he affirms elsewhere that he went to great lengths to track down the students of Quintus.[45] As mentioned above, Pelops had been unforthcoming with Numisianus's anatomical discoveries—"[he] did not expound [Numisianus's works] nor did he show them to anyone, for he preferred that certain theories, as yet unknown, should be attributed to himself" (*Anat. Admin.* 14.1, 232 Simon, tr. Duckworth)—and it is easy to imagine Galen's frustration at being denied access to the discoveries of the greatest anatomist of his time. It is possible that Numisianus died shortly after Galen began to seek him out, and that this explains why Galen apparently never found him. Numisianus was considerably older, perhaps of the same generation as his own teacher Quintus, for "in [Quintus's teacher] Marinus's lifetime [he, Numisianus] had already become pre-eminent in Alexandria" (*Anat. Admin.* 14.1, 231 Simon, tr. Duckworth).

Galen's quest for the intellectual legacy of Numisianus took him, eventually, to Alexandria in Egypt, the city in which Numisianus had achieved

---

45   Von Staden (2004, 206–9) for discussion and references.

fame and where his son Heraclianus still lived. Galen arrived sometime
between 151 and 153 c.e. and would remain until 157. He arrived in autumn.
It was inevitable that his single-minded quest for the best and most brilliant
medical education would take him to Alexandria, which was, in terms of
prestige, the Harvard or Cambridge of antiquity. It boasted an ancient and
famous tradition of medical research, particularly in anatomy. Galen's era
knew no medical schools in the modern sense; he studied with individuals,
not institutions, but Alexandria's glorious reputation attracted the best medical minds. Quintus himself had perhaps studied in Alexandria—Galen links
the location vaguely with Quintus's teacher, Marinus—and for Galen, perhaps intent on reduplicating his famous fellow citizen's career, it was a natural
destination.[46]

Alexander the Great founded Alexandria on the Nile delta in 331 b.c.e.
on campaign against the Persians—Egypt, as it happened, surrendered peace-
fully—and named it after himself. It became the capital city and residence
of the Macedonian dynasty of Ptolemies that ruled Egypt after his death. In
30 b.c.e., after the defeat and suicide of Cleopatra VII, last of the Ptolemies,
Egypt became a Roman province; Alexandria continued to be its administrative capital. In Galen's time its population was probably second only to that
of Rome itself (modern scholars usually estimate, on very little evidence, a
population of about 500,000, while the figures of 300,000 and 750,000 transmitted in ancient sources have no more secure basis). It was famous for its
lighthouse on the island of Pharos—one of the seven wonders of the ancient
world, and its tallest Greek structure, over 100 meters high—for its royal
palaces, its temple of Sarapis, and for the monumental tomb of Alexander,
whose body was transported there after his death at Babylon, purloined, it
was said, by Ptolemy I Soter, who was buried at the same site along with his

---

46   On Galen in Alexandria, see Boudon-Millot (2007a, xxxv–xl); von Staden (2004);
Schlange-Schöningen (2003, 90–99); Grmek and Gourevitch (1994, 1491–1528); Nutton (1993,
11–32). On date of arrival, see Nutton (1993, 12). Autumn: *Trem. Palp.* 8 (7.635K). The association
of Marinus and Quintus with Alexandria, though commonly assumed by modern scholars, is not
clearly attested in any ancient source including Galen, who writes only that Numisianus became
preeminent in Alexandria during Marinus's lifetime. See von Staden (2004, 209–11).

royal successors. But today the archaeological remains of ancient Alexandria are very exiguous. Much of what survived the medieval and Ottoman periods was destroyed to build the modern city in the nineteenth century, and today even the locations of some of antiquity's most renowned monuments—the tomb of Alexander, the Library (see below)—are unknown.[47]

Alexandria's Museum (*Musaion*, "place of the Muses"), with its attached Library—the second Ptolemy's aggressive acquisition of its collection of books was the subject of much comment, anecdote, and legend—was antiquity's first research institution. According to Strabo the geographer, writing in the first century C.E., it had its own grounds and buildings within the royal palaces; the fortunate scholars attached to the Museum, beneficiaries of royal (and later, imperial) patronage, enjoyed communal property rights and free meals for life in the common cafeteria (Str. 17.1.8).

Other Musea existed in the Roman world's great cities, notably the one at Pergamum; but the Alexandrian Museum was the most renowned. However, Galen never mentions it—just as he never mentions the Museum at Pergamum—suggesting that it played little or no role in his education (nor is the Museum mentioned in connection with any of Alexandria's other famous physicians, in any source). Alexandria attracted scholars through its reputation and the very illustrious record of research produced there, which was fueled partly by the Museum, but scholarly activity extended far beyond the narrow group of intellectuals it supported. From early in its history the city had been the center of ancient literary and textual criticism, and it was in Hellenistic Alexandria that many ancient texts took the form in which we know them today, under the scrutiny of early editors and commentators; and it was there that the canon of the Hippocratic Corpus took shape. Galen was himself a prolific and adept editor and exegete of Hippocrates, a skill he

---

47   For references to the population of Alexandria, see Scheidel (2001a, 184–85). The Syriac *notitia* discussed by Alston (2002, 160–62) may suggest a figure closer to Diodorus's estimate of 300,000 than to the higher figure of Josephus, but it is also problematic in several respects. For topography and archaeology, the most extensive ancient description of Alexandria is Strabo 17.1.6–10. We now have an excellent, rigorous survey of ancient Alexandrian architecture in McKenzie (2007). On the disappearance of the ancient remains, see ibid., chapter 1, "How Ancient Alexandria was Lost." Chapters 7 and 8 present the evidence for Hellenistic and Roman Alexandria.

learned from his earliest teachers, but he also mentions the "Hippocratics" at Alexandria (see below).[48]

Very early in its history, Alexandria acquired a reputation for medical research. Under the first two Ptolemies, the physicians Herophilus and Erasistratus became antiquity's most renowned anatomists. Dissections and vivisections of animals had been practiced for some time, notably by Aristotle, who also refers to a treatise of his own authorship, now lost, on *Dissections*. Galen ascribes the first anatomical handbook to Diocles of Carystus, perhaps a rough contemporary of Aristotle, a generation or two before Herophilus.[49]

But Herophilus and Erasistratus not only took the study of anatomy to new heights; they also dissected humans. They were the first, and almost the only, ancient physicians to do this; certainly they were the only physicians of antiquity whose discoveries based on human anatomy were ever published or known. Tradition recounted that they also vivisected humans, and that their victims, condemned criminals, were supplied by the Ptolemies. There is little doubt that Herophilus and Erasistratus, unlike any of the other ancient physicians whose names we know, dissected human corpses (Galen knew of Herophilus's experience with human dissection, having learned this very early in his education; he mentions it in *On the Anatomy of the Uterus*, written while he was still at Pergamum with Satyrus). It is less clear that the vivisections actually happened. Those references that derive from Christian polemical literature—hostile to all scientific endeavor and eager to exaggerate pagan atrocities—are not especially trustworthy. But we also have the more reliable testimony of the first-century Latin author Celsus that live criminals were handed over to Herophilus and Erasistratus for experimentation. (Celsus

---

48   On the lack of references to the Museum in connection with ancient physicians, see Nutton (1993, 14–15); von Staden (1989, 26–27). On the Hippocratic Corpus, see Nutton (1993, 19–22); Wesley Smith (1979, 199–204).

49   Tradition links Erasistratus with Herophilus, but ancient sources do not explicitly place Erasistratus in Alexandria and some scholars argue that he never practiced there. For references, see von Staden (1989, 142). For references to vivisection in Aristotle, see von Staden (1989, 147). On the history of vivisection in antiquity, see Grmek (1997). Diocles' anatomical treatise: *Anat. Admin.* 2.1 (2.283K). On Diocles' date, see van der Eijk (2001, xxxi–xxxviii).

also transmits the rationalization, notorious in modern times, offered by his sources for a practice he considered cruel and unnecessary: that the sacrifice of a few guilty criminals in order to seek remedies for the innocent masses is justified. The most likely sources of this rationalization—though he does not name them—are Herophilus and Erasistratus themselves.) Thus, we cannot exclude the disconcerting possibility (or likelihood) that some of the ancient anatomical knowledge on which Galen relied, and which he transmitted through his own writings down through the centuries to the founding fathers of modern medicine in the Renaissance, derives from the vivisection of live human subjects in experiments that are ghastly to imagine even on animals.[50]

References to human dissection are otherwise very rare. It is unclear why these early Alexandrian physicians could ignore the taboo against cutting open human bodies. This taboo apparently reigned supreme in other eras, although medical writers such as Celsus and Galen not only believed in the value of human dissection but, to Galen, it became a holy grail of sorts. Scholars have suggested that an atmosphere of "frontiersmanship" in the newly founded city of Alexandria was responsible; also perhaps Greek prejudice against native Egyptians, who may have been the subjects and victims of dissection and vivisection, in a society more segregated than would later be possible. (In the Roman period, colleagues of Galen would be allowed to dissect the corpse of a German "barbarian"; see chapter 6.) Also, the native Egyptian tradition of mummification was well-known to Greeks. Social barriers probably prevented any direct transmission of knowledge, for which we have no evidence. Nor is there any evidence that Egyptian embalmers or native Egyptian physicians practiced scientific dissection or vivisection; quite the opposite, for the practice of embalming was itself hedged round with strict taboos. Nevertheless, the Egyptian religious practice may have helped justify what would otherwise have been unthinkable, even as the Macedonian

---

50 Galen mentions Herophilus's human dissections, see von Staden (1989, 142 and T114). Vivisections: Celsus 1 *proem.* 23–26; von Staden (1989, T63a, T144–45). On Alexandria and the anatomical tradition, see also Nutton (2004, chapter 9).

monarchs, in imitation of the Pharaohs, shattered a different taboo by marrying their siblings.[51]

Whatever the reason, human dissection is very poorly attested outside of Alexandria, and there only in the first decades after the city's foundation. But Alexandria retained some of its grisly reputation for experiment on human subjects. Cleopatra VII supposedly tested poisons on condemned criminals (like earlier Hellenistic monarchs, Mithradates VI of Pontus and Attalus III of Pergamum). Much later, Galen saw human bones at Alexandria, where they were used to demonstrate anatomy, a practice he describes with approval, and urges all students of medicine to visit Alexandria for this reason. Galen himself seized every opportunity to observe human anatomy, as when a river overflowed and washed away a tomb with its fully articulated skeleton, or when, by the roadside, he happened across the remains—so the locals told him—of a bandit murdered by his would-be victim. In *On Theriac to Piso*, which may not be genuine, Galen writes that he "often" witnessed executions in Alexandria and, recalling the memory much later as an old man, commented on the swiftness with which the venom of the snakes used for this purpose, possibly Egyptian cobras, took effect. The snakes, he writes, were hurled against the chests of the victims, who were then made to walk around.[52]

The high expectations with which Galen went to Alexandria seem to have been disappointed. He was well received there—by Heraclianus, Numisianus's son, among others. But despite paying assiduous court to the latter over what sounds like a long time, as I mentioned earlier, he never won a glance at Numisianus's written legacy, the books still in his son's possession. Thus, although Galen considered Numisianus the foremost anatomist of his time, he attributes no discoveries or ideas to him—whether out of spite or because he acquired no clear or useful sense of Numisianus's legacy from its

---

51   On "frontiersmanship" and mummification, see von Staden (1989, 29–30, 138–53); and further on the dissection of humans in cultural context, von Staden (1992). On prejudice, see Nutton (2004, 129).

52   On experiments of monarchs, see chapter 1. Cleopatra: Plut. *Ant.* 71. Skeletons and bandit: *Anat. Admin.* 1.2 (2.220–21K). Executions: *Ther. Pis.* 8 (14.237K).

tight-lipped custodians or from the meager selection of his written works that circulated.

Nor does Galen mention any of his teachers at Alexandria besides Heraclianus, either directly or indirectly, with one dubious exception—he knew the Methodist Julian, though Galen disdains to call him one of his teachers. Galen's hostility to Julian far outlasted his student days. Twenty years later, and at a distance, from Rome, Galen continues to rail against the Methodist—then still alive, as he writes—in his massive tract *On the Method of Healing*, recalling a debate in which he humiliated Julian partly by convicting him of contradicting his "grandfather in teaching," Olympicus (a hypocritical remark from Galen, who does not hesitate to criticize his own intellectual ancestors). Presented with Julian's work on the Hippocratic *Aphorisms*, Galen delivered improvised public lectures refuting it over the course of six days, and then, at the insistence of his friends, published his arguments in the extant *Against Julian's Criticisms of the Aphorisms of Hippocrates*. The treatise is not mentioned in *On My Own Books* and may postdate it; if so, Julian had become a lifelong target of Galen's polemics.[53]

As for the other Hippocratic commentators of Alexandria—including those physicians formally calling themselves "Hippocratics"—Galen has nothing flattering to say about them either. He mentions Sabinus, the teacher of his own teacher Stratonicus, and Metrodorus of Alexandria, as execrable interpreters of Hippocrates. Of Metrodorus he adds that his understanding was so flawed that one of his students, Philistion of Pergamum, lost all of his patients after an embarrassing effort to treat a wealthy woman for infertility (after demanding a huge fee he made her eat half-roasted inkfish, which she vomited violently).[54]

To sum up, then, Galen's training in medicine before moving on: This began at age sixteen, with a number of physicians, representing different schools, in Pergamum. After his father's death, Galen traveled to Smyrna, to Corinth, to other undisclosed cities, and finally to Alexandria, all in pursuit

---

53   "Grandfather in teaching": *Meth. Med.* 1.7 (10.54K). *Adv. Jul.*: 18A.246–99K.
54   Sabinus and Metrodorus: *Hipp. 3 Epid.* 1.4 (17A.508K). Philistion: *Hipp. 2 Epid.* 6, 401–2, 404 Pfaff.

of medical knowledge. He especially sought out the students of Quintus, a Pergamene who had practiced in Rome, renowned as an anatomist and as continuator of the tradition of his own teacher, Marinus, whose comprehensive work on anatomy was the equivalent of the standard graduate-level textbook on the subject at the time. Galen learned anatomy through animal dissection and sometimes through human subjects, as when he saw human bones at Alexandria, or observed muscles and nerves through the wasted flesh of disease victims at Pergamum. He also learned Hippocratic exegesis, pharmacology, and especially, clinical medicine from his teachers. From the very beginning of his training, he saw patients, and throughout his life expressed disdain for the "word-doctors" (*logiatroi*) for whom medicine was more about texts and ideas than practice.

Alexandria must have been an experience in itself, not just a place to learn. In Roman times it had a diverse population of which the elite was the exclusive, Hellenized, gymnasium-educated class of Alexandrian citizens, who were alone eligible for Roman citizenship. But the population of resident Egyptians was very large. How much Galen interacted with ethnic Egyptians—people he did not consider Greek—in the city or in the countryside, and how much he observed of native culture, is unclear but seems quite limited. It is unlikely that he could communicate directly with the peasant population, which mostly spoke Egyptian. Galen tells one story of a peasant who was bitten on the finger by a snake "when I was at Alexandria;" the peasant hurried to the city and demanded that a physician amputate the finger, which proved effective (*Loc. Affect.* 3.11, 8.197K). He does not say that he knew the patient or the physician and may have heard the story from a third party.

Galen brought with him to Egypt a theory of the relationship between geographic zone, climate, and race, familiar to all educated Greeks, and expectations about the nature and temperament of the local population: Egyptians should be slender, hot, dry, and hard. He makes no comment on whether his experiences in Egypt confirmed these theories. As he does for other locations, Galen notes dietary practices that he considers unusual: Egyptians eat large quantities of pistachios, with no harmful (or beneficial) effects that he has observed. They are, he writes, also able to eat donkey meat and camel

meat with no ill effects; however, in another passage Galen identifies donkey meat as the cause of Alexandria's high incidence of elephantiasis. This
ancient term "elephantiasis," which Galen describes as a severely disfiguring
skin condition whose victims were shunned as repellent and sometimes driven
to suicide, signifies the disease called leprosy today (see further in chapter 4
below; Galen believed he could control or cure elephantiasis through phlebotomy and snake venom). Galen also observed "some people suffering from
dropsy and many who were splenetic" treating themselves with applications
of Egyptian mud, with good results.[55]

All this reminds us that disease in antiquity, especially in an urban environment and perhaps especially in Egypt, was much more visible than it is
in modern western cities or even in the poorest and most overcrowded cities
of the developing world, where medical and public health advances of recent
centuries have, with the exception of parts of sub-Saharan Africa, expanded
life expectancy far beyond pre-modern parameters. Although Alexandria
had a reputation for healthfulness and although its coastal location probably
spared it some of the endemic diseases of the interior, Egypt was burdened
with innumerable gastrointestinal and respiratory illnesses, fevers, and parasites, and a mortality rate shocking to modern sensibilities, a situation that
did not improve much until the mid-twentieth century.[56]

Alexandria had a large Jewish population and was the center of Hellenized
Jewish culture in antiquity. The most ancient and widely used Greek trans-
lation of the Hebrew Bible, the Septuagint, originated there under Ptolemy
Philadelphus in the mid-third century B.C.E.; according to legend seventy-two

55   Galen on characteristics of Egyptians: *Simp. Med.* 2.20 (11.513–14K); *Comp. Med. Gen.* 4.1
(13.662K); *Hipp. Aph.* 2.14 (17B.597K). For ancient theories of race (including a long discussion
of the term "race"), see recently the introductory chapter and Part I of Isaac (2004). Pistachios:
Aliment. Fac. 2.30 (6.612K). Donkey and camel meat: *Aliment. Fac.* 1.2.8 (6.486K). Diet and elephantiasis: *Meth. Med. Glauc.* 2.12 (11.142K). On Galen's comments on Egyptian food and drugs,
see von Staden (2004, 186–94). Elephantiasis cases: *Simp. Med.* 11.1.1 (12.312–15K) and *Subfig.
Emp.* 10 (75–76 Deichgräber). On the identification with leprosy, see Grmek (1989, 168–73). Mud:
Simp. Med. 9.1.2 (12.177K).
56   Alexandria's healthy climate: Strabo 17.1.7. On disease in ancient Egypt with extensive discussion of comparative evidence from modern Egypt, see Scheidel (2001a, chapter 1). On differences between Alexandria and other regions, ibid. 19–21.

scholars, all working independently in isolation, miraculously produced the same translation. In the Roman era conflicts between the Jewish and Greek populations of Alexandria sometimes became violent, and anti-Semitic feeling among the Greeks seems to have been, at times, intense. "Acts" of Alexandrian martyrs who defied the Romans, often because of their perceived support for the Alexandrian Jews, were popular enough that several examples survive on papyrus. A particularly horrific sequence of events— in which the Alexandrian Greeks with the cooperation of the Roman prefect, Flaccus, rioted against the Jews, looted property, cruelly lynched many victims and drove the entire Jewish population into a single quarter of the city—is well-attested in a surviving speech by the Jewish philosopher Philo of Alexandria, who pleaded the Jews' case to the Roman emperor Claudius. Closer to Galen's time, in the second century, there are hints of violent episodes but we know little about them. It is clear, however, that Jews continued to be a large and vital force in the city. Galen does not mention interacting with Jewish intellectuals at Alexandria, at Rome or anywhere else. He was, however, familiar with Judaism, and also with Christianity. While his comments are typical of references to both religions in other Greek sources and do not necessarily reflect firsthand knowledge (see chapter 5), it is quite possible that he encountered both Jews and Christians at Alexandria.[57]

Wherever he studied, Galen was part of a cohort of other students. Some of them were his friends. At Rome he knew Teuthras, "a fellow citizen and fellow student of mine"; probably they had studied medicine or philosophy together at Pergamum, and both had emigrated to Rome. In the story of the onset of his long illness at Pergamum, Galen refers to "my fellow students" and "my age-mates" as bad influences on his diet—clearly he was spending a lot of time with them and they were eating meals together. When delirious with fever and plucking at imaginary pieces of wool and straw, he remembers speaking semi-lucidly to two friends who were attending him,

---

57   On martyrs, see Musurillo (1954). On Alexandrian Jews and ethnic conflict in Alexandria, see Alston (2002, 219–35); Gruen (2002, chapter 2). On Galen and Judeo-Christian religion, see Schlange-Schöningen (2003, 235–54); Walzer (1949); and chapter 5 below.

and who immediately set about bathing his head. Another story about travel with friends must refer either to Pergamum or Smyrna—Galen and his companions were all still adolescents (*meirakia*) when it occurred. "Traveling in the countryside not far from the city" they fell in with some peasant folk, and, famished, accepted their offer of boiled wheat, which caused all three of the young men severe indigestion. All of this suggests that friendships with young men of his own age, many of them probably fellow students, were important in Galen's early years at Pergamum and Smyrna.[58]

Also at Alexandria: later at Rome, Galen described the diet of "a certain youth who practices medicine at Alexandria," perhaps a friend from his days of study there, in great detail. He was astonished that anyone could maintain health eating only raw foods for four years (this may be an indication that Galen lived in Alexandria for four years, the minimum time that fits the chronology of his life). He also observed the paroxysmal illness of another student, "a certain youth, one of our fellow students in Alexandria, when we first sailed there at the beginning of autumn"; Galen advised and encouraged him, recalling a female patient from his home country with similar symptoms. The cause of the man's illness was eating fresh dates.[59]

Galen himself continued to suffer from the illness whose onset, at age seventeen, had so preoccupied his father near the end of his life.

> ... sometimes I was sick every year, sometimes I would skip a year, until my twenty-eighth year; at which time I came into danger of an abscess in the part at which the liver adheres to the transverse septum, and I forbade to myself the use of all fresh fruits, except figs and perfectly ripened grapes, and even these only in moderation, not like before.
>
> (*Bon. Mal. Suc.* 1, 6.756–57K)

Once again, friendships with his contemporaries are important: "I had a certain companion in this plan, two years older than I. Applying ourselves to

---

58   Teuthras: *Ven. Sect. Eras. Rom.* 1 (11.193–94, 195K); *Ind.* 35. Delirium: *Loc. Affect.* 4.2 (8.226–27K). Boiled wheat: *Aliment. Fac.* 1.7 (6.498–99K).

59   Raw foods: *Aliment. Fac.* 1.25 (6.539K). Paroxysmal illness: *Trem. Palp.* 8 (7.635–36K).

the gymnasium and to not suffering from indigestion, we have remained free from disease until now, for a space of many years." This friendship, like the one with Teuthras, seems to have migrated to Rome and endured a long time. Galen refers to his soundness of health from age twenty-seven again in his treatise *On Healthfulness*. Despite a stressful life of professional obligations and study, "from my twenty-eighth year, after the beginning of my persuasion that there is an art of health, I obeyed its commands for all my life after that, so that I have suffered from no disease, except an occasional daily fever" (*San. Tuend.* 5.1, 6.309K).

In these passages Galen attributes his recovery to regimen, but elsewhere he credits a radical new therapy that he tried for the first time on himself. He was saved by a series of dreams:

> Exhorted by certain dreams, of which two came to me distinctly, I went to the artery in the middle between the forefinger and the middle finger of the right hand, and allowed the blood to flow until it stopped by itself. Not quite a whole pound flowed out. Immediately a chronic pain ceased which was fixed mainly in that part where the liver meets the diaphragm. This happened to me when I was young with respect to stage of life.
>
> (*Cur. Ven. Sect.* 23, 11.314–15K)

Normally only veins were bled; Galen here at the end of his treatise *On Treatment by Venesection* is making a case for arteriotomy, or letting blood from the arteries, in certain circumstances. This incident, he writes, inspired him to use the procedure in other cases. The dream perhaps came from Asclepius: Galen does not say so in this passage, but goes on to tell a story about another patient, a suppliant of Asclepius at Pergamum, saved by similar means as directed in a dream. Later, Galen would tell the emperor Marcus Aurelius that "I had declared myself his [Asclepius's] servant ever since he had saved me from a deadly condition of an abscess" (*Libr. Propr.* 2, 19.18–19K).

It is not entirely certain that all of these three references—the long story that Galen tells in *On Good and Bad Humors* about the onset, development, and resolution of his abdominal illness, and the briefer references in *On Treatment by Venesection* and *On My Own Books* to an abscess from which he was saved by dreams and by Asclepius—recall the same episode.[60] But if they do, I have several reasons for believing that Asclepius's intervention occurred at age twenty-seven and not in Galen's teens as some scholars have assumed. First, had the dream happened while he was still a teenager at Pergamum, Galen would not describe himself as "young," (*neos*); he would call himself an adolescent (*meirakion*), as he does in all other anecdotes about his early education at Pergamum. Galen is consistent and precise in his use of words for the stages of life; as he emphasizes here with the phrase "young with respect to stage of life."[61] Also, in the passage from *On Treatment by Venesection* he refers to the pain of which he was relieved as long-lasting (*chronion*). Further, Galen tells Marcus that he was saved from an abscess; which condition only developed, or threatened to develop, late in the illness described in *On Good and Bad Humors*. Finally, Galen is explicit that his dreams prescribed arteriotomy; this is the whole point of the anecdote in *On Treatment by Venesection*. In the story from *On Good and Bad Humors*, Galen specifically states that in its early stages his illness was treated with phlebotomy, by cutting a vein, not an artery.

Thus we may reconstruct the following story of Galen's illness: he suffered a condition causing him abdominal pain over a period of ten years, beginning at age seventeen. He diagnosed an abscess and attributed its cause to the unwise and immoderate ingestion of fresh fruits. The disease, he believed, would have been fatal, suggesting that his pain was very great; but when he was twenty-seven years old Asclepius, in several dreams and especially in two that made a strong impression, sent signs that Galen interpreted as directing him to cut the artery between his right index and middle fingers. With this—and also with a change of lifestyle, for Galen foreswore most fresh fruit and took up regular visits to the gymnasium—he was cured, and remained in remarkable health for decades afterward. This dramatic change of circumstances is the last dateable event of Galen's stay in Alexandria.

---

60   Cf. Nutton (1999, 138). Galen mentions the incident briefly in *On My Own Opinions*, dating to late in his lifetime, as evidence of the existence of gods.

61   On Galen's words for stage of life, see Mattern (2008a, 105–12).

Chapter Three

THE GLADIATORS

alen left Alexandria in 157 at the age of twenty-seven, returning home to Pergamum. Perhaps he returned overland, on foot; one story suggests that he met a gardener on the way, and treated him with an improvised remedy:

> When I first returned from Alexandria to my homeland, I was passing through the countryside, and I found one of the gardeners choking on a "grape" [a swollen uvula] and [on swollen] fauces and tonsils. He was using a wash of diluted honey, with roses crumbled in it.
>
> (*Comp. Med. Loc.* 6.2, 12.905–6K)

It is unclear whether Galen met the gardener on the road from Alexandria or on an unspecified trip to the countryside, perhaps to visit the estate occupied by his father at his death, which Galen must have inherited. Making use of the materials at hand, he ordered the patient to gargle a reduction of nut-juice and honey. "Observing," he writes, "that an immediate benefit followed," he continued to use the remedy he had improvised on the spot, far from the resources of the city, on the suffering patient whose condition had, apparently, long gone untreated. The story vividly evokes the isolation and poverty of the empire's rural regions.

In the early days after returning to Pergamum, Galen experimented with new drugs for wounded tendons, in a primitive type of clinical trial:

> I gave out each of the medicines I devised to friends who were doctors, not only my fellow citizens but also to those in cities nearby, for the sake of confirming all of them by testing.
>
> (*Comp. Med. Gen.* 3.2, 13.599K)

It was at this point, and just after his twenty-eighth birthday, that Galen was appointed to the post of physician for the gladiators: "I don't know how," he goes on to write, "but the high priest [*archiereus*] of our city decided to entrust to me alone the care of the gladiators, although I was still young as to stage of life. For I had begun my twenty-ninth year."

Gladiatorial games were a Roman tradition and in the East often performed at festivals in honor of the cult of the emperors. They were funded not by the city, but by private citizens, as one of the liturgies on which Greek urban life was founded.[1] The "high priest" that Galen mentions was probably either the high priest of the Emperor Trajan, whose temple on the city's Acropolis was one of its most prominent and beautiful buildings, or he held office at the provincial level, as one of the priests of the imperial cult in Asia; these individuals were also called "Asiarch," and all the most important cities had one. In either case he must have belonged, like Galen's father and like Galen himself, to Pergamum's ruling class—the aristocracy that organized, supervised, and paid for the infrastructure of urban culture, including its public spectacles.[2]

Despite Galen's modest disclaimer ("I don't know how … "), he implies, here and elsewhere, that he was chosen for his medical skill—specifically, his

---

1   Robert (1940, 268–75). On Galen's career among the gladiators, see Boudon-Millot (2007a, xl–xlvi); Schlange-Schöningen (2003, 101–36); Scarborough (1971).

2   Schlange-Schöningen (2003, 111–16). On the prestige of the high priest and inscriptions honoring them or boasting of the gladiatorial games, see Robert (1940, 256–57, 262).

innovative drugs for treating wounds—and not (for example) for his family status and connections, although the latter may have been one factor in reality. Galen had been publicizing his remedies for wounded tendons and immediately goes on, in the passage quoted above, to describe how he applied them to the gladiators in his care.

In another treatise, which survives only in Arabic, Galen offers more details about how he was chosen. "A high priest," he writes, "followed this method (of choosing physicians) when I returned to our city from places which I had set out to visit." Here again, Galen emphasizes that the other physicians were his elders, and that he prevailed despite his youth:

> Although, at that time, I had not yet completed thirty years of my age he entrusted me with the treatment of all the wounded men who had fought duels in combats. Before my time, two or three of the Elders were in charge.
>
> (*Opt. Med. Cogn.* 9, 102 Iskandar, tr. Iskandar)

Here too Galen emphasizes the priest's unusual confidence in entrusting the gladiators to him *alone*. The priest had observed, apparently over some time, Galen's tireless devotion to science and duty (suggesting that despite Galen's protests to the contrary—"Nor did I waste my time or distress myself by visiting men regularly," and so forth—he may have been a friend, and Galen may have owed his selection to his social connections with Pergamum's aristocracy).

The priest had also witnessed an exceptionally dramatic public spectacle. Before an audience that included himself and a number of "intellectuals," Galen performed, as he writes, "many anatomical demonstrations"— implying a lengthy and grueling procedure. At least one of these (as he goes on to relate) was a vivisection; these were exceptionally difficult performances, described more fully in chapter 5, and Galen was under intense pressure to make no mistakes. As the centerpiece of his demonstration Galen chose, with breathtaking audacity, to disembowel a live monkey (perhaps a Barbary macaque, the primate Galen most preferred to dissect). He sliced open its abdomen and emptied its intestines, and then called on "the other physicians who were present" (also called "the Elders of the physicians" in this passage) to replace and secure them back in the abdomen. His rivals, thus challenged, must have been dumbfounded. Replacing the intestines of any animal is extremely difficult; and this was a live, struggling macaque— an animal that Galen would later recommend against vivisecting, so hideous was its suffering to observe.[3] None dared even make the attempt. Galen not only performed the feat, but he went on to demonstrate his skill in treating wounds, severing the monkey's large arteries and challenging his rivals— on the spot, blood spurting from the victim—to offer treatment before it was too late. When they stood paralyzed with indecision, he intervened himself—"making it clear to the intellectuals who were present that (physicians) who possess skills like mine should be in charge of the wounded" (*Opt. Med. Cogn.* 9, 104 Iskandar, tr. Iskandar). (Galen may have ligated the arteries to stop the blood, a procedure he mentions many times when he describes vivisections.)

Galen chose an especially spectacular feat with which to display his skill. At Rome he will go on to perform many similar deeds in public, especially sanguinary vivisections, so astounding in their effects and so difficult to perform correctly. With their combination of skill, daring, danger, and gore, Galen's vivisections bore some likeness to the gladiatorial games whose combatants he treated for several years.[4]

There was a long tradition of physicians serving the state in the Greek East. From classical times, many Greek cities employed public physicians, who might receive a salary and other privileges. In Galen's time, cities selected doctors to be eligible for valuable immunities from Roman taxes and other duties imposed by the imperial government: all doctors had formerly enjoyed these immunities, but an edict of Antoninus Pius in the middle of the second century restricted them to a small number per city. These physicians with immunity are sometimes called *archiatroi*, "chief doctors," on the surviving

3   *Anat. Admin.* 8.8 (2.690K), 9.2 (18 Simon), 11.4 (107 Simon). Cf. Gleason (2009, 113).
4   Cf. Gleason (2009, 108–10), comparing Galen's anatomical demonstrations to the wild beast hunts or criminal executions staged in the arena.

inscriptions that honor them.[5] It is not clear that Galen's appointment to treat the gladiators placed him in this special category, nor do we know whether it was a full-time job that displaced Galen's private practice (this is perhaps unlikely) or whether he received a salary. But Galen's boasting of the recognition he received should be seen in light of the East's long history of the state-honored physician.

Medical contests and demonstrations, including dissections and vivisections, were by now a form of entertainment in the Roman world. I will discuss Galen's performances at Rome in chapter 5; but medicine-as-entertainment was not limited to the empire's capital city. Inscriptions contemporary with Galen's life from the city of Ephesus record the names of victors in medical contests. There were four categories of competition: surgery, medical instruments, verbal composition, and "problems," *problemata*.[6] Some doctors, writes Plutarch of Chaeronea in the late first century C.E., "perform surgery in the theaters in order to attract patients" (*Mor.* 71A); while Dio Chrysostomus describes physicians "who sit themselves in the middle before us," lecturing and demonstrating on the joints, the bones, the *pneuma*; like other "spectacles and processions," the lectures awe and amaze their audience (*Or.* 33.6). While Dio compares these performers unfavorably with the physicians who actually treat the sick, prescribing salutary but sometimes unpopular remedies, it is clear from Galen's stories that no such neat division existed—the same physicians astounding audiences with their virtuosity in dissection or rhetoric were treating patients, writing erudite medical treatises, performing surgery, teaching students.[7]

The chief priest who chose Galen served "at the time of the autumn equinox" in 157 (*Comp. Med. Gen.* 3.2, 13.600K), but Galen was also chosen by the next four successive priests, the first of whom took office in the spring of the following year, "after seven months." It seems that normally priests would serve a year-long term, taking office September 23, the birthday of Augustus; the priest appointed in fall of 157 may have died before his term

5   On public physicians, see Jouanna (1999, 76–80); Nutton (1977); Cohn-Haft (1956).
6   Wankel (1979–84, nos. 1161–69).
7   See Gleason (2009, 89, 100).

was up, so that a successor had to be appointed. A "suffect" priesthood—the appointment of more than one office-holder in a year—is also possible, but causes chronological problems if we assume that each of the five priests who chose Galen served only half a year. It seems that Galen remained in Pergamum until the fall of 161 before setting out for Rome, where he arrived the next year.[8]

Gladiatorial games, Galen writes in his commentary on the Hippocratic treatise *On Fractures*, were held at Pergamum every year, in summer (*Hipp. Fract.* 3.21, 18B.567K)—presumably at an annual festival, but we do not know which one. It seems likely, then, that Galen's first appointment, from fall 157 through the spring of 158, involved the care of a troupe of gladiators who were training for the games and lived permanently in Pergamum.

Gladiators were an ancient Roman institution, so called after the Latin word for sword, *gladius*. In Greek they were called *monomachoi*, "those who fight one [-on-one]." Originally, they fought at funerals—for the first time, according to historical tradition, in 264 B.C.E., when three pairs fought at the funeral of Junius Brutus Pera. As aristocratic families competed ferociously for prestige in Republican Rome, gladiatorial shows honoring their deceased patriarchs became larger and more spectacular and could involve dozens of pairs fighting over several days. More and more, they became obvious political tools—senators up for election to the tribunate or consulship would choose that moment to fulfill their vows honoring relatives long deceased. In this way did the urban population of Rome become accustomed, or addicted, to the bloody spectacles. From the accession of Augustus in the first century B.C.E., most (eventually, all) gladiatorial games in the capital city were sponsored by the emperor and seem to have occurred annually over several days near the end of the year. But gladiatorial games were also staged elsewhere in Italy and in the provinces. The oldest known amphitheater is the one at Pompeii in Campania; the city of Rome had no permanent arena until 30 B.C.E., and the Colosseum—antiquity's iconic amphitheater, and its largest—dates to the reign of Vespasian, in the 70s C.E. Before then the games were staged

---

8   Nutton (1973, 162–64); Schlange-Schöningen (2003, 117–20).

in the forum or possibly in one of Rome's two circuses for chariot-racing. About 272 amphitheaters are more or less attested in the cities of the Roman Empire, and many cities staged games without an amphitheater if massive construction was beyond their means.[9]

Few amphitheaters were built in the Greek East, but not because gladiatorial spectacles, imported from Rome, were unpopular—rather, Greek cities often accommodated the games in the large theaters that already existed. Several of these were also modified in antiquity to accommodate the bloody wild beast hunts—slaughters of exotic animals—that catered to some of the same tastes as gladiatorial contests, with extra barriers to protect the audience from the animals. Even the legendary Theater of Dionysus in Athens, which had witnessed the plays of Aeschylus and Sophocles, hosted gladiatorial games, a circumstance for which Dio Chrysostomus blasted the Athenians in a passage dripping with scorn.[10]

Violent combat sports had long been a staple of Greek culture. Boxing and the *pankration* ("all in"; "total combat") were especially violent, and both had been Olympic sports since the seventh century B.C.E. Boxing gloves in antiquity featured a hard leather knuckle guard, and classical vases depicting boxing contests often show nasty blows to the head and profuse blood. The sport became even more lethal in the Roman period when gloves were often weighted with fragments of metal and glass. (The well-known bronze statue of a seated boxer in Rome, dating to the first century B.C.E., shows cauliflower ears and several bleeding wounds to the face). The *pankration*, fought with bare hands, was less bloody but just as brutal, a form of no-holds-barred wrestling—contestants strangled one another, twisted limbs, bent and broke fingers, and also bit and gouged each other despite rules that theoretically

---

9   Many books in English and other languages have been published on the gladiatorial games. Documents from the eastern Roman Empire are collected and discussed in the fundamental work of Robert (1940). Recommended general introductions in English are Potter (1999; 2012, chapter 26); Wiedemann (1992); the classic essay of Hopkins (1983); and Auget (1972). Most recent and comprehensive, especially for weapons and archaeological remains, is Junkelmann (2000).

10   On gladiatorial contests in theaters, see Gros (1996–2001, 1:342); Robert (1940, 34–36). Dio Chrysostomus: *Or.* 31.121–22.

prohibited this. Both types of contest, like most gladiatorial contests, continued until one competitor signaled surrender.[11]

Thus, Hellenized tastes were not more refined or sophisticated than Roman ones, and gladiatorial contests are well-attested throughout Rome's eastern provinces: not only do authors such as Galen mention them as a normal part of Greek culture, but inscriptions honor the sponsors of games and commemorate gladiators who died, and record financial expenses and local decrees associated with the games. Gladiators and games appear on sculpted reliefs, in mosaics and paintings, in graffiti, on coins. Authors in both Greek and Latin sometimes decried the gratuitous cruelty and perversity of gladiatorial combat; this is a common theme in Stoic and early Christian literature. But Galen makes no moral comment on the institution, and describes his experiences with the gladiators dispassionately, except for the pride he obviously took in being chosen for the post and in his excellent performance.[12]

Pergamum did boast an amphitheater, constructed—like other buildings of the Hadrianic renaissance in that city—in the first half of the second century C.E. Today only a few brick arches survive, on what were (and remain) the outskirts of the city, near the Roman theater, between the ancient Acropolis and the temple of Asclepius. Pergamum's amphitheater was a medium-sized example of such structures, about 136 by 107 meters in overall dimensions, with an arena 51 meters long and seating capacity of about 25,000. Not enough remains to describe it in more detail.[13]

In Galen's time the annual gladiatorial games must have been performed there, as well as the wild beast hunts that took place in Pergamum and cities throughout the Roman Empire. (Galen does not mention treating the wild animal killers for their wounds, although doctors were sometimes assigned

---

11   Good introductions to Greek athletics are Potter (2012) and Miller (2004). On statues of athletes, including the seated boxer, see the recent discussion of König (2005, 102–32); Newby (2005, 88–140).

12   For a fuller discussion of attitudes toward gladiatorial combat, see Carlin A. Barton (1993). On religious and imperialist dimensions, see Furtrell (1997).

13   Golvin (1988, 1: 287). On the Pergamene amphitheater, see also Radt (1999, 265–66).

to them.)[14] Galen does not say where he treated the gladiators. If the troupe was resident in Pergamum all year, they may have trained somewhere other than the amphitheater, possibly in one of the city's wrestling-courts; no barracks like those at Pompeii have been identified. Galen possibly was granted clinic space near their training grounds and in or near the amphitheater. He mentions once, in passing, that cities sometimes provide houses with wide doors, essential for adequate lighting, to practicing physicians, but without saying that he benefited from this at Pergamum or anywhere (*Hipp. Off.* 1.8, 18B.678K).

Who were the gladiators Galen treated? Professional gladiators could be hired individually; or, more commonly, gladiators lived and trained in troupes (called *familiae* in both Latin and Greek) owned by the high priest producing the show, or by a trainer hired to provide them, or by a private investor. Though a *munus* (gladiatorial event) might include a mixture of slaves from a *familia* and freelance professionals, by necessity members of the same troupe often fought each other, no doubt creating interesting psychological dynamics about which we know little. At Pergamum, because the high priest changed every year, it is likely that each priest Galen served sold the troupe to his successor, a procedure also attested in a senatorial decree dating to 177 C.E., regulating expenditures on shows, and in the records of the debate that preceded it.[15]

Notoriously, men of free status who sold their services as gladiators were supposed to take an oath agreeing to be burnt, chained, beaten, and killed with an iron weapon. Their reasons do not survive in their own words; moralizing literary sources usually cite bloodlust or extreme poverty, and both are plausible. The fate of becoming a gladiator was considered especially miserable even for a slave. Masters sometimes sold disobedient slaves to trainers as a punishment. Convicted criminals could also be condemned to combat by the state, although these were not considered gladiators proper, but a separate

---

14   Wild beast hunts are attested at Pergamum in Robert (1940, nos. 264 and 265). On doctors for wild beast hunters, see Wiedemann (1992, 117).

15   On selling troupes to successors, see Robert (1940, 284). On the senatorial decree, see Oliver and Palmer (1955).

and inferior group. Gladiators might also be prisoners of war, although in the East in the imperial period most gladiators had Greek names with no ethnic markers. A few were Roman citizens, and this was more common in the West. Slave or free, many gladiators had social ties. Some left wives (or consorts, for slaves could not legally marry) and children on their deaths, as their epitaphs record. Some belonged to professional associations, *collegiae*, which were mainly social clubs; slaves were eligible to join.[16]

Gladiators were performers in an especially lethal spectacle. True, the shows were not as deadly or as gratuitously bloody as the wild beast slaughters or the ingeniously cruel executions of criminals that often took place on the same day and in the same venue; but the constant specter of death was part of what thrilled the audience. Gladiators could be killed by a deadly (and perhaps accidental) thrust of a weapon; or, defeated, they might kneel and supplicate the sponsoring official for their lives with a raised index finger, the gesture of surrender. At Pergamum this official was the high priest who (probably) also owned the gladiatorial troupe and would no doubt prefer to spare the defeated; but the crowd would roar its support or disapproval, and he hardly dared disappoint them. Reliefs depicting the execution of defeated gladiators show a victim passively accepting his fate, grasping the victor's leg or lying supine on the ground while his opponent thrusts a sword into his throat or back. Gladiators killed in combat or executed on the orders of the sponsor were carried off on stretchers by a slave dressed as the death-god Dis Pater, who dispatched them with a final hammer-blow to the skull. But a gladiator who fought bravely—that is, who put on a good show—might well be spared (*missus*, sent away) to fight another day; an especially brilliant performance might win freedom and retirement for the victor. Some gladiatorial epitaphs attest to long records of victories and *missiones* in the career of the deceased—killed finally in the arena perhaps, or, equally likely, dead later from infected wounds, or of other causes. Some survived to retirement and

16 On the social status of gladiators, see Potter (2012, chapter 26); Wiedemann (1992, chapter 3); Robert (1940, 283–95) . On gladiators as Roman citizens, see Robert (1940, 297). On their wives and families, see Carter (2006) and Robert (1940, 43–44).

lived prosperously afterward. A gladiator's chance of death in any particular contest, either in the arena or later of his wounds, was about one in nine.[17]

Everyone involved had a strong interest in playing dramatically to the crowd and walking away rather than killing or being killed. Victorious gladiators risked death in future contests, and often belonged to the same troupe as their defeated opponents, whom they would face again. The sponsor of the games either owned the gladiators or rented them, and, if he rented, he owed a huge sum for those killed. Many gladiators boast on their epitaphs of having harmed none of their opponents, and this may have been expected and honorable conduct: thus some complain that they were killed by deceit or betrayal, and one epitaph even records the revenge-killing of a renegade gladiator who unnecessarily slew his opponent.[18]

Gladiatorial combat was not, then, a free-for all: gladiators fought according to rules of engagement in which they were skillfully trained, and which were enforced by referees at every contest. They fought one pair at a time— that is, in duels—and a typical combat lasted about fifteen minutes.

They were bulky men, fattened on a special high-carbohydrate, vegetarian diet. On this point the evidence from an extraordinary find—the skeletons of sixty-eight gladiators recovered from a cemetery in Ephesus, discovered by archaeologists in 1993—confirms Galen's own observations on their diet:

> The gladiators in my homeland eat mostly this food [a concoction of fava beans and boiled barley] every day, becoming fleshy in the condition of their body—but the flesh is not compacted and dense, like pig's meat, but rather somehow more flaccid.
>
> (*Aliment. Fac.* 1.19, 6.529K)

Pliny the Elder wrote that gladiators were also called *hordearii* after their diet based on barley (*hordeum*: *NH* 18.72). The fat they accumulated offered

---

17   On the gesture of surrender, see Carter (2006, 102–3). On mortality, see Junkelmann (2000, 142); Ville (1981, 318–25). On the god of death, see Junkelmann (2000, 140–41).

18   On the survivability of gladiatorial combat, see Carter (2006). For the revenge-killing, see Carter (2006, 109–10); Robert (1940, no. 34).

insulation from serious injuries, while allowing for showy surface wounds: bleeding from a gaping gash that affected no major nerves or muscles, the gladiator fought on undaunted while the crowd went wild. They wore special costumes. The *retiarius* wielded net and trident against his opponent, the *secutor*, with his fishlike helmet; the "Thracian," the "knight," and roughly a dozen other types each had their own set of offensive and defensive weapons, most fighting half-naked, bare-chested and in loincloths. Individual gladiators seem to have trained specifically in one technique and identified as that type, even on their epitaphs. Like modern entertainers, they exuded glamor and sex appeal even as their marginal social status drew contempt.[19]

From Pergamum and the territory nearby a few gladiators' epitaphs survive. Chrestinus, from Nicomedia, was slain by Achilles. His tombstone depicted two victory-crowns and his dog, named Mourdon. The wife of a gladiator named Stephanus set up his tombstone; he had survived eighteen fights. Chrysomallus's tombstone bore only his name and a sculpted relief: dressed as a *retiarius*, he grips his trident with both hands.[20]

Although gladiators aimed to put on a good show without necessarily killing their opponents, serious wounds did happen. Many of the skeletons recovered from the cemetery at Ephesus suffered cranial injuries, some of which had healed over time while others were lethal. Some were blunt force blows caused by the gladiator's own helmet, when hit on the head in combat; some show the sharp punctures of swords or tridents; three skulls show massive, fatal trauma, perhaps crushed by an opponent's shield and full body weight; and four distinctive fatal blows are attributable to the Dis Pater's hammer. Some healed wounds had obviously been treated by doctors.[21] Gladiators were extraordinarily expensive—the value of some professionals could run to 15,000 sesterces, the price of a small public building, and their owners invested in their medical care. It was Galen's job to treat them, and at this he excelled.

---

19   On diet, see Curry (2008, 28–31). On glamor, see Hopkins (1983, 22–23); Carlin A. Barton (1993, 47–89). On the cemetery, see further Kanz and Grossschmidt (2006).
20   Robert (1940, nos. 260–63).
21   On the cemetery in Ephesus and gladiatorial injuries, see Kanz and Grossschmidt (2006).

Galen used his new formula for the treatment of wounded tendons. He applied it, as he writes, to wounds at the lower front of the thigh, apparently common in gladiators. Previous physicians and trainers (*didaskaloi*, who taught the gladiators combat skills) had treated wounds by bathing them in hot water and applying a plaster of wheat flour boiled in water and oil, a procedure Galen excoriates—"[the patients were] not treated, but rather destroyed, for very few of them were saved, and those became lame." Galen himself omitted the hot water and used frequent applications of oil together with a remedy of his own invention, the concoction he tested on his own patients and those of other physicians in the early days after his return to Pergamum. With this therapy, as he claims, he saved all the gladiators in his care in the first year of his practice, although in previous years many had died. In another passage Galen describes his method of treating severe wounds in more detail; gladiators were most often wounded in summer, as he relates, because that is when the games were held, and in his view keeping the wound moist was of great importance. He soaked linen cloths in wine and placed the folds on the wounds, covering the cloths in soft sponges which he moistened day and night. He even devised a method to collect the excess wine that dripped down from the wound in an empty skin and re-use it. The ethanol and acidity in wine can kill many microbes (though only those causing foodborne illness have apparently been tested), especially if it is applied full strength, continually and over a long period, as Galen describes; although his re-used wine was probably not as effective as the fresh liquid. For Galen, however, who knew nothing of pathogenic microbes, the aim was to keep the wound moist, as I have mentioned.[22]

Transverse (crosswise) wounds to the thigh had to be sutured, because the muscles, when severed, would separate (whereas, as Galen writes, a bandage is sufficient to close a vertical wound). One gladiator, a "knight" (these fought on horseback with lances and, when dismounted, with swords) had such a deep and broadly gaping gash across his lower thigh

---

22   *Comp. Med. Gen.* 3.2 (13.564–65K, 599–600K); *Hipp. Fract.* 3.21 (18B.567–69K). On wine as disinfectant, see Waite and Daeschel (2007), with review of previous literature.

near the kneepan that Galen was forced ("I dared") to exceed anything he had witnessed his teachers accomplish in drawing the muscles together, suturing deep layers of muscle and stripping the covering (he may mean the epitenon) off of the severed tendons before joining them with extreme care.[23] Here Galen criticizes those physicians who stitch together only the skin or the most superficial layer of muscle when treating deep wounds; reasonably, for deep sutures are necessary to align the wound edges and reduce tension in the wound.

Gladiators often acquired wounds on the hands and feet, like soldiers. Also like soldiers and hunters, they might suffer severed arteries and veins, sometimes so serious that the vessel had to be ligated with a loop of thread.[24] One gladiator was wounded in the abdomen and nearly disemboweled. The omentum, the folded membrane that protects the small intestines, projected from the wound and turned livid, and Galen had to remove it: "almost the whole thing," as he writes, suggesting a large and gruesome wound. The patient survived, but ever afterward was constantly cold and had to keep his abdomen wrapped in wool (*Usu Part.* 4.9, 3.286–87K). Later, Galen would describe techniques of "gastrorrhaphy"—by which he meant replacing intestines prolapsed from wounds to the abdomen and repairing the wound surgically (the word is still used, but has a somewhat different meaning in modern surgery)—in his treatise *On the Method of Healing.* Galen was not the first to write on this topic, but his discussion of suturing methods differs greatly from that of the only earlier surviving example, a passage from Celsus, writing in Latin in the first century C.E., whose seventh book of his treatise *On Medicine* is the most important discussion of surgery to survive from antiquity. This divergence suggests that Galen's advice reflects his own experiences and most probably his long stint treating gladiators. The techniques he describes approximate what would now be called block-and-tackle sutures and mattress sutures; he recommends full-thickness sutures for abdominal repair (this would also be done today), rather than the suturing in layers he

---

23 *Comp. Med. Gen.* 3.2 (13.601–2K). On "knights," see Junkelmann (2000, 123–24).
24 Hands and feet: *Anat. Admin.* 3.1 (2.345K). Ligation: *Usu Puls.* 3 (5.160K).

may have used for wounds to the thigh (his description is not specific enough to determine this).

It is likely that by this time Galen owned a large number of medical instruments, both for treating patients and for anatomizing animals. The graves of physicians from Rome's European provinces (most of them were associated with the army) and the detritus of the houses buried by Mount Vesuvius preserve a staggering variety of scoops, spoons, spatulae, hooks, forceps, scalpels, shears, needles, probes, vaginal and rectal specula, catheters, bone saws, trephines, chisels, levers, cupping vessels, cauteries, and so on, so precious and familiar to their owners that many were buried with them. Doctors typically seem to have owned many instruments, sometimes dozens, and Galen will later write that he lost the prototypes for instruments of his own design in the fire that consumed Rome in 192.[25] But of surgical instruments he mentions in his passage on gastrorrhaphy only the "syringotome," a type of knife ("fistula-knife"), which he contrasts with double-edged or pointed knives, and the suturing needle. He does not refer to retractor hooks, of which many examples have been preserved, and Celsus mentions them; Galen instead instructs that a skilled assistant retract the wound with his hands.[26] Galen also does not, in this passage, say what material he used for suturing. In another, much-cited location from the second half of the same work *On the Method of Healing*, written much later, he discusses ligatures for arteries, when arteriotomy is necessary as a treatment; he prefers a substance called "Gallic" in Rome and imported from Gaul (we do not know what he means). Since this is not widely available outside the capital city, silk is second-best and can usually be procured from wealthy women; failing that, anything that does not decay easily will do, for example, famously, dried gut (*Meth. Med.*

25   On medical instruments, see especially Baker (2004, chapter 5); Cruse (2004, chapter 6); Bliquez (1994); Künzl (1983). On Galen's lost instruments, see chapter 8 below.

26   On gastrorrhaphy: Galen, *Meth. Med.* 6.4 (10.411–20K). The edition of Johnston and Horsley (2011) adds drawings and commentary, in translation, from Witt (2009). "Syringotome": 10.415K. Hands: 10.416K. Celsus: 7.16. Papavramidou and Christopoulou-Aletra (2009) offer a helpful modern perspective despite misunderstanding of the nature of some ancient sources.

13.22, 10.941–43K). It is not clear what material Galen in fact used to stitch up the gladiators, or for the surgeries he performed later in life.

Galen also saw wounds to the heart. He describes them in *On the Affected Parts*, written several decades later (5.2, 8.304K). If one of the ventricles was perforated, he writes, the victim bled to death immediately, especially if it was the left ventricle. Some wounds reached the cardiac muscle but did not penetrate to the interior of the ventricle. These gladiators might live through the day and perhaps the following night, but soon died. (Galen notes that they remained lucid until death, incidentally disproving the Aristotelian notion that the heart is the seat of reason.) Galen reports these events dispassionately, as always—he is very consistent in expressing no sympathy, fear, pity, disappointment, attachment, or any other emotion for his patients. But as this last example demonstrates, he talked to the dying gladiators. He clearly spared no effort or ingenuity in treating their wounds. And, in contrast with his merciless scorn for heavy athletes (whom he seems to consider quite separately from gladiators, never mentioning the two in the same discussion), no word of criticism for this despised and servile class survives in his work.[27]

The passage from *On the Affected Parts* suggests that Galen witnessed many fatalities among the gladiators and lost many patients; but this is not what he writes elsewhere. In his first two years, as he claims, no gladiators died in his care. Elsewhere, in a passage that contradicts this, Galen writes that he lost two gladiators in his first year, but none under a later priest who also appointed him: though his predecessors had lost sixteen gladiators.[28] In any case Galen clearly took great pride in his record and in the fact that five successive priests honored him with the position at which he proved so superior. What happened after this we do not know. Perhaps the sixth priest chose someone else. In any case Galen's term as physician to the gladiators came to an end in autumn of 161, and by the following autumn he was in Rome.

---

27   For a recent discussion of Galen's views on athletes, expressed at most length in *Adhort. Art.*, see König (2005, 274–300) and further in chapter 5 below.

28   *Comp. Med. Gen.* 3.2 (13.600K); *Opt. Med. Cogn.* 9 (104 Iskandar).

Later—when giving reasons for his flight back to Pergamum in 166—
Galen will complain that he had to wait for *stasis*, or civil conflict, in his
homeland to end; but we know neither what sort of trouble he was referring
to, nor when it broke out (this may well have happened when he was already
at Rome).[29] Some have speculated that the disruption caused by the war with
the kingdom of Parthia, to the east across the Euphrates—for one of the
emperors, Lucius Verus, invaded it in that year 161—caused the *stasis* and
Galen's departure; but the effects do not seem to have reached Pergamum, nor
did Parthia invade the Roman provinces, and in any case the Greeks never
used the word *stasis* to signify a foreign war.[30] It is much more likely that
Galen refers to political discord in Pergamum, perhaps akin to the rioting and
lynchings described by Dio Chrysostomus, when the ire of the people (and
its own wealthy rivals) turned against one of its leading families. But all of
this is speculation. We do not know why Galen stopped treating gladiators
and decided to try his fortunes in the empire's sprawling capital. It may simply have seemed the right time to fulfill an ambition of long standing. Like
it had drawn Quintus, Satyrus, and other aristocratic Pergamenes aspiring
to fame and pretending to culture, Rome, the center of power, prestige, and
influence, drew him into its vortex.

---

29   *Stasis*: *Praecog.* 4 (14.622K): 9 (14.648K).
30   Nutton (1973, 164–65); Schlange-Schöningen (2003, 133–36).

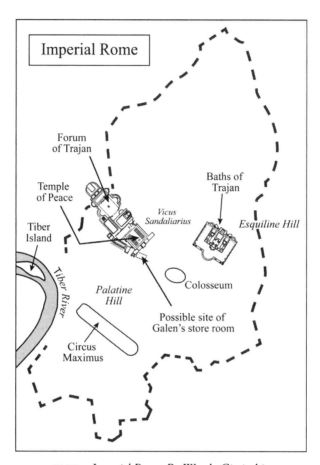

MAP 3: Imperial Rome. By Wendy Giminski.

Chapter Four

ROME

alen's last term as physician to the gladiators probably ended in late summer of 161. He was in Rome a year later, by the early fall of 162, and before his birthday in that year, still thirty-two years old.[1] It is perhaps at this juncture, after his departure from Pergamum and before he set out for Italy, that he journeyed to Lycia on Turkey's southern coast, to Palestine (Roman Syria Palestina or, as it was sometimes called in Greek, Syria *Koile*, hollow Syria), and to the copper mines of Cyprus. (These journeys may date to his return to Pergamum in 166–68, however.[2]) Galen sought rare ingredients for his drug recipes.

1   In *Ind.* 34, Galen writes that he arrived in Rome at the age of thirty-two. By the time of the final showdown with Martianus on bloodletting, the speech transcribed by Teuthras's slave (see below), he was thirty-three (*Libr. Propr.* 1, 19.15K). The easiest fit with the evidence (assuming that Galen's memory of dates is always accurate, which is not necessarily the case) is that Galen arrived in Rome some time before his birthday (which was in the early fall; see chapter 1, n. 31) in 162 and that his confrontations with the Erasistrateans and treatment of Eudemus (which occurred over the course of a winter) happened later that year and in early 163. Schlange-Schöningen (2003, 139–42) points out that based on *Praecog.* 2 (14.609K) Galen must have been at Rome by early fall of 162, when he treated an anonymous patient for quartan fever; and nothing excludes an earlier arrival. For a recent discussion of this chronology, see Boudon-Millot (2007a, liv–lvi).

2   The timing of these journeys is very uncertain. Nutton (1973, 169) places them in 161–62; Boudon-Millot (2007a, li–liv) takes no position. I am not impressed by Galen's failure to mention

> I sailed along the whole of Lycia in a small boat for the sake of inquir-
> ing into the things there. From Syria Koile [Palestine] I brought back
> many black crustaceous rocks and rocks which, when exposed to fire, emit
> a meager flame [i.e., asphalt], found in the eastern part of the highlands
> surrounding the so-called Dead Sea, where there is also bitumen.
>
> (*Simp. Med.* 8.2.10, 12.203K)

Returning from Palestine, he encountered a camel caravan carrying Indian
lycium—catechu, extract of acacia—directly, as he believed, from India;
questioning the merchants, and convinced that they had no knowledge of
how to counterfeit (*notheuein*) the drug, and since the requisite materials were
not to be found in the area, he acquired some (*Simp. Med.* 8.3.8, 12.216K).
(Galen himself was perfectly skilled in the art of preparing counterfeits of
rare drugs, including this one, as he writes in the same passage.) Galen offers
no further details about his visit to Syria and Palestine; but later, in Rome,
a native of that region—the ex-consul Boethus—would be one of his most
valued friends.

Cyprus produced a pyritic ore, which had to be roasted and then smelted
to extract the copper, a process that resulted in several by-products. Here
Galen acquired the mineral substance he calls diphryges, which he considered
the most effective medicine against malignant tumors; and cadmeia (usually
identified as calamine by modern scholars, although calamine is now a defunct
term for two separate minerals). Galen thought cadmeia, like diphryges, was
normally a by-product of copper smelting, but that it occurred naturally on
Cyprus. In Galen's time the Roman state owned most mines and adminis-
tered them through procurators, who were often imperial freedmen or (as
in the case of the "prefect and procurator" of the mine at Soli, which Galen
visited) men of equestrian rank; and sometimes military officers. These either

---

his friend Flavius Boethus, who was governor of Syria Palestina in the late 160s and whom Galen
might have been expected to visit if the journeys had occurred at the later date; I do doubt, however, whether Galen would have undertaken these arduous journeys at a time when the "great
plague" raged through the region (see chapter 6).

managed the mines directly or leased operations to private individuals or corporations, who paid half the revenue to the state.

Mining was notoriously noxious and deadly work. The labor force might be condemned criminals (including Christians) or especially unfortunate slaves; sometimes, as in Spain, forcibly relocated and coerced natives; sometimes free lessees or employees of the state; sometimes soldiers. The laborers Galen saw at Soli were chained slaves, probably condemned criminals. Today the heaps of slag produced by smelting in Spain and also on Cyprus are perhaps the Romans' most chilling and impressive legacy: for they exploited the mineral resources of their subjects with special rapacity and mined on a massive scale. The Greenland ice sheet preserves the record of elevated levels of lead released into the atmosphere by Roman-era silver smelting. From Cyprus they extracted several hundred tons of copper a year.[3]

The copper mines of Soli made an impression on Galen, whose description borders on the surreal. The mine was about 30 stades (around 7 miles) from the town. A "large building" or "large house" stood directly adjacent to the mine, with an entrance near the right-hand wall (that is, to the left of those approaching the house). In the mine Galen saw "three belts"—three layers of slag—"extending extremely far, one on top of the other." The procurator, boasting of the abundance, offered Galen whatever he wanted from the slag heaps and Galen accepted "a huge quantity."[4] He brought it all first to Asia, and then to Rome when he moved there; thirty years later, writing the later books of his treatise *On the Mixtures and Powers of Simple Drugs*, he still had a supply of the minerals acquired in Cyprus, of which cadmeia was the one most prized by the friends he shared it with.[5]

Adjoining or facing the other side of the house was an underground passageway, as broad as three men, high enough for a tall man to walk upright.

---

3 On cadmeia: *Simp. Med.* 9.3.11 (12.219–20K); on diphryges: *Simp. Med.* 9.3.8 (12.214K). On Roman administration and workforce, see Hirt (2010); Healy (1978, 103–38). On forced relocation and miners in Iberia, Hirt (2010, 228–32). On Greenland glaciers, see Hong et al. (1994).

4 *Simp. Med.* 9.3.21 (12.226–27K). On the distance to town: *Simp. Med.* 9.3.8 (12.214K).

5 *Simp. Med.* 9.3.11 (12.220K), 9.3.21 (12.227K).

It led downhill to an underground lake or pond "about a stade long" (a stade was about one-eighth of a mile). The lake was full of thick, warm, pale green water. The water collected, as Galen explains, by condensation at a rate of about eight Roman amphorae per day, or forty-eight gallons. The temperature in the passageway reminded him of the changing-rooms at the baths—that is, it was hot, but not with the intense heat of a sweat room. The stench was insupportable: "the smell of the air seemed stifling and difficult to bear, smelling of copper and verdigris." Slaves, naked and chained at the feet, traversed the passageways, fetching the water to the surface where they poured it into square ceramic pools in front of the building. There it was allowed to evaporate, and the copper sulfate—*chalkanthos*, as Galen calls it—was collected.

So dense was the air in the tunnel, as Galen writes, that it was nearly impossible to keep the lamps that lined its walls burning. The slaves did not linger in the tunnel but raced down and back as quickly as possible. They had excavated the tunnel, as Galen learned, over many years, gradually expanding it if it seemed that the supply of water was dwindling, and fatal accidents were not unusual: "Sometimes the excavated part collapses suddenly ahead, so that every one of them is killed."[6]

Galen was relentlessly inquisitive and tirelessly committed to his craft and, no less than this, to being the foremost and best practitioner of his profession. Perhaps nothing illustrates this more vividly than the lengths to which he traveled; for his education, as I have already described, but also to procure a store of precious medicaments that must have been—and surely this was his intent—unparalleled. One could also acquire rare items from friends traveling to the provinces as governors, or from friends native to the region, "as you have seen me doing" *(Antid.* 1.2, 14.8K). Only by these methods could one be quite certain of getting the genuine item, for the adulteration and substitution of ingredients, the local imitation of expensive imported items like nard, and other, similar practices were very common.[7]

---

6 *Simp. Med.* 9.3.34 (12.238–40K). See Schlange-Schöningen (2003, 284–89) ("Sklaven in der Kupfermine von Soloi").

7 On adulteration and substitution, see Nutton (1985, 142–44).

The visit to Cyprus must have taken weeks, including the sail in either direction, the trek from the town to the mine and Galen's protracted negotiations with the procurator, by whom he was well received and who may have been a friend or acquaintance. (He may have visited Cyprus on the return from Syria Palestina, although he made that trip partly overland, when he encountered the camel caravan.) Galen not only toured the mine, collecting oxides and sulfates that we cannot accurately identify today but that were known and distinguishable to him; he descended the suffocating passageway; he tasted the water; he interrogated the chained slaves. He also interacted with the local peasantry enough to comment on their diet: they use polenta instead of wheat to make bread, "which I myself have seen peasants do in Cyprus" (*Aliment. Fac.* 1.11, 6.57K).

Later, he would make two separate trips to the island of Lemnos, off the western coast of Turkey, to procure signets of its famous earth prepared specially by the priestess of the cult of Philoctetes, the legendary hero of the Trojan War era who was cured of snakebite there. These signets were compressed medallions stamped with an image of the goddess Artemis, to guarantee their authenticity, and were thought to have great medicinal value for healing abscessed wounds, snakebite, animal bites, rabies, and poison.[8] I discuss Galen's visits to Lemnos here because they illustrate two of the themes of this chapter, namely the hardships of travel, and the acquisition of exotic drugs. Galen made his first trip to Lemnos during his second journey to Italy from Pergamum, when he was recalled in 168. The visit was unsuccessful because, as Galen writes, although he managed to talk the ship's captain into making a special stop at Lemnos, the ship put in at the wrong town. Galen did not know that there was more than one important town on Lemnos but had assumed that (like many Aegean islands) it had only one. A return journey from the other direction, at some indeterminable later date (but perhaps

---

8   Lemnian earth has been much studied and analyzed in modern times, most recently by Hall and Photos-Jones (2008), who identify the substance as a combination of two clays (montmorillonite and kaolin), alum, and hematite, and discuss potential medicinal benefits. They also collect and discuss ancient references to Lemnian earth. See also Nutton (1985, 143–44).

later in life, in the 190s), was more successful. Here Galen records particulars for the edification of others who might wish to imitate it: from Philippi in Thessaly he descended 120 stades to the sea; from there he sailed 200 stades to Thasos, and thence 700 stades to Lemnos, and then an equal number of stades from there to Alexandria Troas in Asia. The name of the city he sought was Hephaestias, after a hill sacred to the blacksmith-god Hephaestus, which produced the sacred earth with its special qualities.[9]

On this second visit, Galen observed the priestess preparing the signets himself; his object was to learn the recipe for the mixture (although he writes elsewhere that he had, as an adolescent, learned exactly this recipe among others from a highly paid teacher). He asked the locals whether it was possible that goat's blood had been mixed with the soil, explaining its red color (as he had read in the famous medicinal catalog of Dioscorides and other sources). This question provoked universal laughter. Galen then procured, from one of the town's prominent citizens, a book about Lemnian customs, which included information about the medicinal uses of Lemnian earth; this man, as Galen writes, made extensive use of the material and asserted (among other things) that it cured rabies if drunk with wine and placed on the bite wound. Galen left Lemnos on this second occasion with 20,000 of the signets and knowledge only obtainable through exhausting and inconvenient travel and the close interrogation of local sources (*Simp. Med.* 9.1.2, 12.171–75K; Dioscorides 5.97).

Galen's trips to Lemnos illustrate some of the more obscure challenges of travel in antiquity, not least of which was the difficulty of knowing exactly where one was going and how to get there, in an era when gathering any type of specialized information was an art requiring subtlety, ingenuity, and fortitude.[10] While sailing could greatly increase the speed (but not necessarily the convenience) of travel at certain times of year, it was also riskier and could be harrowing; shipwreck was not uncommon. Galen himself seems to

---

9   On the visits to Lemnos, see *Simp. Med.* 9.1.2 (12.171–75K); 9.3.9 (12.216K); *Antid.* 1.1 (14.8K). On the chronology and routes of these journeys, a vexed subject, see Nutton (1973, 167–69) and Boudon-Millot (2007a, xlvii–l).

10   See Brodersen (2001, 7–9) on this passage.

have traveled back and forth to Rome largely or mostly overland and on foot—that is, he walked. The most likely itinerary for his journey to Rome in 161–62 took him overland through Thrace and Macedonia on the Roman road, the *Via Egnatia*; he mentions "traveling on foot through Thrace and Macedonia" (*Simp. Med.* 9.1.2, 12.171K). On his second journey he sailed, as we have seen, from Alexandria Troas to Lemnos and also from there to Thessalonike, but probably proceeded the rest of the way on foot; and on his later trip east, the one on which he acquired the Lemnian signets, "I crossed from Italy into Macedonia and traversed it almost entirely by foot" as far as Philippi, on the border of Thrace, before embarking for Thasos and then Lemnos (ibid., 12.172K).[11]

On his rushed departure (or flight) from Rome in 166 (see chapter 6), Galen was obliged first to journey overland to Brundisium in southern Italy (he covered by telling everyone he was going to visit his country estate in Campania) before embarking for Cassiope on Corcyra; from there he must have sailed to the Greek mainland, but proceeded, apparently, on foot as far as Corinth and from there by carriage to Athens (on the way he saved two slaves from being murdered by their master) before, perhaps, embarking for Asia, or he may have made the rest of the journey overland.

Thus, Galen traveled by carriage at least once, between Corinth and Athens, like his patient Pausanias, who was injured with three paralyzed fingers after a fall from a carriage (or, in one version of the story, off a horse).[12] But this is his only reference to travel by carriage. In most of his stories about the hardships of travel, Galen is traveling on foot. Once he was so exhausted he walked a whole stade in his sleep "seeing dreams; nor was I awakened until I tripped over a stone" (*Motu Musc.* 2.4, 4.435–36K). On another occasion "I was traveling through so much snow, that no bare part of the earth was visible." (Heavy snowfall is rare in most of the Mediterranean world; Galen may

---

11 On the logistics of Galen's trips between Rome and Pergamum, see Nutton (1973, 167–69). For another case study of the hardships of travel in the Roman Empire, based on the experiences of Galen's contemporary Aelius Aristides, see Mitchell (1993, 1:165–67).

12 Pausanias's fall: *Anat. Admin.* 3.1 (2.343–45K); *Loc. Affect.* 1.6 (8.57K) and 3.14 (8.213–14K); *Opt. Med. Cogn.* 9 (106–8 Iskandar).

be walking through Macedonia in this anecdote.) "The air appeared completely pure" and what he perceived as the *pneuma*, or vapor, of snow in the air was so cold that it froze ("bit") one's whole face, not just the eyes or nose, and likewise a hand, if extended outside one's cloak (*Simp. Med.* 4.2, 11.625K). One of his patients, caught in heavy rain and wind while traveling, became so chilled around the neck when his cloak was soaked that he damaged nerves and lost feeling in his head (*Loc. Affect.* 4.7, 8.258–59K). On the other hand, another patient became so overheated and dried by a journey "which was entirely sandy and dusty, under a hot sun," and also by insomnia when he tried to sleep at an inn, and by other factors, that he developed a dangerous fever and nearly died (*Meth. Med.* 10.3, 10.671–73K). The exhaustion and constant movement of travel could also cause fever and wasting.[13]

Travel overland was slow, and Galen's journey from Pergamum to Rome would have taken months. Inns, when they could be found at all, were notoriously uncomfortable and treacherous; Galen claims, in all seriousness, that some innkeepers serve their guests human flesh and call it pork (*Aliment. Fac.* 3.2, 6.663K). Whether or not this is true, "mystery meat" was probably not an unusual experience, and travel was hard on the digestive system in other ways. As a teenager, Galen was traveling with other friends his own age "in the countryside, not close to the city" (the "city" is most likely Pergamum or possibly Smyrna, for he is still a *meirakion* in this passage), they became very hungry ("of course, because we were traveling and famished") and shared a meal with some peasants who offered them food. The peasants themselves had run out of bread, so the women made a porridge of boiled wheat, which Galen and his friends were entirely unable to digest and suffered from gas, headaches, and blurred vision (*Aliment. Fac.* 1.7, 6.498–99K).

Galen never describes being attacked by bandits, but he was lucky. It goes without saying that he never traveled alone. He mentions falling in with other wayfarers—his acquaintance from Crete, the peasants who offered boiled wheat—as a normal practice. It is fair to assume even in passages where Galen mentions no companion that he is accompanied by his own slaves,

---

13   *Hipp. 6 Epid.* 4.20 (17B.281K); *Hipp. Aph.* 2.28 (17B 519–20K).

whose presence is hinted at in many stories though he rarely speaks of them directly.[14] Banditry and fear of bandits are attested in all periods and regions of the Roman Empire, even in Italy, although it was part of the empire's claim to glory and legitimacy to have made its roads safe to travel. Galen mentions banditry several times, reflecting a world in which it was pervasive (imperial propaganda and the flattering claims of obsequious orators eager to please an emperor with praise of Rome, or of himself, notwithstanding). Once, by the side of the road (he does not say in which part of the world) Galen saw a naked skeleton: the body of a bandit, as he learned, killed by one of his would-be victims. None of the local inhabitants had wanted to bury him, but "from hatred" had allowed the birds to devour his flesh until only the bones remained "like a lesson for anyone wanting to observe a skeleton" (*Anat. Admin*. 1.2, 2.221–22K). Galen thus includes the corpses of "bandits lying unburied on a hillside" among opportunities to observe human remains (*Anat. Admin*. 3.5, 2.385K). Arguing a point, he writes that old men and young ones fleeing bandits will run at different speeds—the old man will be slower—but the old man fleeing bandits will run faster than a young man in no hurry (*Caus. Puls*. 1.7, 9.17K), and indeed much faster than he might be able to in normal circumstances (*Caus. Puls*. 3.2, 9.158K). Eudemus, Galen's famous patient (about whom more below), compares Galen's professional rivals in Rome to the gangs of bandits who, apparently, infested the highlands near Pergamum (*Praecog*. 4, 14.622K). Finally, to cure a patient of debilitating anxieties a doctor masquerades as the ghost of the patient's dead friend, killed by bandits in the cemetery just outside the city gates (*Hipp. 2 Epid*. 2, 207–8 Wenkebach and Pfaff).[15]

Travel was, then, a dangerous process but also a slow one that afforded many opportunities for observation. It took Galen into the countryside and is the likely occasion of many of his remarks on rural life and culture, as for example that on Cypriot grain above. In the fields of Thrace and Macedonia

---

14   See Mattern (2008a, 139).

15   On banditry and its pervasiveness in the Roman Empire, see the classic article of Shaw (1984).

Galen saw a grain similar to what was called *tipha* in his home region of Asia; asking the natives, he learned that they called it *briza*, and the exact spelling and declension of the word (*Aliment. Fac.* 1.13, 6.514K). Wine, he writes, is different wherever one goes, and often unsuitable for export, therefore unknown beyond its specific region (*Bon. Mal. Suc.* 11, 6.806K); and Galen makes frequent comments on local foods and dietary habits in his treatises on foods, often introduced by the phrase "I have observed" or something similar, though it is often difficult to tell which of his comments on food taboos are based on first-hand observation and which on rumor or tradition. Thus, all Greeks eat snails every day, as he tells us, but Egyptians eat "wood worms, vipers and other snakes" (*Aliment. Fac.* 3.2, 6.668–69K). To consume the meat of old donkeys, horses, and camels—or, even worse, lions, leopards, and dogs—Galen considers uncivilized, though "some people" or "some tribes" do eat them; but hunters (hunting was an elite pastime) in Pergamum sometimes eat fox meat in autumn, when the foxes have become fat on ripe grapes and their meat is especially tasty.[16]

It was not only travel that brought Galen into the countryside, for he also owned at least two rural estates: the property near Pergamum he had inherited from his father, who retired to the countryside before his death; and later, a house in Campania, in southern Italy. In this region many aristocrats living mainly in the city of Rome, like himself, owned bucolic retreats that were also working farms. Galen also hunted, an activity typical of the leisure class, and this too brought him into the countryside (*Simp. Med.* 10.2.22, 12.299K). All of this brought him face-to-face with the peasant population of the empire's rural regions. Galen's references to peasants are numerous and convey a surprisingly clear picture of his impressions of them and of their lifestyle. He was most familiar with the area around Pergamum, and many or most of his observations on the peasant diet and peasant life are located in "our country."[17] "Among us," for example—that is, in the area around Pergamum—it is a custom among the peasants to be bled every spring. One

---

16   *Aliment. Fac.* 3.2 (664K). Cf. Wilkins (2003, x–xi).
17   See Wilkins (2003, xiv); Nutton (1995b, 363–65).

peasant youth (*agroikos neaniskos*) came into town to be bled and stayed in lodgings in the city; an incompetent doctor cut an artery, and Galen had to treat the wound (*Meth. Med.* 5.7, 10.334–35K).

The picture of peasant life that emerges from Galen's descriptions is one of poverty and isolation: disfiguring conditions may continue long without treatment, as in the case of the gardener whose story is told at the beginning of chapter 3. A fifteen-year-old boy has suffered from a parotid fistula in his face—the result of a tumor or abscess—for six months by the time Galen sees him; "he was shown to me in the field." Galen used a swine's hair to plumb the fistula, which was very deep, and he gave the patient as much medicine as he had on hand, a plaster of lead monoxide mixed with a sauce of oil and vinegar. Two months later he met the boy in the city and was surprised to find him cured (*Comp. Med. Gen.* 1.7, 13.402–3K). (In fact, parotid fistulas usually resolve on their own; no modern doctor would, of course, prescribe a plaster of lead, on which see more below.) Peasants suffered from crushed and stubbed toes, wounds, scurf, pains in the ears caused by cold or other factors.[18] In the absence of less offensive drugs readily available in the city, Galen might treat them with urine, ordering his patients to piss on their own wounds, a remedy he considered repellent but effective (*Simp. Med.* 10.2.15, 12.285–86K). (Human urine inhibits or kills some kinds of harmful bacteria and is used in traditional Indian medicine on wounds today.[19]) Peasants might have to prepare their own medicines, following Galen's instructions (*Comp. Med. Loc.* 6.3, 12.917K); urban patients, wounded while journeying through the countryside, will be treated with makeshift bandages and slings until they can return to the city to have their broken bones or dislocations properly set (*Hipp. Off.* 2.7, 18B.8744–45K). Similarly, physicians in the country must make do without most of the drugs available so easily in Rome.

---

18   Toes: *Simp. Med.* 10.2.15 (12.285–86K). Ears: *Simp. Med.* 11.1.49 (12.367K), *Comp. Med. Loc.* 3.1 (12.600K). Wounds: *Simp. Med.* 6.4 (11.866K, a sickle wound); *Simp. Med.* 10.2.9 (12.271–72K, two cases); *Simp. Med.* 11.1.1 (12.322–23K); *Comp. Med. Gen.* 3.2 (13.582–84K, 592, three cases); *Comp. Med. Gen.* 3.6 (13.633K). Scurf: *Comp. Med. Loc.* 1.8 (12.466K).

19   See, e.g., Kayne (1968); Ramesh et al. (2010).

If he happens to be in a village and not carrying any of the drugs he (often) prescribes for the treatment of patients in the town, he [the skillful physician] should be able to find whatever he may need for therapy from flowers, fruits, roots, barks.... You have seen me doing this many times.

(*Opt. Med. Cogn.* 12.3, Iskandar 124, tr. Iskandar)

Many stories from Galen's pharmaceutical works illustrate this exact point. He treated the wounds of one "man of the field" with a fresh cheese and leaves of patience dock; but if the latter are not available, Galen writes, grape leaves will do (*Simp. Med.* 10.2.9, 12.271–72K). The cheese that Pergamenes call *oxygalactinos* (very sweet) is especially effective, and "when a peasant (*agroikos*) had a large wound it cemented [the wound] when applied" (*Simp. Med.* 10.2.9, 12.272K). He used viper flesh on another wound with nerve damage, "and the nerve hardly suffered any phlegm, but the man was hard and rustic.... Many doctors before me have written that it is necessary for them to mix in frankincense or myrrh for this use, but I had neither of those things, being outside the city in the fields" (*Simp. Med.* 11.1.1, 12.322–23K). Euphorbia is the medicine on which he relies most for damaged nerves, but since he has often encountered these "while traveling, on ship, in the field, or in the city but far from my own house" he has often had to improvise; he treated one farmer "in the field" with fresh bee glue from the farmer's property (*Comp. Med. Gen.* 3.2, 13.582–83K, 592K). He uses spurge to treat another peasant, found growing near his patient's courtyard (*Comp. Med. Gen.* 3.2, 13.583K). Pitch, vetch flour, dove dung, or oak leaves can all be pressed into service in a pinch when practicing "in the field."[20]

Galen also reports on rural remedies that he has observed. To treat ear pain, some country doctors—Galen has seen this—use oil crushed from the pillbugs that breed under the jars in which peasants store water in their houses (*Simp. Med.* 11.1.49, 12.367K). He has seen peasants treat frostbitten

---

20 *Comp. Med. Gen.* 3.2 (13.583–84K); *Comp. Med. Gen.* 3.6 (13.633K); *Simp. Med.* 6.4 (11.866K).

ears with oil warmed in hollowed-out onions, set in ashes (*Comp. Med. Loc.* 3.1, 12.600K). He has met a vinedresser who cut off his own finger after it was bitten by a snake, and it healed perfectly (*Loc. Affect.* 3.11, 8.198K). He saw another man, "one of those who work in the field," treat himself for colon pain by cinching himself up with a belt, eating bread and garlic, and drinking nothing but unmixed wine at night, a very successful cure (*Meth. Med.* 12.8, 10.865K).

Country therapy could be disgusting, as in the urine remedy that Galen recommended for wounded toes. A country doctor he knows, or has heard of, uses goat's dung mixed with vinegar to treat snakebite and other venomous bites, hazards of country life: again, Galen normally eschews this medicine and has never used it on his "urban and famous" patients, but

> sometimes such things are useful, as on a journey, or when hunting
> or staying in the country, when none of the better medicines is available,
> for the peasant man is also hard-bodied, similar to an ass.
>
> (*Simp. Med.* 10.2.22, 12.299K)

The peasant is, as this passage implies, almost a different species, exceptionally "hard-bodied," hard laboring, constantly exposed to sun and air, living on a meager diet, unaccustomed to bathing, and prone to accumulation of the hot, dry, bilious humor; while his urban counterpart (enjoying shady baths once or even twice per day, eating plentifully and exercising in the gymnasium) is much more likely to accumulate phlegm. Peasants often require harsher remedies than urban patients, remedies that women, children, and other especially soft-bodied people would never endure.[21] However, Galen's attitude toward the peasantry is not as harsh as it may seem in the passage quoted above. When he compares peasants to donkeys this is not necessarily deprecatory, as Galen often compares humans to animals when discussing

---

21 Peasants vs. women and children: e.g., *Comp. Med. Gen.* 7.11 (13.1009K). On peasants in Galen, see Mattern (2008a, 104–5, 127, 130–31). Galen contrasts urban and rural types, e.g., in *Hipp. 1 Epid.* 1.3 (17A.2100211K). On baths: also *Hipp. Fract.* 1.41 (18B.394K).

questions of temperament (one's "mixture" of qualities) and constitution. Thus, one urban, aristocratic patient is "slender and muscular ... like a dog" (*Meth. Med.* 10.3, 10.671K). Although he often mentions peasants, no passage that I am aware of betrays condescension, contempt, or any of the hostile attitudes Galen so often gives vent to when discussing athletes, "sophists," wealthy and luxury-loving patients, women (very occasionally), or, of course, his medical rivals, living and dead. Galen appears to respect the peasant's life of self-sufficiency and backbreaking labor, or at least he describes it without derision. He compares the conditioning of peasants favorably with that of bulked-up, overfed athletes (*Hipp. Aph.* 1.3, 17B.363K).

It is furthermore clear that Galen, scion of the Greek aristocracy and surely one of the Mediterranean world's most highly educated physicians, was not too proud to treat the rural folk he encountered while traveling, although their lifestyle and their appearance and some of their customs were alien to him. He treated them ingeniously, without making the excuse that most of his tools and remedies were unavailable, nor was he above rummaging through their homes, gardens, courtyards, and workshops in search of items that might be useful. Indeed he mentions this many times, as though it were entirely normal to find him on a farmer's property, devoting his intensely focused effort to its owner's problem. Galen bragged about treating peasants and did not disdain to advertise this as part of his claim to professional excellence. Some of these patients had gone untreated for a long time and were probably very glad of his attention. Here one is reminded of Galen's attitude toward gladiators, also men of humble status on whom he lavished his best efforts, and about whom he writes, quite surprisingly, with no hint of disrespect.

Galen arrived in Rome in the spring, perhaps, of 162 c.e.[22] As to what he found there—perhaps those who have visited a gargantuan ex-colonial city like Delhi are in the best position to imagine. Although the size of its population and of its monuments could not equal what has been attained in the last centuries, in squalor and lethality Rome far exceeded any modern city and

22 On the date, see Schlange-Schöningen (2003, 139–42).

probably most ancient ones. That is, Galen practiced medicine for decades in one of human history's most unhealthy environments.

Public sanitation in the city was horrific by modern standards. Rome had, however, a unique and critical advantage over most premodern cities: fresh water. Its system of eleven aqueducts brought in a continual supply of it, day and night, in staggering quantities (perhaps exceeding what is available per person in Rome today), and from remote locations (that is, Romans did not rely on water from the pestilential Tiber river).[23] The water was collected in cisterns and flowed from there to public fountains and to public (and, in wealthy houses, private) baths. Roman water struck Galen as clean and high in quality: "In Rome, just as there are many other advantages in the city, also there is the goodness and abundance of fountains and the water of none of them is smelly, toxic, muddy, or hard, just as it is not in my city of Pergamum" (*Hipp. 6 Epid.* 4.10, 17B.159K). Fountains and baths were continually fed and must have drained by overflow, which could have helped wash waste into the sewers and out into the Tiber River. This probably reduced the risks of diseases spread by contaminated water, although fountains could still be contaminated in the short term in all of the usual ways, by the people using them or by animals. (Leeches might certainly be found in them, one of which made its way up the nose of a patient of Galen's). Water could also be contaminated at home where it was stored in unsterile containers at ambient temperature.[24]

Rome had an additional public-health advantage besides its system of water supply: the grain dole received by the plebeian class, which may have alleviated malnutrition. But there are important reasons not to exaggerate the benefits of the grain dole. The plebeian class was not Rome's poorest class—slaves and noncitizen immigrants did not qualify, the number of recipients was fixed and hereditary, and spots that opened up due to attrition had to be purchased. The total number of recipients of the free grain dole was probably 200,000 people, a fraction of Rome's total population. But for political reasons, emperors also took other measures to ensure the grain supply and to

---

23 For a brief recent summary of the system of aqueducts, Lo Cascio (2006, 61–62).
24 Scheidel (2009). Leech: *Loc. Affect.* 4.8 (8.266K).

control prices; these included massive construction at Rome's harbor, Ostia (unsuccessful under Claudius, but successful under Trajan); the diversion to Rome of much of the grain tax levied on Egypt and Africa; and an administrative office, the prefect of the grain supply. Again, it is not clear whether these measures helped the very poor, and they did not eliminate food crises in the city if the harvest was bad, or if war or epidemic disease prevented the cultivation of grain or its transport, or if fire or flood destroyed the city's stores. Two major food crises are attested at Rome in Galen's lifetime. Nevertheless the urban populace of Rome was less vulnerable than many others to malnutrition and to its exacerbating influence on disease.[25]

But in other ways Rome was a dangerously unhealthy place, probably much more than its rural surroundings. The river, for example, was contaminated, as in other cities. Galen warns against eating fish from sources near cities, and especially from the rancid Tiber:

> The worst fish live at the outlets of rivers which clean out the sewers, the taverns, and the baths, and the stuff used to clean clothes and linens.... The flesh of the moray eel ... is worst in the outlets of rivers like these, such as the one that flows through Rome.[26]

The Tiber flooded every four or five years, temporarily contaminating the water supply. These floods also exacerbated the health hazards from the corpses, garbage, and feces that polluted the city (see below), and added to them the dead bodies of people drowned in the flood, and ordure washed up into the streets from the sewers, which lacked valves to prevent backflow.[27]

Rome's population is difficult to estimate, but it was very densely inhabited, and historians often cite a figure of one million as a best guess.[28] Of these

---

25 Garnsey (1988, part IV).

26 *Aliment. Fac.* 3.29 (6.721–22K). See also *Bon. Mal. Suc.* 9 (6.795K) and Nutton (1995b, 364–365).

27 Aldrete (2007, 141–54 on disease; 71–81 on frequency). He estimates one major flood every twenty years and "lesser but still significant" floods every four to five years.

28 For a review of evidence on Rome's population density, see Lo Cascio (2006, 59–60).

million or so residents, large numbers lived in *insulae*, multistory apartment complexes. In antiquity these are known only in Rome and its port city Ostia, but in Rome the number of them attested is huge: the *Regionaries*, a description of the city's fourteen regions dating to the fourth century C.E., counts no less than 46,000 *insulae*, an implausibly large figure. The poor lived on the upper stories and rented, it seems, by the day. Or they lived in one-room or multiroom shops; in boarding houses; in shanties and huts built up between portico columns or against aqueducts; in tombs; in cellars and stairwells; and on the street. They inhabited Rome's unhealthiest areas, the low-elevation valleys between hills and near the Tiber. The poor have left no records of their complaints, but we occasionally find shocking descriptions of Roman living conditions even in the literary works of the wealthy—such as a famous letter of Cicero, Rome's greatest orator and slumlord, congratulating himself on his philosophical indifference to the collapse of two of his properties (even the mice, as he writes, have fled).[29]

Edicts of Augustus, Nero, and Trajan limiting the height of structures in the city were probably aimed at the often precariously constructed *insulae*, but they seem to have had little effect (as their repetition suggests); and in any case even Trajan's revised code allowed buildings of sixty feet, a perilous height considering the building techniques used. Some *insulae* were structurally sound, such as the Casa di Giulio Romano, the only one that remains at Rome, built of brick-faced concrete, and the *insulae* at Ostia; but it is precisely the shabbier structures that do not survive for us to examine. (The Casa di Giulio Romano is in any case taller than seventy feet, the legal limit at the date of its construction.) Many *insulae* probably had weak walls with rubble and clay cores, common building practice at Pompeii (the only location where fragile structures are preserved), and many probably used sun-dried clay bricks with timber framing, a technique well-attested for cheap buildings in the Roman world. Sources including the architect Virtuvius and the

---

29   *Ad Att.* 14.9; cf. Aldrete (2007, 106); MacMullen (1974, 86). On *insulae*, see Scobie (1986, 404–7).

philosopher Seneca, and the satirists Juvenal and Martial, attest to cracked foundations, split joints, and crumbling walls.[30]

Floods of the Tiber caused many residential buildings to topple— unfired bricks and clay infill dissolve when exposed to water, and some ancient descriptions of Tiber floods note exactly this effect.[31] Floods also weakened foundations in the long term, when cheap construction methods were used.

The air in the city's poorly ventilated dwellings was foul. One child's embalmed and mummified corpse, with some soft tissue preserved, shows evidence (at the age of only eight years) of "rather abundant" anthracosis, carbon accumulation in the lungs today most commonly found in coal miners. In this case it was probably caused by indoor air pollution from oil lamps, cooking, and indoor fires of wood or dung. The girl died of pleuritis, or inflammation of the lining of the lungs; this could have been caused by tuberculosis or another disease, but foul indoor air has been blamed for the pleuritis that left traces on the 162 corpses so far recovered from Herculaneum (a town near Pompeii, buried in the same eruption of Mount Vesuvius in 79 C.E.), and conditions at Rome were certainly no better.[32]

Little is known about Rome's sewer system. There were public latrines, but very few homes were connected to the sewers. Some houses and apartment buildings had unflushed private toilets or cesspits. Even if cleaned out periodically by the professional waste removers who (most likely) sold their contents as fertilizer to farmers, these pits were still health hazards if vermin spread the microbes to other parts of the house. The baths offered public latrines drained by the sewers, but they were inconvenient and many people emptied their excrement into the street or relieved themselves in the streets, on heaps of garbage or in doorways. Laws prohibiting the throwing of feces,

---

30   On building techniques and building codes, see Scobie (1986, 404–7); Aldrete (2007, 102–18).

31   Aldrete (2007, 117).

32   On the Herculaneum bodies, see Capasso (2000). The Roman mummy came originally from a grave 5 miles outside Rome along the Via Appia and dates to the second century C.E. (Ascenzi et al. 1996, 205–18). The body was probably mummified in Rome.

animal carcasses, and human corpses into the street would not have been necessary if there were not a problem, and the city lacked a good method of enforcing these ordinances. Butchers and tanners threw blood and refuse into the streets.[33]

At least eighty people, conservatively estimated, died on an average day (free of epidemics and disasters) in the city of Rome.[34] If even a small percentage of these corpses—the poorest 5 percent, say, mostly beggars living in shanties or in the streets—went unburied, this would have burdened the city with 1,500 human corpses per year. In the late Republican period many of them were ended up in open, mass burial pits, some dozens of which have been found and excavated on the Esquiline Hill outside the original city gates. The Esquiline was closed for this purpose around 40 B.C.E., when Maecenas, future advisor of the emperor Augustus, famously built suburban pleasure-gardens over the burial pits. It is not clear where the unburied dead were brought in Galen's time; they were probably cremated in public pyres. But not all corpses were successfully collected and burnt. Literary sources tell us that unburied bodies ended up in the Tiber, in garbage pits, or in the streets, carrion for dogs and vultures. Suetonius relates an anecdote in which a street dog appeared at the future emperor Vespasian's breakfast table carrying a human hand.[35] Abandoned infants also fell prey to dogs, which in turn might be killed and eaten by the poor or skinned as a source of cheap leather. Sick and aged slaves were abandoned to die in the streets or on Tiber Island, the more traditional location.[36]

Galen and his patients visited the public baths daily or even twice daily (although the wealthiest had private baths in their houses). Baths abounded in the city, from the grand Baths of Trajan with its magnificent reduplication of rooms and facilities to humble establishments on street corners. Bathing was considered civilized life's greatest pleasure, and the imperial baths were surely Rome's most elegant, beautifully lit and luxuriously decorated public

---

33   Scobie (1986, 407–22).
34   For what follows, see Bodel (2000, 128–51).
35   *Vesp.* 5.4; Bodel (2000, 129); Scobie (1986, 418).
36   Scobie (1986, 419–20).

buildings.[37] But they also spread bacteria and disease. Most were probably drained by overflow (little is known about bath drains), so that to some extent the water was replaced over time; but no means of disinfecting the water were known or used. Bathing was a normal part of therapy for illnesses of all kinds, including diseases now known to be infectious (dysentery, leprosy, respiratory problems); this is very obvious in Galen as in other medical sources, and Hadrian supposedly reserved baths for the sick before 3 P.M.[38] The heated water of the warm pool offered ideal conditions for microbes to flourish, and many ancient writers comment on the filthiness of bathwater (to the references usually cited I might add Galen's overlooked testimony on urinating in the baths, from chapter 1). Celsus warned that if an open wound is exposed to bathwater "it usually becomes malignant" (5.26.28, *cancrum transitus esse consuevit*). Cockroaches were abundant at the baths (Pliny *Naturalis historia* 11.99). Air was often of poor quality, smoky from the furnaces, and could cause patrons to faint.[39]

Rome was, then, an ideal environment for any disease spread by vermin, flies, mosquitoes, feces, dogs, or (because of its densely packed population) through the air, as well as for respiratory illnesses caused by indoor air pollution. One of its most dangerous, pervasive, and characteristic illnesses was malaria. Epitaphs show that deaths in the city surged in late summer, a fact susceptible to different interpretations (all of them reflecting dismally high mortality rates), but it adds to other evidence that malaria was endemic. This seasonal mortality affected both children and adults of all age ranges (though the elderly were also likely to die in the winter, probably of respiratory infections).[40] There are four strains of the malaria parasite, of which the

---

37   Dunbabin (1989, 6–46).

38   On baths, see Mattern (2008a, 50–52, 58–59, 140–43); Fagan (1999, 85–103); Scobie (1986, 425–27); SHA *Hadr.* 22.7. Leprosy: see Galen *Simp. Med.* 11.1.1 (12.314K) = *Subfig. Emp.* 10 (77 Deichgräber). Coughing up blood: *Meth. Med.* 5.13 (10.369K).

39   Fainting: Galen *Usu Resp.* 4 (4.494K), *Hipp. Aph.* 2.41 (17B.540K). Smoke: Fronto *M. Aur. Caes.* 1.3.4 (1.86 Loeb). See Fagan (1999, 186–87).

40   On diseases in the city of Rome, also with discussion of seasonal mortality and references to previous studies, see Scheidel (2009); id. (2003, 158–76); Sallares (2002, chapter 8, "The City of Rome").

most lethal—*P. falciparum*—may lurk behind the ancient concept of "semi-tertian" fever, which recurred every two days but was distinguished from tertian fever by an exceptionally long period of paroxysm with a short remission. In Galen's view this type of fever is both especially dangerous and the disease most characteristic of the city of Rome, as later, from early modern times through the nineteenth century, the city was to be connected so closely in the western imagination with the disease by then called "malaria" and attributed to the city's "bad air." As Galen writes:

> That this type of fever [semitertian] occurs as I have said, there is no need for the testimony of Hippocrates or the word of anyone else, when we see it every day, especially at Rome; for as other [diseases] abound in other places, this ill abounds in that city.[41]

Conditions in much of the city were ideal for breeding malaria mosquitoes, as sources of stagnant water abounded: the *impluvia* that caught rainwater under the open roofs of entryways to upscale homes; the vegetable gardens among and between houses that provided some of the population's food; and no less than 1,204 ponds or lakes attested in ancient catalogues of the city.[42] Overflow from fountains and baths also would have created pools of stagnant water, as well as a great deal of moist, microbe-rich mud as it mixed with the filth in the streets. Cases of malaria may have spiked in flood years, as the receding floodwaters created new breeding grounds for mosquitoes.

Immigrants to the city, without immunity, were especially vulnerable to falciparum malaria. Stories come down to us of newcomers who succumbed to disease soon after their arrival: the German and Gallic troops brought to

---

41   *Morb. Temp.* 8 (7.435K). Also "semitertian fever arises, especially in Rome, for it is most familiar to the people of that city," *Hipp. 1 Epid.* 2.25 (17A.121–22K). See Sallares (2002, 222). On "semitertian fever" and *P. falciparum*, see Sallares (2002, 14–15), with a quotation from Celsus; and in Galen, see, e.g., *Typ.* 3 (7.464K). Galen and other physicians hotly debated the definition of "semitertian fever" among other things, and there is, of course, no one-to-one correspondence between this and falciparian malaria; see Mattern (2008a, 64 with note 57). On malaria in Rome, see also Scheidel (2003, 163–69).

42   On gardens, see Sallares (2002, 211); lakes, ibid. 215.

the city by the usurper Vitellius in the chaotic year 69 c.e., and Alaric, the Goth who sacked Rome in 410 c.e.[43] Less deadly forms of malaria in conjunction with typhoid fever and tuberculosis, diseases most typical of adolescence and young adulthood, also probably carried off many victims. Death and mortal illness, in Rome, was not especially associated with old age (and very few of Galen's recorded patients are old), nor even necessarily with childhood. While the life tables commonly used by historians to reconstruct patterns of mortality usually predict very high infant and child mortality at the lower ranges of average life expectancy, scholars are now more aware of the problematic (and mostly theoretical) nature of data in these ranges. That is, life tables tend to exaggerate child mortality relative to adult mortality (and these factors can fluctuate independently of each other). In the city of Rome, sudden death could occur at any age.[44]

"Fever" was the disease par excellence of the Hippocratic *Epidemics* and also in Galen, who devoted several specialized works to fever, and it is the condition he describes most frequently in his stories about his patients. For Galen, fever was not mainly a symptom but a disease—characterized by recurrent, paroxysmal fits of heat, rigors, and sweating; digestive problems, tension in the body, insomnia, and headache; and often chills, vomiting, and delirium. This constellation of symptoms does not overlap perfectly with those of malaria, but is very suggestive that his own idea of fever, and that of the previous generations that influenced him, arose in a world where malaria was common. Galen and other sources also describe cases of concurrent infection with different intermittent fevers, which can happen in malaria patients.[45]

Other diseases, of course, abounded in the city. The microbial DNA analyses that would confirm the presence of tuberculosis and leprosy, bacilli closely related to each other, have yet to be done on remains from the city and its surroundings; but both have been found in the provinces, adding to the

---

43   Sallares (2002, 225–26). I would not rest conclusions about the hyperendemicity of falciparian malaria on the single passage of Galen that he cites; but it is a possibility, as conditions in Rome could probably support it.
44   See Scheidel (2003) and (2001).
45   On fever in Galen, Mattern (2008a, 64 with n. 57 and 155–58).

skeletal evidence already known for these conditions, and many people seem to have been infected with both microbes. Greco-Roman medicine recognized a disease it called *pthisis*, a wasting condition with cough, which probably reflects centuries of experience with tuberculosis. Tuberculosis is well-attested in ancient medical literature and its skeletal form sometimes left traces on bones; it is reasonable to assume that Galen saw many cases, and that it was a major cause of mortality in the city (at its peak in the early nineteenth century, tuberculosis was the leading cause of death in the western world). Fatalities from tuberculosis often occur in young adulthood, and like malaria, it probably created an environment much more lethal for young adults than life tables predict and than historians are accustomed to imagining.[46]

Leprosy has a close reflection in the ancient idea of elephantiasis, which seems to have developed in the Roman era. Rufus of Ephesus, a contemporary of Galen, offers the most detailed clinical description of elephantiasis; the facial distortions, ulcerations and putrescence of the skin, and shedding of fingertips that he describes all evoke leprosy, suggesting that this disease was common in the Greco-Roman world around that time. Some sources of the first century C.E. (Pliny the Elder, Celsus) describe elephantiasis as a disease new to Italy, perhaps arriving along with massive numbers of immigrants from the provinces to the center of power; Pliny also adds that it died out in Italy, but he was almost certainly incorrect, as later sources including Galen are familiar with it. Galen mentions elephantiasis many times and treated patients for it, although he writes that it is most common in Alexandria, attributing this to a diet rich in producers of black bile. It is rare, he writes (without basis in firsthand observation) in Germany and, as he adds oddly, in Mysia (*Meth. Med. Glauc.* 2.12; 11.142K), though several of his stories about elephantiasis patients are set in Asia Minor. In Galen's world it was a loathed and much feared condition; one victim lived alone in the countryside, shunned by his friends; another, a philosophical type, decided on contracting

---

46   On co-infections in first-century Israel and Roman-era Egypt, see Donoghue et al. (2005). For an analysis of recent genetic research on the history of leprosy and tuberculosis, see Stone et al. (2009). On *phthisis*, see Grmek (1989, 193–94); on bones, ibid., 177–80; Dubos and Dubos (1987, 8–10).

it that he did not wish to live. (Galen, however, claimed to be able to cure elephantiasis with snake venom). Rome's dense and largely impoverished population and unsanitary conditions could easily have supported leprosy as an endemic disease.[47]

This is, of course, only a small sample of the diseases that plagued ancient Rome. It is a good guess that diarrheal diseases, hepatitis, typhoid, and tetanus were rampant. Galen's reference to jaundice (below) suggests leptospirosis, transmitted by pigs, dogs, and rats. Tapeworms and other parasitic worms were likely very common. Finally, Pliny the Elder singled out for special mention among diseases new to Italy a skin condition he calls *mentagra* (or *lichen* in Greek), "painless and not life-threatening, but so disgusting that any sort of death is preferable," transmitted by kissing and thus (as he states) confined to males of the upper classes; it would arise on the chin and spread to the entire face, neck, chest, arms and hands (*Naturalis historia* 27.1). Pliny's description long led scholars to suspect endemic syphilis, a nonvenereal form of syphilis; but bone analyses show no conclusive evidence of diseases caused by bacteria of the genus *treponema*, which include syphilis and related illnesses, in the Old World before Columbus. (Such evidence is abundant in the pre-Columbian New World, leading to the hypothesis that it was imported to Europe from there.) Celsus, however, describes a variety of warts and lesions of the genital region, some sounding quite dire, and suggesting that other sexually transmitted infections were common (*De medicina* 5.28, 6.18).[48]

Galen also describes at least two patients with gout, probably including the patient from the preface to this book, whose "chalkstones" Galen relieves with a plaster of rancid cheese; although he does not diagnose this patient

---

47   On leprosy, see Grmek (1989, 152–76). Rufus of Ephesus: Oribasius 45.28. Pliny: *Naturalis historia* 26.5. Most of Galen's references to specific cases of elephantiasis occur in Pergamum, but three are probably set in Rome (the augur and the snake-catcher: *Simp. Med.* 11.1.1, 12.314–314K = *Subfig. Emp.* 10, 77–78 Deichgräber; also *Hipp. Aph.* 6.47, 18A.80K, a patient Galen treats over years).

48   For a recent review of scholarship on syphilis in antiquity, see Harper et al. (2011). The classic article of Baker and Armelagos (1988) is still important. On sexually transmitted infections in antiquity, see Grmek (1989, chapter 5).

with *podagra*, perhaps because his lesions did not occur on the foot (*pos*, the more classic location). Gout is a complaint well-attested in Roman-era writings, including Galen's own works: in one passage a street huckster is peddling a cure for it, "and while he was speaking someone suffering from gout was standing right there, who was affected only moderately so that he could still walk"; Galen challenged the quack to cure the patient, but his remedy only made the condition much worse (*Simp. Med.* 1.29, 11.432–33K). Scholars have long speculated that the apparently high incidence of gout among the Roman aristocracy may reflect heavy metal poisoning from the lead that was widely used for plumbing and household cooking and storage containers, also medicinally and on the face, by women, as a skin whitener. Galen does not know that lead is toxic or describe lead poisoning, although other ancient sources suggest this idea. In particular a poem on poisons, the *Alexipharmaca* by the physician Nicander of Colophon, dating to the second century B.C.E., more or less accurately describes the effects of an overdose of cosmetic white lead (*psimythion*), if ingested.[49] Skeletal studies show levels of lead in some areas of the Roman world (including Italy) much higher than in prehistoric populations (which show almost no lead accumulation) and higher than levels normally seen today. A review of skeletal lead in twenty population samples from Roman-era Italy shows that lead content increased by about tenfold from 200 B.C.E. to 200 C.E. The teeth of adult skeletons from Rimini (ancient Ariminium) and Ravenna, dating to the first through third centuries, contained on average 85.5 to 92.5 mg/g of lead; by comparison, 1990s studies of dentine lead levels from cities in Germany, Canada, Mexico, and northern Israel only in exceptional cases found lead levels half this high. While acute lead poisoning may or may not have been a health hazard for ancient Romans, it is possible that "insidious" low-level lead poisoning explains the prevalence of gout and some of the bone lesions described below. But the effects of lead poisoning are diffuse and many symptoms are neurological and behavioral. It is therefore hard to point to specific evidence, but the very obvious high levels of

---

49   See Jacques (2002, vol. 3, *ad* lines 74–86, pp. 8–9 with commentary, pp. 82–84).

exposure in bones and teeth from Roman Italy suggest that lead poisoning was a significant cause of suffering.[50]

Some chronic conditions left traces on ancient skeletons that can be detected today. Chronic nutrient deficiencies and anemias caused by malnutrition or dysentery, infection with parasites, malaria, and other diseases can leave traces today, causing porosity of the bones above the eyes in the cranium, and in the skeleton generally; the same stressors can also cause malformations of dental enamel. Studies of Roman-era skeletons show especially poor health close to the capital city (whereas skeletons from Britain, for example, are relatively healthy). Rates of *cribra orbitalia* (porosity of the bone above the eyes) approach a staggering 80 percent in some locations close to Rome. Recent research suggests that common causes of *cribra orbitalia* were megaloblastic anemia caused by vitamin B_{12} deficiency, rickets, and scurvy, all of which imply terrible chronic suffering in those affected.[51]

Scholars have long debated the healthfulness or unhealthiness of the city of Rome, and I find the darker portraits far more convincing than efforts to rehabilitate an idealized view. That said, mortality and disease probably varied widely by region. While some Roman suburbs were pathologically unhealthy, as noted above, two show rates of *cribra orbitalia* under 20 percent (still very high from a modern perspective, or even a premodern one). Within the city, inhabitants of higher regions—the famous "hills"—were probably spared some of the ravages of malaria and may have enjoyed longer life expectancy. The variable topography of health in the city is a very obvious theme

---

50   When lead poisoning became a major focus of medical attention in the 1970s, scholars such as H. A. Waldron and J. O. Nriagu scrutinized ancient literary, material, and biological sources for evidence of its effects; see, e.g., Nriagu (1983a, b). Nriagu's arguments about the effects of lead on the Roman imperial family and on the political stability of the Roman Empire, however, are highly speculative. On skeletal lead levels in Roman Italy, see Aufderheide et al. (1992). On dentine lead in Ariminium and Ravenna, see Facchini, Rastelli, and Brasili (2004). On 1990s lead levels, see Tsuji et al. (1997, table 2). The authors attributed elevated lead levels in the Ontario population to lead shot in wild game.

51   Facchini, Rastelli, and Brasili (2004, 132); Scheidel (2009, 11; 2010a, 7–8). For a recent discussion of the etiologies of porotic hyperostosis and *cribra orbitalia*, which are different although both conditions are caused by nutrient deficiencies, see Walker et al. (2009).

in early modern and modern literature, and some ancient sources also tell us that high ground was especially healthy and low areas near the Tiber especially noxious. Similarly, people living in less crowded districts and those better served by the public water supply were probably healthier than others.[52] Aristocrats who could afford to leave the city during the summer months also may have lived longer, although probably not by much: a demographic analysis of emperors and their families (whose lives are well-documented) suggests that among Rome's most privileged class, even those lucky enough to die of natural causes could expect on average to live only about twenty-five years at birth. For most people in the city life expectancy was probably shorter, perhaps under twenty years, in which case Rome's population could not have reproduced itself: the city was a population sinkhole, a phenomenon well-established for early modern London. That the Roman plebs, despite its generous daily allotment of grain, did not reproduce itself is evident in laws allowing the sale of vacant grain entitlements (the number of recipients was allowed to remain steady, but the privilege was inherited). Attracting to it hordes of immigrants, many of whom died immediate or statistically accelerated deaths, the empire's capital city has been described as a voracious consumer of flesh, exacting a kind of grim tax in human bodies on its subjects.[53]

It is difficult to imagine the impression that the city must have made on Galen. He had lived in Pergamum, and in Alexandria; but Pergamum, according to Galen's best guess, had a citizen population of some 40,000 and a total population (with women and slaves, but perhaps excluding children) of about 120,000. Rome was larger by an order of magnitude, and probably,

---

52   On these factors, see Sallares (2002, 201–34), noting that ancient Rome was much larger than the medieval and early modern city, with presumably more habitation of its unhealthier low-lying regions. On lower rates of *cribra orbitalia* in some suburbs, Scheidel (2009, 11).

53   On life expectancy of emperors, see Scheidel (1999). On early modern London, see Wrigley (1967). On the plebs, see Lo Cascio (2006, 67–68). On Rome as grim reaper, see Scheidel (2003, 174–76). Lo Cascio (2006) questions the assumption that all premodern cities were population sinks and reviews the arguments for this view and criticisms of it, and in this he is perhaps correct. But I find it hard to believe, based on the current state of evidence for sanitation and disease in the city, that Rome was not an exceptionally lethal environment. In particular, Lo Cascio's dismissive attitude toward the evidence for malaria in ancient Rome is unwarranted and the argument that follows somewhat contradictory.

with its million or so inhabitants, the largest city in world history at the time. It struck Galen as huge, anonymous, teeming with the sick: "a city with such a throng of people, that the rhetor Polemo praised it by calling it the epitome of the world" (*Hipp. Artic.* 1.22, 18A.347K); "this populous city, where daily ten thousand people can be discovered suffering from jaundice, and ten thousand from dropsy" (*Purg. Med. Fac.* 2, 11.328K). Rare dislocations of the arm, never described by Hippocrates, Galen has seen five times—four at Rome; "because of the large number in the city of the Romans, you will ask not why I saw these cases, but why I did not see more of the same type of dislocation" (*Hipp. Artic.* 1.22, 18A.347–49K).

The social atmosphere was ruthless. Reputation, on which medical success depended, was hard-won there, and doctors could slip under the radar as nowhere else: "One peculiarity of Rome, which is not shared by other cities, is that not even neighbours, let alone other inhabitants, know how a patient has died, or by whom he has been treated. This is because the city is great and populous."[54] In Rome, unlike Pergamum, one might deny or disguise a lower-class background, a tactic of which Galen accuses his rivals (*Praecog.* 14, 14.623K). Competition in the city is cutthroat: physicians might round on a newcomer like a gang of bandits, exploiting the slightest error to their advantage (*Praecog.* 14, 14.622K); they might even plot poison, as they had murdered one newcomer together with two of his servants, ten years before Galen's arrival (*Praecog.* 14, 14.623–24K). Thus warns Eudemus, Galen's compatriot, teacher, and first notable patient, whose story is told in more detail below.

Medical specialization was possible at Rome as nowhere else—there were dentists, ear-doctors, proctologists; specialists in many kinds of surgery, for hernias, kidney stones, or cataracts (*Part. Med.* 2.2, 2.26 Lyons). In a well-known passage, Galen writes of a doctor at Pergamum (named Eudemus, but certainly not the same Eudemus as Galen's patient), who applied a harsh astringent called the "plaster of Isis" directly to the naked

---

54   *Opt. Med. Cogn.* 1 (46 Iskandar, tr. Iskandar); see also *Praecog.* 14 (14.622K).

meninx of patients after trepanning their skulls; Galen writes gingerly that he might have tested this method if he had continued practicing in Pergamum, but "since I have spent most of my time in Rome I follow the custom of the city, leaving most deeds of this kind to those who are called surgeons" (*Meth. Med.* 6.6, 10.454–55K).

Rome's size, its teeming population, its social complexity—Galen comments on all of these. But what must have impressed him too, or maybe most of all, although he does not say so, was its sheer physical splendor. The capital's public buildings and monuments were like those in Rome's lesser cities, but gargantuan in scale. Its amphitheater held 50,000 spectators on four levels of marble-faced brick and concrete, with thirty-two entrances. The nearby colossal statue of the nude emperor Nero, after which the amphitheater eventually came to be called, stood 120 Roman feet high; by Galen's time it had been converted into a statue of the sun god Sol, with a crown of rays twenty-three Roman feet long and a base seven meters on each side. The forum of Trajan, constructed early in the century, dwarfed the other imperial fora and surpassed even Vespasian's Temple of Peace in magnificence and complexity. His bathing complex sprawled over almost thirteen acres of vast courtyards and soaring, vaulted roofs, niches, rotundas, apses, and exedras all faced in fine brick, stuccoed, presumably covered in paintings, mosaics, marble paneling, and metal coffering, and crammed with sculpture and other artwork. And these are just a few of the splendid structures that loomed over the crowded, festering city. They defined public life and they form the backdrop for some of Galen's stories—the baths of Trajan (which he calls the "gymnasium of Trajan") where patients bathe and exercise and take massages, or where a philosopher lectures; the Temple of Peace, where his enemies call him out every day, challenging him to an intellectual duel. Finally, the streets were noisy and crowded with the business of everyday life, lived mostly outdoors in Rome as in its Mediterranean provinces: vendors hawked their wares, schoolteachers and butchers plied their trade; an argument breaks out over the authenticity of a book just purchased, with Galen's name on it; a rival insults one's knowledge of Hippocrates; a quack, as we have seen, collects a crowd by touting his gout remedy and, when challenged by one of his audience, demonstrates it on a patient.[55]

Galen did not arrive in this intimidating city friendless and without resources. Teuthras, a very old friend ("my fellow citizen and fellow student"), was probably already there when he arrived: he witnessed one of Galen's first cases in the city ("When I first came to Rome"), that of a twenty-one-year-old woman with suppressed menstruation, cough, dyspnea, and a red face; all signs, as Galen believed, indicating bloodletting. Her doctors, followers of the teachings of Erasistratus, refused to do this. It was not Galen's case: he was still young and new in town; the patient's regular doctors were older and their relationship with the woman's family was long established. Galen does not say how he became involved, but sickness in wealthy families could be a very social, almost public, event. The patient died suffocating and coughing up blood, and her case became the subject of open debate, together with several others who were being treated by the same Erasistratean physicians.

When the argument nearly became violent, Teuthras had to restrain Galen physically—seizing his raised arm—and calm him down. The next day Galen's friend publicly read case histories from Erasistratus's works illustrating patients who had died, on Teuthras's interpretation, because they had not been bled. When someone in the audience asked the (apparently redundant) question whether Erasistratus had been right to avoid phlebotomy, Galen stepped in with a response so eloquent that Teuthras later sent one of his slaves to transcribe it; this is the extant treatise *On Venesection against Erasistratus*, and Galen tells the story of its generation in his companion treatise *On Venesection against the Erasistrateans at Rome*, written a few years later, when he returned to Rome after a sojourn in Pergamum.[56]

---

55   An excellent reference on Rome's architecture is Richardson (1992). On the decoration of public baths, see Dunbabin (1989). On Roman architecture in Galen's stories, see Mattern (2008a, 49–53). Temple of Peace: *Libr. Propr.* 2 (19.21K). On noise and crowds, see MacMullen (1974, 57–87). Book: *Libr. Propr. praef.* (19.8–9K). Rival: *Praecog.* 4 (14.620K). Gout: *Simp. Med.* 1.29 (11.432–33K).

56   The story: *Ven. Sect. Eras. Rom.* 1 (11.187–95K). Teuthras is the addressee of *On the Pulse for Beginners* (*Puls. Tir.* 1, 8.453K).

As this story suggests, while Galen had friends in Rome, he did not take long to make enemies. One he mentions by name is the aged and much-respected physician Martianus. The latter appears in a slightly different account of the story told above, which Galen wrote much later, in the 190s, in his treatise *On My Own Books* (1, 19.13–14K). In this version Galen was speaking publicly on Erasistratus's work *On Bringing Up Blood*, and a passage was chosen at random with a stylus for exegesis and commentary, apparently a common game. Galen spoke pointedly on the passage, aiming his barbs specifically at one "Martialius," an Erasistratean physician probably identical with the detested Martianus, who will appear below in the story of Eudemus ("Martialius" is probably a copyist's error in the poorly transmitted *On My Own Books*). This Martianus must have been one of the senior Erasistrateans who treated the plethoric young woman so incompetently. He was one of Rome's most well-established and prominent physicians, the author of well-regarded works on anatomy; Galen describes him as "malicious and contentious," adding that he was, at that time, some seventy years old. A friend then had the lecture transcribed; Galen does not name Teuthras here, but must be referring again to the treatise *On Venesection against Erasistratus*.

Galen was then, as he writes, in his thirty-fourth year; that is, it was 162 or 163 C.E. He had already become a public figure, a vocal advocate against a particular school of medicine (the Erasistratean school) and bitter rival of Martianus, whom he challenged both fearlessly and publicly. Teuthras would die of smallpox when the first epidemic wave hit Rome in 166 C.E. (see chapter 6). Galen, for his part, will later write that he withdrew from the public arena, perhaps as a result of this confrontation: "I wanted to escape the slanderous tongues [of my rivals], neither saying anything beyond what was necessary among the patients, nor teaching in public, as before, nor performing demonstrations" (*Libr. Propr.* 1, 19.15K). Perhaps he found the episode exhausting—or, more likely, the decision to withdraw dates to later in his career; the passage is ambiguous, as I shall describe in the next chapter.

Galen's first socially prominent and well-connected patient in the city was the Peripatetic philosopher Eudemus: a man of his father's generation, sixty-three years old at the time. The story of Eudemus took place in the winter of 162/163, starting "at the beginning of winter" (*Praecog.* 2. 14.610K), and it is Galen's longest anecdote, running to some ten modern pages. It opens his autobiographical treatise *On Prognosis*, which traces, through a series of case histories, Galen's career in Rome to its pinnacle, the point where he became one of the physicians on retainer to the emperor Marcus Aurelius. Galen wrote *On Prognosis* around 178 c.e.—long after he had become established in Rome, fled home to Pergamum, and been recalled by the emperors; long after he had been hired by Marcus to provide him with his daily dose of theriac, and to treat his young son; at a time when his memories, especially of the earliest episodes, were much shaped and enhanced by recollection and retelling. The stories must be read with these cautions in mind.[57]

Deeply implicated in the story of Eudemus is another friend, named Epigenes, to whom Galen addressed *On Prognosis*. Epigenes may, like Teuthras, have been another Pergamene who preceded Galen to Rome. Certainly Epigenes knew Eudemus better than Galen did: Galen will demur and avoid giving Eudemus medical advice based on his unfamiliarity with the patient, while Epigenes pipes up without hesitation (*Praecog.* 2, 14.606–7K). Epigenes witnessed the whole story of Galen's first high-profile case: "You were present throughout the whole illness of Eudemus the Peripatetic philosopher, from start to finish" (*Praecog.* 2, 14.605–6K).[58]

Eudemus's relationship to Galen is difficult to unravel. He apparently knew Galen's father; at least, he had heard about the fateful dream that precipitated Galen's change of career (*Praecog.* 2, 14.608K). Galen calls him his "teacher" (*Praecog.* 3, 14.613K), suggesting that Eudemus may be the unnamed Peripatetic with whom Galen studied as a teenager at Pergamum, although Galen continued to seek out philosophical education throughout his life. If Eudemus was one of Galen's first teachers in Pergamum, he would have had

---

57 Galen lost all copies of this treatise during his lifetime in the fire of 192 c.e., but it appears that extant manuscripts preserve a copy that survived without his knowledge. An excellent edition and translation of *On Prognosis* with extensive commentary is Nutton (1979). See pp. 48–51 on the date of composition.

58 For the story of Eudemus: *Praecog.* 1–2 (14.599–613K). On the case, see Schlange-Schöninge (2003, 150–55).

good reason to know of Nicon's dream, although he did not know that Galen had become a professional physician and thought he was a philosopher who studied medicine "as a sideline" (*Praecog.* 2, 14.608K).

Galen and Eudemus, fellow countrymen of good family and refined education, moved in the same circles in a highly social world. Galen mentions casually at the beginning of his story that it was Eudemus's custom to visit him every day (*Praecog.* 2, 14.606K); and Galen, in turn, is part of Eudemus's entourage, visiting the baths with him and a crowd of others, and also visiting him twice daily during the winter of his illness (*Praecog.* 3, 14.613K). Galen and others of his class and standing moved always at the center of a crowd: of followers, friends, servants, and students, for whom they in turn also formed part of the crowd that distinguished and defined them, a phenomenon that explains Eudemus's and Galen's relative unfamiliarity with each other despite daily contact. In many places, including in *On Prognosis* (1, 14.599–600K), Galen professes disdain for the custom of *salutatio*, the flattering round of visits that Roman aristocrats performed as part of their connection to one another and to their betters; but Galen's relationship to Eudemus clearly has some of this character. That Eudemus's friends, not all of them professional physicians, would take intense interest in his health and even offer medical advice is also typical of Galen's milieu. Sickness was a social event; it was the duty of one's friends to visit and care for the patient and to advocate for his best treatment, and it was fashionable for aristocrats to attain a fairly high level of medical knowledge, as I will discuss further in the next chapter.[59]

The story of Eudemus begins as the philosopher is on his way to the baths with Galen, Epigenes, and (apparently) several other people. Suddenly he asks Epigenes (was the latter a doctor, or simply an educated aristocrat proud of his medical knowledge?) whether he ought to bathe, given certain feverish symptoms: he had experienced a fit of chills three days previously, and in accordance with popular medical wisdom had avoided eating and bathing at "the suspect hour" on subsequent days. Galen will eventually diagnose Eudemus with quartan fever ("quartan" in this case means recurring every

59   See Mattern (2008a, 21–27, 84–87).

three days, as ancient doctors counted inclusively); a tentative modern diagnosis is malaria of the relatively benign type caused by the *P. malariae* strain of the protozoon. Epigenes thought nothing of Eudemus's symptoms, like "all the others present" (*Praecog.* 2, 14.606K), but Galen was silent and offered no opinion. Upon questioning, Galen admitted that he suspected quartan fever; that is, he predicted a recurring attack later that day. Eudemus begged him to take his pulse; Galen did so, but since, as he stated, he was unfamiliar with Eudemus's natural pulse, he could offer no definitive diagnosis. Galen spent much of the rest of the day with Eudemus and Epigenes, but in the evening had to leave to visit another patient. After he had left, Eudemus experienced a second episode—this time a sensation of heat throughout his body.

The signs of illness were still subtle. Galen uses the word *anomalia* (*Praecog.* 2, 14.606K), a vague sense of something wrong. The disease was creeping up on Eudemus, or lying in wait, but no less potentially lethal for that reason. The Eudemus case illustrates the anxiety that any symptom in the general constellation of what Galen calls "fever"—rigors, chills, sweats, sensations of heat—generated in its patients. Fever in Galen, as I have mentioned, is a recurrent, paroxysmal, and highly dangerous condition diagnosed through subtle changes in the pulse;[60] and he is unwilling to pronounce his patient free from it (*apuretos*). He was proved right: Eudemus soon "began clearly to be feverish" and to praise Galen as the sole accurate prognosticator among his entourage of friends and physicians (*Praecog.* 2, 14.608K).

In the grip of the paroxysm, Eudemus "gathered together the best doctors in the city" (*Praecog.* 2, 14.609K). Galen again demurred and modestly stood aside, "not wishing to contend with them through words," but he was present when they prescribed a dose of theriac (a complex drug, discussed in detail in chapter 6) on the morning of the next expected attack. Galen disagreed—privately, when the other doctors had departed, he told Eudemus and Epigenes that their prescription would only make the disease worse. Eudemus found it too awkward, however, to raise Galen's objections with the illustrious doctors he had consulted, and when they returned in the morning

60   Mattern (2008a, 155–58).

to administer the drug, he took it. The paroxysm recurred at its accustomed time and the doctors—who waited in attendance, to see what would happen—reassured the patient that the drug might take some time to have an effect, and then left. But the paroxysm recurred again, and not on the fourth day; it recurred (apparently, there is some confusion in the text here) on the same day. Eudemus's doctors returned in the morning and gave him another dose of theriac, with the result that Eudemus experienced two paroxysms again that day.

On Galen's interpretation, Eudemus now had two quartan fevers—the original, plus one produced by the effects of the first untimely dose of theriac—and, after asking Eudemus to save the urine he passed overnight and inspecting it the next day, he confidently predicted a third, to attack that very morning. This in fact happened, and the timing was good. Two of Eudemus's most influential friends were visiting, and he had been discussing Galen's prediction with them at the time. The guests included the former consul Flavius Boethus, who will be discussed in the next chapter. Eudemus, astounded at the accuracy of Galen's prediction, praised him to Boethus and all of his visitors.

The patient was, in the meantime, worn out (*kataponoumenos*) by the three quartan fevers, and the other doctors pronounced his case hopeless. Galen may have privately shared their pessimism, but he continued to treat Eudemus out of obligation: "I myself, however, had of necessity to respond to him when he called twice a day, for he was my teacher, and because I happened to live nearby" (*Praecog.* 3, 14.613K). For this he was ridiculed; especially by one Antigenes, a student of Quintus, and thus an older, more established heir to the same illustrious medical tradition as Galen himself. Antigenes, writes Galen, "treated all the most powerful people" (ibid.). He mocked Galen publicly and mercilessly, before Galen's "supporters" (literally "praisers"), both professional and lay: it was mid-winter, and Eudemus was sixty-three years old, and Galen meant to cure him of three quartan fevers: absurd!

The patient was in fact cured, and Galen accurately predicted the remission of each of the three quartans. His predictions were publicized and awakened, in sequence (as he writes), wonder, astonishment, and "no small reputation, not only for my prognoses but for my therapy" (*Praecog.* 3. 14.614K). For the case had generated much drama and tension over time: while Galen skillfully avoided direct confrontation with Rome's foremost physicians, his predictions were all made public, either by the patient himself who advertised them to his crowds of visitors, or by Epigenes, who "continually proclaimed my predictions … and my therapy" (*Praecog.* 3, 14.614K) or, paradoxically, by Galen's rivals, who openly mocked him. As the disease resolved step by step exactly according to Galen's prognoses, his enemies "prayed to the gods that [he] would miss the mark" (*Praecog.* 3, 14.614K).

In the event, Antigenes was "all but demolished" (ibid.), and so, as Galen writes, was Martianus, the illustrious Erasistratean, who now enters the story of Eudemus for the first time. Martianus went so far as to accuse Galen of divination—by augury, as he would reply when questioned further, unable to get his story straight; or animal entrails, or omens, or astrology.

Martianus visited Eudemus on the day Galen had calculated for his release from the third and last quartan fever. Eudemus was, at the time, in the throes of his final and especially acute paroxysm, and Martianus left feeling cheered at the likely failure of Galen's prediction. A second, a third, and even a fourth doctor visited, with the same result. But Eudemus began to feel better, and when he finally succeeded in summoning the busy Galen and demanding another reading of his pulse, he heard good news: Galen pronounced that his disease would resolve that very night. Eudemus questioned him urgently and pointedly, and a medical discussion of some sophistication ensued. Eudemus, in the end, proclaimed Galen a rival of Pythian Apollo in the art of prophecy.

The conversation regarding the pulse must have happened, as other events in this episode, before a crowd of Eudemus's visitors; for Martianus got wind of it. Visiting Eudemus and finding him in perfect health, he could not contain his vexation but challenged Galen openly when he encountered him by chance in the *vicus Sandaliarius*, the district Galen calls the "Sandaliarion." The second book of Hippocrates' *Prorrhetics*, said Martianus, apparently returning to his accusations of divination, specifically states "I do not prophesy (*manteuomai*) about these things" (*Praecog.* 4. 14.620K; Galen slightly misquotes the Hippocratic text, which uses the future form of the verb). Galen responded that he did not consider this book to be a genuine work of Hippocrates and refused to engage Martianus ("I answered only, 'You heard it [my prediction] from Eudemus, not from me,' and I immediately moved on").

Another of Galen's well-known cases (well-known today because, much later in the 190s, he wrote an especially engaging account of it in his grim, pithy diagnostic treatise *On the Affected Parts*) may date to about this same time, perhaps shortly after the cure of Eudemus, as it reflects Galen's newly minted reputation as a diagnostician of almost supernatural ability. Galen introduces the case of the Sicilian physician, friend of Glaucon, with words similar (but not quite identical) to those with which he opens the story of the young woman treated by incompetent Erasistrateans: "When I first came to Rome" (*Loc. Affect.* 5.8, 8.361K). Galen identifies Glaucon only as "the philosopher Glaucon" without saying how he knew him; but apparently Glaucon was a friend. Galen had been walking about the city with him a few days earlier when they had met a Sicilian physician, apparently a friend of Glaucon's, and Glaucon had introduced them. Now, encountering Galen by chance in the street, Glaucon explains that his Sicilian friend has fallen ill. "Taking my hand in his, he said, 'We are near to a patient, whom I have just seen.'" Glaucon is not, however, a physician, or not yet; in the event, Galen will be so successful that Glaucon becomes his student, and recipient of his treatise *On the Method of Healing to Glaucon*. But at this point Glaucon has a low opinion of the medical profession. He has heard from two friends, whom he names (Gorgias and Apelas), that Galen's prognoses and diagnoses were "more like divination than medicine"; and Glaucon will use the opportunity, as he explains, to test whether the art of medicine can in fact diagnose and prognosticate in this case.

Galen deferred the question with a vague reply and hoped for the best. "As you know," he writes to his unknown addressee, "I have often said that sometimes conclusive signs happen to appear for us, and at other times it is all ambiguous" (ibid. 8.362K). But this was the young physician's lucky

day. As he entered the house he passed someone, no doubt a servant, carrying a bedpan from the sickroom. The gruesome contents—a watery, bloody
fluid "like newly slaughtered meat"—immediately suggested a disease of the
liver. Galen pretended he hadn't seen it, and proceeded into the bedroom
with Glaucon. The patient explained that he had just moved his bowels and
offered his hand so that Galen might feel his pulse; Galen did so and reached
the conclusion that the liver was inflamed. At this point a second stroke
of luck occurred: the patient had prepared for himself a concoction of hys-
sop and honey, which Galen noticed in a small pot. This was a remedy for
pleurisy, and Galen deduced that the patient felt pain in area of the false ribs
(the *nothai pleurai*) on the right side, as a result of his liver disease.[61]

He now had all the information he needed to impress his audience, both
the physician and the philosopher: "Realizing that fortune had presented me
a way to achieve a good reputation with Glaucon," he put on the best show
he could. He took the patient's hand and placed it over his false ribs on the
right side, telling him that he felt pain there; the patient agreed with this. To
Glaucon, it appeared that Galen had made the diagnosis by the pulse alone,
an especially impressive feat because making distinctions in the pulse was a
subtle skill; Galen did possess this skill exquisitely, but, of course, was not
relying solely on it in this case.

Galen went on to inform the patient that he suffered from a cough, which
he then described: "You will agree further that the urge arises for you to
cough, and that you cough at moderate intervals a slight dry cough, spitting
up nothing." Hearing this, and perhaps influenced by the power of suggestion, Glaucon's friend coughed *in exactly that way*. Glaucon could restrain his
astonishment no longer and began to shout enthusiastic praise of Galen. But
Galen was not finished. Assuring Glaucon that the art of medicine could
prophesy even more than he had already done, he went on to describe the
patient's sensations on drawing a deep breath: increased abdominal pain, a
heaviness in the hypochondrium. Now Glaucon's friend, astounded, also burst

---

61   On the pain and other symptoms that Galen associated with inflammation of the liver, see
Loc. Affect. 2.10 (8.124–25K).

out in praise, he and Glaucon expressing noisy appreciation at the same time. Galen pressed his advantage further: based on his diagnosis, he predicted a drawing-down of the collarbone, but hesitated this time to say anything definite, fearful, as he writes, of losing the reputation he had just acquired. He spoke in more qualified terms, suggesting that the patient would experience this sensation if he had not already. Again he hit the mark. But Galen had one more trick up his sleeve: he knew that the patient believed himself to be suffering from pleurisy. "Seeing that the patient was greatly astonished, I said, 'I will offer one more prophecy in addition to what I have said already. I will tell you the patient's opinion of the disease from which he suffers'" (ibid. 8.365K). Galen's correct guess once again produced expressions of admiration from the patient and also from his attendant, mentioned for the first time here (unless he is the same person who removed the bedpan early in the story), and who had applied oil to the patient's chest as though for pleurisy; he was thus a confirming witness to the accuracy of Galen's guess. As for Glaucon, "from that time he has held a high opinion of myself and of the entire art of medicine, of which previously he had thought nothing much" (ibid. 8.366K).

I hasten to emphasize that although Galen's aim here is to impress his audience and he thus arrives at his diagnosis backwards—by telling the patient his symptoms rather than listening to him—his observations are acute and thorough, and the patient's oral responses are critical: as I shall explain in chapter 7, interrogation of the patient was a normal and important part of Galen's practice. Note, in this story, the details Galen provides about the patient's stool, cough, and pain: his description of the stool in particular (watery, bloody, bright red like newly slaughtered meat) is specific enough to suggest a modern diagnosis of food-borne illness. But Galen was also sensitive to questions of reputation and the impression he made on observers, and skilled in the theatrical aspects of his craft. Other passages in his work confirm this story's message, to take opportunities to win the admiration of the patient and, perhaps more importantly, those around him or her. The patient's pulse might betray the guilty anxiety of disobedience (as in the case of the boy Cyrillus); first make sure that the problem is not just the agitation of being examined, and then confidently pronounce that the patient has disobeyed your instructions: with luck most of the audience will be disbelieving at first, but some one among them will know the patient's transgression and inform on him (*Praesag. Puls.* 1.4, 9.250K). Listen carefully to what the patient and those around him let slip about the patient's history and course of illness; by correctly guessing the patient's experiences, as in the case of Glaucon's friend, the physician will capture their admiration (*Hipp. 6 Epid.* 2.47, 17A.998f). All of this will, of course, ensure the respect and the compliance of one's patients (*Hipp. Prog.* 1.2, 18B.3K). But it was also by such means that Galen gained reputation and rose to prominence in Rome, a vast and chaotic environment but one that was still largely "face-to-face" in character and, of course, highly competitive.

Galen concludes the story of Eudemus with a moral diatribe on life in the great city. At the patient's house, after his exchange with Martianus, Galen and Eudemus commiserated about the hostile and competitive atmosphere of the city. Galen's experience is typical, in Eudemus's view: the wealth and opportunities available in the empire's great capital attract men of low character who will do anything to get ahead, and whose crimes go unnoticed or unpunished in a way not possible in smaller towns. They will not believe Galen, says Eudemus, when he proclaims his intention to return to his homeland as soon as the turmoil there—*stasis*—has abated. They will assume that he, like themselves, came to Rome seeking fame and especially fortune, and will do their best to run him out, either with slander or, if they have to, with poison—indeed ten years ago, Eudemus recalls, a young doctor and two of his servants had been poisoned in just such circumstances. "I shall depart from this great and populous city," Galen replies in this conversation recalled years later, "for my small and scantly populated one, in which we all know each other, from what family we come, and what sort of education we have and property and character and way of life" (*Praecog.* 4, 14.620K). To the end of his days Galen remained a Pergamene and made at least one sincere attempt to make good on his vow to return home (see chapter 6). But there is no question that he spent most of the rest of his life in the teeming, seductive, pernicious, and deadly city of Rome.

Chapter Five

ANATOMY AND BOETHUS

In the Rome at which Galen arrived in 162, medicine was intellectually fashionable. Ancient Roman prejudices against what some had perceived as the decadence and mercenary nature of Greek culture, including medicine, had (for the most part) given way to a more cosmopolitan view. Every educated Roman, every gentleman, should be master of a number of intellectual disciplines, including medicine. Thus, Plutarch believed that every gentleman should be "physician-friendly" and count doctors among his entourage;[1] and Aulus Gellius considered it a disgrace that anyone pretending to education would be ignorant of the difference between his veins and his arteries (*Noctes Atticae* 18.10). It was also becoming more difficult to draw lines between Greek and Roman high society, although some people, like Galen himself and probably his friend Boethus, identified strongly as Greek and others as Roman. But Marcus Aurelius, the senior Roman emperor (about whom more in the next chapter), for one, was a renowned Philhellene and wrote his *Meditations* on Stoic philosophy in Greek. Roman aristocrats without exception spoke Greek, sometimes as their first language; and we have no evidence that Galen, despite many decades of

---

1   *Moralia* 122B–E. See Boulogne (1996).

residence in the city, ever learned Latin, for he cites no Latin author directly.[2] Some aristocrats practiced medicine without identifying as professional doctors; this included, later in Galen's lifetime, the emperors Severus and Caracalla, praised for their skill in healing in the perhaps spurious *On Theriac to Piso* (*Ther. Pis.* 2, 14.218–19K).

Galen's entourage of friends and students included many of these aristocratic amateurs, whom he does not formally distinguish from his colleagues or professional students, calling all of those in his company his "friends" or "companions." Galen wrote educational works "for beginners" addressed to them; he taught them dissection; he wrote technical treatises for them; and he brought them along when he visited patients.[3] His social and professional relationships were not distinct but, like Socrates, his friends and companions learned from him by virtue of the time they spent with him. He never mentions accepting money from students and may not have done this. In his mind and in his circle, medicine was not a discipline primarily learned or practiced in order to make a living; it was cultural capital.

Recall that Galen presented himself—and was perceived, as he writes, by others, like Eudemus—as a philosopher and physician both (*Praecog.* 2, 14.608K). Galen promoted a view of medicine as a queenly discipline of the same rank as philosophy, astronomy, mathematics, or music—all of which the truly educated physician should know, just as any truly educated gentleman, any *pepaideumenos*, would know medicine. This attitude seems to have been common, although perhaps not universal, among the Greco-Roman elite; although we should also remember that Galen was holding his profession aloft in a city and world where it was also practiced by slaves in the households of the rich, or by freedmen, or by rough-and-ready graduates of apprenticeships. With these types Galen had virtually nothing in common and he barely mentions them, although he probably counted professional assistants among his own household slaves.[4]

---

2   Nutton (2009, 24).

3   On Galen's pedagogical works, see especially Boudon (1994).

4   On medicine and Roman high society, see Mattern (2008a, 21–27), and more recently Johnson (2010, chapter 5). The classic essay is still Bowersock (1969, chapter 5, "The Prestige

All this is by way of introducing one of Galen's most illuminating relationships, namely his friendship with the senator and ex-consul Flavius Boethus. Galen knew Boethus for only three years before the latter departed to govern his native province of Syria Palestina, where he died; but Boethus was nevertheless perhaps the most important relationship in his life, the one that brought him fully into Roman high society and eventually into the emperor's circle, and the one that inspired not only a sequence of anatomical handbooks but his masterwork *On the Usefulness of the Parts*, his encomium to the artistry of Nature in seventeen books.

Flavius Boethus was a native of the city of Ptolemais in modern Israel, near the border of Lebanon, in the Roman province of Syria Palestina, an ancient Caananite/Phoenician settlement also (and later) called Acre, and given its Greek name by one of the early Ptolemies in the third century B.C.E. The former province of Judea had only a generation previously been shattered by the revolt of Simon bar-Kokhba, which Emperor Hadrian repressed with extreme brutality, expelling the Jews from Jerusalem and refounding the city as the Roman colony of Aelia Capitolina; it was at this time, too, that the name of the province was changed. We know nothing about Boethus's ancestry, but ethnically he most likely considered himself Greek, as his name suggests; Galen does not mention any Jewish, Samaritan, or other identity in connection with him, although this is not conclusive. Boethus's full name tells us that an ancestor was granted Roman citizenship by one of the Flavian emperors, in the first century C.E., possibly in connection with the Jewish revolt of 66–70. By the time Galen met him he had already held the consulship, the empire's highest magistracy. Galen met him through Eudemus, who was only one of the philosophers in his entourage, for Boethus was an intellectual, and a philosopher himself: Galen mentions also Alexander the Peripatetic (about whom more below), who tutored Boethus in the tradition of Aristotle, and Eudemus was also a Peripatetic.[5]

---

of Galen"). For the legal status of known medical practitioners at Rome in tabulated form, see Korpela (1987, 110–11).

5   Biographical details on Boethus are collected in Halfmann (1979, no. 95), but do not exceed what Galen tells us himself; see Nutton (1979, 164). Boethus's native city: *Anat. Admin.* 1.1 (2.215K).

Eudemus, in the course of his illness, had praised the miraculous prognoses of his young new physician to all his friends, including two that Galen mentions by name—(Lucius) Sergius Paulus, who had already held the consulship once, and would hold it again in 168 and become prefect of Rome, the official in charge of hearing judicial cases in Rome and Italy;[6] and Boethus. Boethus and Paulus, together with "[Marcus Vettulenus] Barbarus, the uncle of the junior emperor Lucius, then prefect of the place called Mesopotamia [no doubt as a commander in Lucius' then-ongoing war with the Parthians]" and "[Cn. Claudius] Severus, consul and enthusiast of Aristotelian philosophy" would also be early spectators of Galen's anatomical demonstrations in Rome. Both of these men are known from other sources, Barbarus as a friend of the renowned Athenian sophist Herodes Atticus, who may have spent time in Pergamum and known Galen or his family; and Severus later married the daughter of the emperor Marcus Aurelius.[7]

Nor are these the only noteworthy names dropped in the story of Galen's early career in Rome: one of his first Hippocratic commentaries, on the treatise *On Regimen in Acute Diseases*, written (along with eight other such commentaries), as he claims, while his library of books was still in Asia (*Libr. Propr.* 9, 19.34K), is addressed to C. Aufidius Victorinus. Victorinus was the son-in-law of Fronto, the emperor's friend and tutor, and would later hold the consulship and the prefecture of Rome. Galen claims that he wrote the commentary only after Victorinus had pestered him for it repeatedly, as though they knew one another well.[8]

Galen's pre-existing connections with Eudemus and perhaps with Barbarus partly explain his rise to prominence in Rome. But his success was also—and Galen himself emphasizes this factor above all others—a result

---

His and Galen's mutual friendship with Eudemus: *Praecog.* 2 (14.612K). Ex-consul: ibid. and *Libr. Propr.* 1 (19.13K). Aristotelian philosopher: *Praecog.* 5 (14.627K) and *Libr. Propr.* 1 (19.13K). His friendship with Eudemus and with Alexander the Peripatetic: *Anat. Admin.* 1.1 (2.218K); *Praecog.* 5 (14.627K).

6   *Praecog.* 2 (14.612K) on Paulus, see Nutton (1979, ad loc., 163–64). Galen mentions Sergius Paulus as one of Boethus's companions also in *Anat. Admin.* 1.1 (2.217–18K).

7   *Praecog.* 2 (14.613K). See Nutton (1979, 166–67).

8   Mattern (2008a, 20 with n. 61).

of his medical skill and erudition, that is, his mastery of the practical, as well as the literary and philosophical, aspects of his discipline. This he displayed in very public, high-stakes contests (like the cure of Eudemus, or his conflict with the Erasistrateans over the therapy of the female plethoric patient; both episodes are discussed in chapter 4) in a society where medical skill and knowledge commanded high prestige. Galen was in a position to teach something that many members of the Roman ruling class wanted very much to learn. He could enlighten them on the textual tradition and the correct interpretation of Hippocrates, as he did with Victorinus; he could cure them of malaria, as he did with Eudemus. But his appeal to Boethus was his skill in anatomy.

Boethus knew Galen by reputation, even before Eudemus mentioned him to his friend. Galen must have begun performing public dissections and vivisections almost as soon as he arrived in the city, and in fact may already (and temporarily) have renounced them. In *On My Own Books* he appears to make a curious statement suggesting that, during his first year in the city, he dropped out of public life. As I have mentioned, he makes this statement after describing his showdown with Martianus and other Erasistrateans on the necessity of bloodletting, which Galen (and his sidekick in this episode, Teuthras) defended in the case of two female patients and other patients (*Libr. Propr.* 1, 19.15K). The conflict had culminated in the treatise against Erasistratean doctrine that Galen had dictated and given to Teuthras, the extant *On Venesection Against Erasistratus*. Galen's demonstration for Boethus and his friends, described below, was a "private" affair in Galen's understanding of the term and not necessarily inconsistent with a decision to avoid public life. Nevertheless, it is difficult to know what to make of his supposed renunciation given the many references to lectures, anatomical performances, demonstrations, audiences, and the humiliation of rivals adduced in the pages below. It is possible that all of Galen's stories either preceded his decision to avoid demonstrations, or refer to performances for private audiences, or took place after he was dragged back into public life to refute critics of his masterpiece *On the Usefulness of the Parts*, who were saying unspeakable things about it (see chapter 6). There is also another possibility toward which I lean myself (and other scholars have also made this point);[9] it may stretch the meaning of Galen's passage—though not so much of the Greek words themselves—but it makes much better chronological sense. In *On My Own Books*, after telling us about his public lecture and the treatise he gave to Teuthras, Galen writes:

> Then I don't know how, but when I came a second time to Rome [in 169; see chapter 6], recalled by the emperors, he [Teuthras] who had received the book had died, but not a few people had the book, which had been composed for the sake of the rivalry (*philotimia*) of the moment, when I was speaking in public, and moreover I was still young when I did this, being only in my thirty-fourth year. *From that time* I decided neither to teach any longer in public nor to perform demonstrations."
>
> (*Libr. Propr.* 1, 19.15K)

From what time? Galen moves back and forth over several years in this paragraph: from his first year in Rome, at age thirty-three, to his return from Pergamum some six years later—and further on in the paragraph he will revert to the earlier time period ("Having spent three more years in Rome, when the great plague began … "). But it is at least possible that Galen gave up on public demonstrations only after his return from Pergamum and as a direct result of finding out that his book *On Venesection against Erasistratus*, composed informally and in a spirit of competitiveness (it is highly polemical, even "venomous," in tone), had circulated without his knowledge. Otherwise, there is no obvious reason why Galen should have made such a drastic decision; his confrontation with Martianus had, after all, ended very successfully. On the other hand, the book's publication seems to have horrified him, perhaps partly because it implied a vague betrayal by an old (and now deceased) friend. It had been composed in the heat of the moment and not intended for general circulation; and it had apparently been so persuasive that, in his work *On Venesection Against the Erasistrateans at Rome* (composed after his

---

9   Boudon-Millot (2007a, 188 n. 5); Schlange-Schöningen (2003, 204 n. 136).

return in 169), Galen was obliged to modify his views, pleading with the new Erasistrateans to have mercy on their patients and scale back their use of bloodletting.[10]

In *On Prognosis*, Galen tells us that when he returned to Italy from Pergamum, he avoided city life and the malice of his rivals, following the emperor's son, now in his charge, around the countryside (*Praecog.* 9, 14.650K). It is possible that this passage and the passage from *On My Own Books* refer to the same time and the same decision, rather than to two separate periods of withdrawal. In either case, I am not sure how seriously we should take Galen's protestations that he shunned the spotlight.

To return to Boethus, however: the ex-consul was an avid spectator of dissections. He had, as Galen writes, an intense passion for anatomical displays (*Anat. Admin.* 1.1, 2.215K). Galen had won his position as physician to the gladiators by publicly vivisecting a monkey; he found in Rome, it seems, a thriving culture of anatomy-as-spectacle. Into this he flung himself with his usual intensity and confidence bordering on (or venturing well into the territory of) arrogance. On hearing Eudemus mention Galen's name, Boethus was especially delighted—because, based on Galen's reputation as an anatomist which had perhaps followed him from Pergamum, he had already invited the physician to perform a demonstration on the organs of speech and the breath. As it happens these particular demonstrations—a series of vivisections, described below—were among the most spectacular and gruesomely entertaining in Galen's repertoire and Boethus had perhaps requested them for this reason.

It is no accident that dissection appealed especially to followers and enthusiasts of Aristotelian philosophy. Aristotle had pioneered animal dissection and, indeed, the science of comparative anatomy and of biology, zoology, and taxonomy generally. And Aristotle's teleological approach to science—his wonderment at the order he discovered in the bodies of animals, which he interpreted as evidence for a benign and intelligent creator; his insistence that

---

10 *Ven. Sect. Eras. Rom.* 1 (11.194–95K); here Galen specifically exonerates Teuthras from blame, but this confirms that it was something that had occurred to him. "Venomous:" see Brain (1986, 103).

"Nature does nothing in vain"—brought an intellectual, even mystical dimension to dissection. Galen would later consider his own teleological works, on "causes," or on "usefulness," to be most worthy of, and appealing to, a philosophical audience. But his relationship to Aristotle was ambiguous: as often as Galen praises him among the "Ancients" who combined philosophy and dissection, inventor of founding principles of logic that Galen considered essential to medical science, and proponent of the theory of four elements in which Galen unflaggingly believed; as much as Galen shared and staunchly upheld Aristotle's commitment to the visible evidence (the phenomena) and belief in the artistry of Nature, he just as often excoriates his distant predecessor and, especially, the latter's present-day followers for their ignorance and mistakes. Some of these were very obvious: on the seat of intelligence (for Aristotle, the heart rather than the brain); on reproduction (especially, the surprisingly persistent belief that female seed was excreted through the bladder and did not contribute to reproduction; upheld even by Herophilus, who discovered the Fallopian tubes); on the heart (which in Aristotle has only three chambers); on the nerves (which, according to Aristotle, originated in the heart); on the brain (whose function, as Aristotle believed, was to cool the heart); and on a long list of other subjects. Galen did not revere Aristotle in the same way he revered Hippocrates or, to some extent, Plato (the former was virtually never wrong; the latter was wrong only very occasionally); and yet his intellectual debt to Aristotle was perhaps greater than to either of these.[11]

Around this time—after the cure of Eudemus—came Galen's first introduction to the royal palace: a slave of Charilampes the "chamberlain" or "bodyguard" (*doryphoros*), the emperor's chief domestic servant and certainly either a slave or freedman himself, had suffered from an injured nerve or tendon that the palace physicians were unable to cure. Galen was summoned to the case by Epigenes, his personal friend and the addressee of *On Prognosis*, though he does not mention how Epigenes knew the chamberlain or his servant. Galen also mentions treating an "orator in the Sandaliarion,"

---

11   For a concise recent discussion of Galen's relationship to Aristotle, see van der Eijk (2009, 261–81). See also Rocca (2003, chapter 2).

Diomedes, about whom nothing else is known; but he was apparently close to the imperial household, for once again the "court physicians" had failed to cure this patient (*Praecog.* 5, 14.624–25K). These are the oblique beginnings of Galen's competition with the imperial physicians, a circle he eventually joined (see chapter 6).

To prepare for Galen's grand demonstration, Boethus collected the victims, pigs and young goats—"a large number (*pleionas*)," as Galen writes. These animals are best suited for demonstrations on the voice, as Galen explains, because their voices are very loud (see also *Anat. Admin.* 11.4, 106–7 Simon). It is not clear where the demonstration took place, but it is likely that Boethus's house had at least one capacious open courtyard, and this is a possible venue—aristocratic houses were designed to accommodate crowds. Galen's audience included, besides Boethus himself, an intellectual coterie of "Stoics and Peripatetics," and Galen calls the performance a "contest," presumably one in which he would meet the challenges posed by his very erudite spectators, though this first attempt proved too abortive to merit the term properly. Among these intellectuals was one of Boethus's teachers, Alexander of Damascus, whose views were Peripatetic but also tinged with Platonism. Galen also mentions two very prominent sophists of his era—Adrian of Tyre, whose biography is included among those written by Philostratus in the third century c.e., and who would go on to hold the chair of rhetoric at Athens and eventually at Rome, both of these special appointments in the gift of the emperor; and Demetrius of Alexandria, pupil of the famous androgynous orator Favorinus and member of the Museum at Alexandria.[12]

Alexander was, in Galen's word, especially *philoneikos*—"conflict-loving," competitive, a charge that Galen often (and hypocritically, to modern readers) levels at his enemies. It goes without saying that not only Alexander, but every other intellectual in the room including Galen himself, throve on competition, which was warp and weft of the fabric of their culture. But it would not do to appear too eager for battle, and Galen was master of the strategy of seeming aloof. He made a friendly overture to Alexander by inviting him

---

12   On Demetrius and Adrian, see Nutton (1979, 190–91).

to participate as commentator on the demonstration—to be "our teacher in drawing conclusions from [what is apparent from anatomy]"—hoping thereby, as he represents, to defuse Alexander's competitive streak and stave off an ugly dispute. Galen then proposed to demonstrate the function of the recurrent laryngeal nerves—"the finest nerves, a pair of them like hairs," as he writes, proud of his ability to locate minute anatomical structures.[13] They were his own discovery, unknown to his predecessors, and he also emphasizes the startling power of these delicate threads: for when cut, they would silence the animal without damaging it in any other way. This demonstration was, then, to be performed on pigs and goats before Boethus and his audience of glitterati. But it was cut short when Alexander piped up with the objection, "should we first agree with you that we should trust the evidence of the senses?" Disgusted, Galen stalked out in a huff, muttering that if he had known there would be vulgar Skeptics in the audience (*agroikopyrrhoneioi*), he would not have come. (Fig. 8 illustrates this scene in a sixteenth-century edition of Galen's works.)

This feud between Alexander and Galen may have already had a history and may have lasted a long time. Galen had a lifelong enemy in the philosopher Alexander of Aphrodisias, known from Arabic sources, also an Aristotelian—who disputed endlessly with him in person and in print, and called him "mule head" (possibly, according to one source, because Galen had a big head). This Alexander challenged Galen on questions of causality and also of time, which Galen believed, contradicting Aristotle, must be defined independently of motion. It is possible that these two Alexanders are identical. Both held the imperially appointed chair of philosophy at Athens: Alexander of Damascus, as Galen writes in *On Anatomical Procedures*, eventually received that position (*Anat. Admin.* 1,1, 2.218K), which Alexander of Aphrodisias is known to have occupied from 198. According to the Arab tradition, Galen and Alexander of Aphrodisias shared a teacher named Herminos; Galen does not mention this teacher elsewhere, but if the information is true, the two already had an acquaintanceship and intellectual rivalry

---

13   *Anat. Admin.* 8.4 (2.669K); *Usu Part.* 7.14 (3.576–77K); *Loc. Affect.* 1.6 (8.53–54K).

of long standing. Alexander's was, then, possibly one of the familiar faces Galen encountered when he moved to Rome.[14]

To return to the scene of Galen's dissection: his audience was disappointed and insisted—together with the consulars Severus, Paulus, and Barbarus, who had not been present at this original, abortive demonstration—that he repeat the performance. Galen agreed, and over a number of days, performed a series of vivisections demonstrating the muscles and nerves involved in breathing and in the voice. He describes several of these experiments in his treatise *On Anatomical Procedures* (of which the surviving text was written later, in three stages).

Here he describes how to cut open the pig, taking great care to avoid rupturing the pleural membrane; severing the intercostal muscles on both sides will cause the pig to lose its voice, as it becomes unable to exhale forcefully enough to make a sound. A better effect, however, is achieved by ligating the intercostal nerves, which paralyzes the muscles. Hooking the individual nerves out of the thick spinal muscle, without perforating the pleural membrane, is, as Galen writes, very difficult and he is specific about the type of hook required. Ligating the nerves with a needle and thread, one can (with the help of assistants, so that the nerves may all be tied off quickly) extinguish and revive the animal's voice at will, to the wonderment of spectators; the skillful anatomist avoids crushing or cutting the nerve, so that the voice is restored when the thread is loosened. This experiment, as Galen explains, is of his own design, unknown to his teachers (*Anat. Admin.* 8.3, 2.663K). "Many have often observed it, but few are able to do it" (*Anat. Admin.* 8.3, 2.665K); it must be practiced on a dead animal before it can be attempted on a living one (*Anat. Admin.* 2.662K). Galen also describes further experiments on breath and the voice: cutting out the rib of a living animal; severing the spinal cord; ligating the recurrent laryngeal nerves—here he recalls an occasion on which he had publicly demonstrated the anatomy of the thorax, over several days (this is perhaps the same event as the one he describes in *On Prognosis*, but not necessarily). He had invented a special scalpel allowing him

14   Nutton (1984b: 315–24; 1979, 189); Temkin (1973, 74–76).

to slice through the spinal column of a young pig at a stroke, without excising the vertebrae (*Anat. Admin.* 8.6, 2.682K).

Galen's demonstrations on the breath and voice for Boethus and his friends were, then, a grueling series of performances involving very delicate surgery on live, struggling animals, and spanning several days, in which his audience expected him to perform perfectly and make no mistakes. No doubt they caused the death by vivisection of a small herd of animals (perhaps the same supply collected by Boethus for the first demonstration, that never happened). The technical difficulty of the procedures was not the only challenge but also the demands of the audience; for in performances of this type the spectators were also active participants, a point I return to below. Alexander's outburst was out of bounds because its epistemological absurdity totally undermined the demonstration, not because challenges from the audience were unexpected.

Galen threw himself into the discipline of anatomy with characteristic obsessiveness and ferocity. He seems to have performed a staggering number of dissections and vivisections, not only before large audiences, but he labored over these investigations more privately too—although we must imagine that even his private experiments involved servants, slaves, and friends or "students." His fanatical diligence emerges in many offhand comments from his anatomical works. Slicing through the peritonea of his victims, for example, he observed peristalsis "in innumerable (*myriakis*) living animals" (*Nat. Fac.* 3.4, 2.157K). Unlike his teachers who left the flaying of dead animals to their assistants, he flayed them himself, and thereby discovered eight new muscles (*Anat. Admin.* 1.3, 2.231–33K). An animal too long dead (and no doubt repulsive to see and smell; Galen mentions no way of preserving a body) could be revivified with hot water or kneading, so that the motions of the tendons might be observed (*Anat. Admin.* 1.5, 2.243–44K).

The animals that Galen mentions most often in his experiments are pigs, goats, cattle, and monkeys. He considered monkeys anatomically most similar to humans, and especially valuable in dissection for that reason. Barbary macaques and olive baboons are the monkeys best represented in skeletal remains from the ancient Mediterranean world and, imported to Rome from

Egypt or the western African provinces (at great expense? through influential contacts? Galen would have spared no effort to acquire his victims), they were probably the ones most often dissected by Galen. Hamadryas baboons, green monkeys, guenons, and patas monkeys, depicted in the art of dynastic Egypt and attested in Late Period cemeteries, may also have been available.[15] Galen preferred macaques: he specifies that the monkeys most resembling humans have an upright posture, round faces, and large thumbs, lacking prominent canine teeth and a tail; by most of these measures the Barbary macaque or *Rhesus sylvanus* (which has only a stump tail) outshone the monkey called "dog-faced" (that is, the baboon; *Anat. Admin.* 6.1, 2.532–35K). But Galen's discussion of the merits and drawbacks of different species of monkey suggests that his anatomy is based on an amalgam of these and of other mammals— that is, he did not set out deliberately to describe the Barbary macaque. It is unlikely that Galen knew of or dissected any true apes, which do not appear in the art or literature of the ancient Mediterranean.

Besides these animals Galen also dissected many others, including (as he tells us) cats, dogs, mice, snakes, fish, and birds—specifically the crane and the ostrich, animals with long necks, which he dissected to investigate the mystery of the recurrent laryngeal nerves. (This pair of nerves, which descends from the vagus nerve to the thorax and then rises back up to the larynx, inspired ancient meditations on the design of creation, as it has also done in modern times).[16] He never, as he humbly acknowledges in a comment revealing about the lengths to which he drove his anatomical experiments, tried to dissect "ants, mosquitoes, fleas, and other such tiny animals" (*Anat. Admin.* 6.1, 2.537K).

Galen twice mentions dissecting an elephant, and it is unclear whether he refers to one event or to two. In *On the Usefulness of the Parts* he describes

---

15   Bailey et al. (1999); Goudsmit and Brandon-Jones (1999, 2000). Two guenons were also preserved at the Saqqara catacombs. A colony of barbary macaques lives wild in Gibraltar today, but they were apparently not native to Europe in Greco-Roman antiquity (Delson 1980, 18, 25). Hamadryas baboons, olive baboons, green monkeys, and patas monkeys are attested in Dynastic Egyptian art and in Late Period cemeteries (Osborn with Osbornová 1998, 32–42).

16   *Anat. Admin.* 11.4 (108 Simon). See Sandys-Winsch (2009), in which Richard Dawkins observes the dissection of the recurrent laryngeal nerves of a giraffe and explains their evolution.

dissecting an elephant's trunk, which he much admired as an example of a useful tool (for grasping and also for breathing underwater) and of nature's providence (*Usu Part.* 17.1, 4.348–49K). In *On Anatomical Procedures* he tells of another (or perhaps the same) dissection, in this case a spectacle attended by many physicians in the city. Galen maintained that they would find a bone in the animal's heart, against his rivals who argued that the heart has no bone. Galen claims easily to have found the bone with his companions, while his bungling competitors were unable to locate it; later he sent one of these companions to beg the bone from the imperial cook, who was, apparently, to prepare the heart as a royal dish. Galen kept the bone as a reminder of the occasion (*Anat. Admin.* 7.10, 2.619–20K). We can guess that what Galen actually felt in the elephant's heart was its fibrous skeleton, but we cannot know what structure, recovered by Galen's obedient friend from the emperor's kitchen, graced his collection of specimens: for the elephant's heart has no bone. Galen himself correctly held that while all mammalian hearts have a supporting cardiac skeleton, not all have a true bone. The heart bone or *os cordis* is present in large ruminant animals and (apparently) in otters but not in the elephant, although Galen's misconception that it exists in elephants, and generally in larger mammals but not smaller ones, is still common today.[17]

These are the animals that Galen explicitly claims to have dissected himself, although he mentions many more in discussions of comparative anatomy, including camels, horses, lions, mules, donkeys, dolphins, seals, whales, bears, and weasels. He dissected the fetuses of goats still in the uterus, using a reed to inflate the organ (*Anat. Admin.* 12.6, 154 Simon); and once dissected a "great number" of pregnant animals in sequence to prove the thesis that the uterus is always found wrapped tight around the embryo (*Sem.* 1.2, 4.515–16K). He even vivisected pregnant goats, explaining how to strap them down on their backs and shave the fur before slicing open the abdomen with a single bold stroke, and then incising the uterus itself. In these experiments he would test the function of the umbilical cord and observe the fetus's movements and its method of breathing: ligating the umbilical cord will cause the fetus to jerk in

---

17   Fowler and Mikota (2006, 317). On otters: Egerbacher, Weber, and Hauer (2000, 485–91).

distress.[18] On one occasion Galen delivered a goat fetus by Caesarian section from its dying mother; it proceeded to walk and scratch with no instruction, to the wonderment of his audience (*Hipp. 6 Epid.* 5.4, 17B.245K).[19]

For a vivisection of the heart, an especially spectacular demonstration, the animal should be placed on its back on a board with holes drilled through it, and bound to the board with ropes passing through the holes. Once the heart has been exposed, it is possible—after ligating the blood vessels to prevent exsanguination—to undo the animal's bonds and observe it running, eating, and drinking as though unharmed. One can also touch the heart, either with the bare hand or—because the beating muscle may leap out of the fingers—with tongs.[20]

For such procedures young animals are preferable as easier to slice through, but for the dissection of dead animals, especially monkeys, it is better to use old ones as they will have less fat to impede observation. One could even starve monkeys before killing them, to reduce the amount of troublesome fat. Galen killed his animals by drowning them, to avoid damaging any structures, although strangling them was an alternative. On the other hand, one could conveniently purchase an ox brain for dissection from any urban butcher; the latter can also supply bovine tongues and larynxes. And for observing the delicate structures of nerve foramina in the bones, it is best to bury a monkey in moist earth for at least four months, so that the bones are clean but not desiccated. "For I have always at hand a large number of specially prepared bones of [monkeys]."[21]

The brain, too, could be dissected in a living animal. Galen prefers pigs or goats for this experiment, again because some of the demonstrations were

---

18   *Anat. Admin.* 12.6 (151–54 Simon); cf. *Usu Part.* 6.21 (3.510K).

19   The etymology of the term "Caesarian" is murky but most likely relates to the Latin verb *caedere*, "to cut." Pliny the Elder writes that an ancestor of Julius Caesar's was born this way and that this is the origin of the cognomen Caesar (*Naturalis historia* 7.47), but this story may not be true. The Caesarian section was probably not a survivable operation until the nineteenth century, and before this was performed only as a last-ditch effort to save the fetus after the mother's death. See Todman (2007).

20   Tongs: *Anat. Admin.* 7.13 (2.635–36K); *Plac. Hipp. Plat.* 1.5, 5.186K.

21   *Anat. Admin.* 14.9 (229–30 Simon), tr. Duckworth. Young animals: *Anat. Admin.* 7.12 (2.627–28K), 7.13 (2.635–36K); also 8.8 (2.690K). Old animals: *Anat. Admin.* 5.4 (2.500K),

most effective on animals with a loud voice; and also because he did not like seeing the expression on the face of a monkey that was being vivisected. This last is a rare comment on the ethics of vivisection.[22] For the most part, Galen was ruthless. He drowned animals, starved them, inflicted unimaginable suffering by vivisecting them, without hesitation or apparent remorse; the pain, and the animal's screams, were part of the show. He might slaughter one animal after another, a whole herd of them, to prove a point; and he often emphasizes the need for bold and merciless strokes.

The vivisection of the brain requires an especially dispassionate approach, as the anatomist must slice through ("without pity or compassion") at a single stroke the skin and pericranial membrane of the animal to expose the skull, which may cause torrential bleeding (*Anat. Admin.* 9.11, 19 Simon, tr. Duckworth). The anatomist must then cut away the top of the skull without damaging the meninx. The latter is then raised off the surface of the brain with hooks and sliced through without touching the brain itself, and then peeled back, exposing the entire brain—an operation that must only be performed in the summer, as Galen writes, or failing that, in a specially heated room, for the animal will expire if its brain is exposed to the cold. By pressing on each of the four ventricles of the brain in sequence and releasing the pressure, the animal can be reduced to different levels of debility and revived. It can be blinded by pressing on the anterior ventricles in the region of the optic nerve root.

These are just a few of the ingenious and grisly experiments in vivisection, some of his own invention, that Galen performed. These displays were not only noisy, but also bloody. In brain experiments, for example, the hemorrhage that follows the first incision into the skull can be so catastrophic that many experimenters will lack the heart to go on; one must summon the courage to continue (*Anat. Admin.* 9.10, 18 Simon). Some of the animals (pigs) were large, and monkeys in particular were wild animals with long, sharp canines (no wonder Galen preferred the smaller canines of the macaque

---

8.3 (2.661K). Starving: *Anat. Admin.* 11.3 (94 Simon). Drowning and strangling: *Anat. Admin.* 1.3 (2.233K), 8.10 (2.701–2K), 13.4 (191 Simon). Butcher: *Anat. Admin.* 9.1 (2.708K), 14.6 (259 Simon).

22   *Anat. Admin.* 9.10 (18 Simon); also 11.4 (106–7 Simon).

over those of the baboon). Galen knew or used no method of sedating them. Avoiding injury during a vivisection was probably a major element of the challenge involved.

Anatomy was a skill of the highest order, which Galen practiced exhaustively, demonstrated, and taught.

> Of those who have seen the parts of a body shown by a teacher, none is able having seen it once or twice to remember it accurately, but it is necessary to see it many times.
>
> (*Comp. Med. Gen.* 3.2, 13.608K)

Anatomy was a tradition that depended on the transmission of prior knowledge from master to student; and this, along with its dependence on animal anatomy and the only very exiguous tradition of human dissection in Greek science, explains the bizarre errors (difficult to believe in a man who, for example, discovered the interosseous muscles of the hand and the bulbar conjunctiva of the eye, and described seven pairs of cranial nerves) woven into the fabric of Galen's anatomical work. One of the most notorious is the twin-chambered uterus or uterus with two cavities;[23] the double uterus is found in many animals (and in a small percentage of humans) and remained a tradition uncorrected even by Herophilus, who dissected human reproductive organs. Galen believed, following Hippocrates, that human females were gestated in the left part of the uterus. Similarly the retiform plexus, a web of small blood vessels at the base of the brain, is found in cattle, goats, sheep, and pigs, but not in primates or humans. First described by Herophilus, Galen considered this structure an exceptional example of the delicate craftsmanship of Nature.[24]

Galen believed the pulse to be an action of the heart and arteries, which breathed by means of the pulse, absorbing *pneuma* from the air through the

---

23 *Usu Part.* 14.4 (4.150K); *Sem.* 2.5 (4.634K).

24 Uterus: *Usu Part.* 14.4 (4.153K); *Sem.* 2.5 (4.631K); *Loc. Affect.* 6.5 (8.436–37K). Retiform plexus: *Usu Part.* 2.10–11 (3.696–97K); cf. Rocca (2003, 202–19; 2008, 253–54).

skin. This *pneuma* was an ethereal, almost mystical substance very prominent in Stoic philosophy, as the spirit that animates the body; according to Galen and some of his predecessors it took two separate forms in the human body, vital *pneuma* produced in the heart's left ventricle, and psychic *pneuma* produced in the brain, mainly through the refinement of vital *pneuma* in the retiform plexus. The impulse of pulsation began in the heart and was transmitted to the arteries through their coating and was not a result of the heart's pumping function, which Galen never recognized. A difficult vivisection designed to prove this, in which he inserted a reed into an artery and then pressed the artery's coating flat against the reed, cutting off (as he saw it) the pulse to the rest of the artery on the opposite side from the heart, must have failed; or his observations were biased toward his own view against that of Erasistratus, who had argued that the pulse was caused by the heart pushing vital *pneuma* through the arteries that distributed it to the body.[25]

Erasistratus's physiology was the dominant theory at the time, but Galen rejected parts of it—the arteries, he declared, patently contained blood and not only vital *pneuma*, as several of his vivisections demonstrated. *Pneuma*, as Galen argued, was absorbed not only or mainly through the lungs, but also through the skin into the small terminal arterial vessels and directly into the brain through the mouth and nose. The purpose of the lungs in Galen's system was mainly to ventilate the heart and thus regulate innate heat—an entity emanating from the heart and present from birth (it gradually diminished with age), which, cooking the blood as it arrived from the veins, injected it with vital *pneuma* that the arteries then distributed around the body. Neither Galen nor his predecessors postulated the circulation of the blood, although he argued that blood passes from the arteries to the veins through a system of invisible capillaries and from the right side of the heart to the left via the pulmonary artery and pulmonary vein. He also believed that venous blood passed directly from the right side of the heart to the left through perforations in the septum. It was not until the seventeenth century

---

25   *An Arter. Sang.* 4 (4.733–34K); *Anat. Admin.* 7.16 (2.646–49K).

that William Harvey would explain the structure of the heart and the nature of the pulse by postulating the circulation of the blood.[26]

Galen described a three-part physiological system based on the liver, heart, and brain, deeply influenced by the *Timaeus* of Plato, who had divided the human soul into three parts located (roughly) in these organs.[27] The liver was the central organ of nutrition, receiving food from the stomach and turning it into venous blood, which was then distributed throughout the body through the veins; in Galen's system, the liver was the source of the veins. Some of this blood passed from the right side of the heart to the left as mentioned, where it received essential *pneuma* transferred from the lungs; this vitalized arterial blood was then dispersed throughout the body through the arteries, of which the heart was the origin. The brain was the source of reason, voluntary motion, and sensation, communicating with the body through the system of nerves, which originated there, and receiving its own crucial supply of *pneuma*, stored in its four ventricles (which, rather than the gray matter, Galen considered the source of the brain's function), through the arteries or directly from the nose and mouth. The brain's ultra-refined psychic *pneuma* traveled throughout the body through the nerves, allowing sensation and movement; delivered from the anterior ventricles through the optic nerves to the eyes and radiating out through the pupils, it was also the substance allowing vision.[28]

Most of Galen's physiological ideas were long traditional by his time, although rival schools of thought competed. The system he describes or

---

26 English translations of Galen's four treatises *On the Usefulness of Respiration, Whether the Arteries Naturally Contain Blood, On the Usefulness of the Pulse,* and the extant summary of *On the Causes of Respiration,* with a succinct discussion of Galen's theory of respiration and its place in ancient medical thought, are available in Furley and Wilkie (1984).

27 In fact Plato says nothing specific about the heart or liver, although Aristotle and the Stoics identified the heart as the seat of reason. Cf. Donini (2008). On Galen's ideas of the soul, its anatomy, and its relationship to the body, see Gill (2010, chapter 3); Tieleman (2003); von Staden (2000); and Hankinson (1991b).

28 For a brief introduction to Galenic physiology, see Debru (2008). The most important treatises are *On the Usefulness of the Parts, On the Doctrines of Hippocrates and Plato, On the Natural Faculties,* and *On the Usefulness of Respiration.* All are available in English translation: May (1968); de Lacy (1980–84); Brock (1916); Furley and Wilkie (1984, 71–134).

implies, piecemeal in several different treatises, was not original to him and (partly as a result) not elegant or even especially coherent. Galen had no revolutionary insight into the function of the body, although his early and lifelong fascination with respiration and the voice inspired new experiments. But he was antiquity's greatest anatomist, and the intricacies of what he saw in his subjects filled him with awe. Galen believed in a providential creator and vigorously defended this position against those, like the Erasistrateans or the Epicureans, who took a more mechanistic or skeptical view. Galen's masterpiece on this subject is *On the Usefulness of the Parts*, written for Boethus shortly before the latter's death and discussed further below.

Galen's anatomical demonstrations were not only instructive, although this was their main purpose, but they were also a form of entertainment, at which he excelled. The bloody, controlled violence of the vivisections, and their incontrovertible proof of man's mastery over animals, resembled the wild beast hunts so popular in the Roman arena—and especially in the capital city itself, where the most exotic animals were killed in huge numbers in festivals twice a year, testimony to the wealth, power, and authority of the Roman emperor and his people. Besides this, the structure of Galen's demonstrations recalled the performances of the sophists; and like them, Galen usually called his public dissections and vivisections *epideixeis*—"exhibitions" or "displays"—rather than "demonstrations" proper (*apodeixeis*, in Greek).[29]

Like these masters of rhetoric who enthralled huge audiences (sometimes filling theaters, or even amphitheaters and stadia) with their virtuoso displays of on-the-spot improvisation, Galen might also improvise in a demonstration, taking suggestions from the audience about what to dissect. The sophists called these challenges from the spectators *problemata*, things "thrown forward," and so does Galen, who writes of taking on *problemata* as though this were routine. Thus, Martianus, his notorious rival, becomes spiteful "having learned that, regarding an anatomical problem (*anatomikon problema*), my speeches and my public teachings were greatly praised by all who followed

---

29   On the performative aspects of Galen's demonstrations and their relationship to the Second Sophistic, see Gleason (2009); von Staden (1997a); Debru (1996); von Staden (1995). On beast hunts, see Gleason (2009, 108–110); Wiedemann (1992, 55–67).

them" (*Libr. Propr.* 1, 19.13–14K). On another occasion, discussed in the previous chapter, the "problem" was a work of Erasistratus, *On the Bringing Up of Blood*: "the discussion of Erasistratus's *On the Bringing Up of Blood* was proposed (*problethentos*) to me in public, and a stylus was stuck in it, in the customary manner;" that is, a passage was chosen at random for Galen's commentary (*Libr. Propr.* 1, 19.14K). Here Galen is lecturing and not also anatomizing, but a similar performance later on—some time after Galen's return to Italy from Pergamum in 169—explicitly includes impromptu dissections. On this occasion he assembled the scrolls of the anatomical works of all of his predecessors before him and challenged the audience to name *any part for dissection*—Galen would not only locate the relevant passages among the mountain of scrolls but, by immediate demonstration on an animal, prove that his ideas were correct and theirs were wrong (*Libr. Propr.* 2, 19.22K).

Like those of the sophists, Galen's displays depended on audience participation and considerable audience pushback for their effect; they were not set pieces, but interactive demonstrations of superiority. Every performance thus risked catastrophic humiliation, not only if a difficult vivisection were botched but also if a challenger could manage to stump or wrong-foot or otherwise embarrass the performer. Galen himself was a master of this, and especially of exposing the technical incompetence of rival anatomists—those unable, in his view, to demonstrate the truth of their theoretical claims. Galen might challenge an adherent to the physiology of Erasistratus or Aristotle to expose an animal's heart and test the effects of ligating the pulmonary artery; when his hapless rival inevitably severs the animal's pleural membrane, and it expires immediately, Galen presents a second and a third, exposing one beating heart after another until his shaken competitor finally admits defeat.[30] An Erasistratean who proclaimed that he could demonstrate that the aorta contained no blood is similarly pressed to prove his claims—this time by friends or students of Galen, who had learned his techniques. They proffered animals and, when the physician demanded a huge fee of 1,000 drachmas for the demonstration, they put down the money on the spot. The poor man

---

30   *Anat. Admin.* 7.13 (2.635–36K); cf. Gleason (2009, 93–94).

was forced—"by all those present," that is, before a crowd—to take up the scalpel and attempt the very delicate procedure of exposing the aorta without killing the animal. "He was found to be so practiced [sc. so poorly practiced] in anatomy that he cut into the bone." One of his companions—"another of the same chorus"—then made an attempt, but cut arteries and veins, and the animal bled to death. Galen's friends then performed the experiment correctly, ligating the aorta in two places and, on the death of the animal, showing the artery between the ligatures to be full of blood (*Anat. Admin.* 7.16, 2.641–43K).

Galen does not tell us where these contests took place, but they seem improvised and informal, and probably happened in a public place. The implication, in the last story discussed, that he or his students could be found wandering the streets of Rome with a small herd of farm animals, a huge supply of silver coins (1,000 silver *denarii*—Galen calls them drachmas— perhaps transported by slaves in a chest?), a stash of medical equipment and an entourage of assistants, friends, and supporters, ready to truss and vivisect their victims on a moment's notice and presumably splashing spectators and the city's streets with gore, may seem far-fetched, but it is hard to see how else to interpret this passage. None of these incidents involved Galen alone; he did not declaim, debate, publicly anatomize or indeed do anything, including treating patients, without his entourage of friends and supporters. His enemies had their own friends, like those of the incompetent Erasistratean whose entourage Galen calls his "chorus." The audience took sides; friends or followers might be won or lost at any time.[31]

Galen was then a fixture in Roman public life, like the sophists and philosophers who declaimed and debated in the booksellers' district (the *vicus Sandaliarius*), at the Temple of Peace or at the Baths of Trajan, all of which Galen himself describes as likely locations for this kind of activity; and Galen himself did not just anatomize publicly, he also discoursed on philosophy, language, health, and presumably many other subjects. *Ad hominem* insults, dirty looks, stalking off in a huff (as Galen did in his confrontation with

---

31   See Mattern (2008a, 14–21).

Alexander), aggression, tears, and even violence were normal features of these public displays. Thus, a debate on the vocabulary of the pulse in front of the Temple of Peace might involve eight or more interlocutors and end in a fistfight (*Puls. Diff.* 1.1, 8.494–95K).[32]

Sometimes Galen would raise the stakes in these contests by posing a problem for his rivals in advance, undoubtedly with much public fanfare, and challenging them to produce a response in a set time:

> I ... allowed the followers of Asclepiades and Epicurus to seek out how, if they themselves stood in the place of the shaper of animals, they would have bestowed nerves on the aforementioned muscles. For I am accustomed to do this sometimes, and to concede to them not just days, but as many months as they wish for reflection.
>
> (*Usu Part.* 7.14, 3.571K)

He challenged self-proclaimed philologists to comment on the meaning of words in Celtic, Thracian, and other languages; when they could not, he presented them a simple word in Greek and, when they offered a definition, countered that the word meant something else in Thessalian dialect (*Thras. Med. Gymn.* 32, 5.868K). He might deliberately create tension by insisting that Platonists, Epicureans, Stoics, and Peripatetics all be present at some philosophical debate (*Anim. Peccat. Dign.* 5, 5.91–93K). The displays Galen describes sound like back-and-forth dialogues between performer and challenger, and sometimes between their factious entourages of friends.[33]

Also like the sophists, Galen taught students "in private": that is, Galen trained others in anatomy, who learned the way he had learned it himself, through continual practice and demonstration. Galen takes evident pride, in some of the anecdotes recounted above, in the skills of those who learned anatomy from him—the students who challenged the Erasistratean for 1,000 drachmas or the ones who felt the bone in the elephant's heart. On

---

32 Mattern (2008a, 9–11); see especially *Diff. Puls.* 2.3 (8.571–74K) and *Meth. Med.* 2.5 (10.112–14K).

33 E.g., *Diff. Puls.* 1.1 (8.484–95K), 2.3 (8.571–74K), 3.3 (8.653–57K).

yet another occasion a rival had been spreading false interpretations of the experiment on the aorta described above; but "those who had observed the procedure [done] by me" challenged him to perform it, producing a live goat for that purpose. The rival demurred, forced to admit that he lacked the skill to perform the demonstration, which the challengers then did themselves, before the assembled spectators (*Anat. Admin.* 7.16, 2.645–46K). As I have mentioned, Galen does not normally or consistently distinguish between students and "friends" or "companions," which is what he calls them in these stories—clearly they are people whom he trained in anatomy, but he emphasizes his social relationship to them, not his professional one, or rather he imagines these as intertwined.

Galen's dissections and vivisections had a spoken, rhetorical aspect—the running commentary he voiced as he proceeded. These commentaries he often wrote up or caused to be transcribed and are the origin of many of his lost anatomical works and several surviving ones. The anatomical works, that is, were intended as practical guides for dissection and vivisection, and were meant to accompany live demonstration and hands-on experience, and not to substitute for them. Galen argued that many of his predecessors saw no reason to write anatomical treatises because, in his view of medical training in the morally and professionally superior past, they had anatomized since childhood, as part of their earliest education at home, and had no need for written memoranda. (He maintained this view despite very little evidence for animal dissection before Aristotle and perhaps intended it to explain this lack of evidence.) Written treatises, then, came about of necessity, as the profession declined (*Anat. Admin.* 2.1, 2.280–81K). As I have mentioned, before even coming to Rome, Galen wrote a treatise *On the Motion of the Chest and Lungs* for a fellow student who wished to be able to perform the demonstrations on his own; Galen usurped the role of teacher in this case.[34] He often wrote for specific individuals who had seen the demonstrations performed. Thus, after witnessing Galen's series of demonstrations on the thorax and voice, Boethus, desperate to preserve Galen's commentary, sent slave secretaries to transcribe

---

34   *Libr. Propr.* 2 (19.17K); *Anat. Admin.* 1.1 (2.217K).

it. This may be the origin of Galen's lost work *On the Voice*, in four books, and of *On the Causes of Respiration*, originally in two books, of which the brief surviving treatise by the same title (4.465–69K) may be a summary; both were addressed to Boethus (*Libr. Propr.* 1, 19.13K).[35]

A passionate lover—this is the language Galen uses—of anatomical spectacles and follower of Aristotelian philosophy, Boethus was Galen's most important addressee, even though Galen knew him for only a few years before he left Rome on the journey from which he never returned. Besides the works already mentioned, Galen wrote several other anatomical treatises for him: *On the Anatomy of Hippocrates, On the Anatomy of Erasistratus, On the Anatomy of Living Animals*, and *On the Anatomy of Dead Animals*. None of these has survived. He also composed two books on *Anatomical Procedures*, which were lost when Boethus died in his province of Syria Palestina, and Galen's own copies perished somehow. He rewrote the work, and when finally complete—but not before the last books had also been lost in the fire of 192, and had to be rewritten—this second version of *On Anatomical Procedures* ran to fifteen books, and Galen considered it much better than the original. That first, lost work he calls "memoranda"—*hypomnemata*, the word he uses to designate his dictated notes on demonstrations, so called because they were aids to remembering what the recipient had actually witnessed. That is, it arose out of Galen's performances, spectacles that Boethus had observed himself, and was intended as a pedagogical tool.[36]

Boethus, then, was a zealous student and follower of Galen, a devotee of his public demonstrations and a generous sponsor of them. He was Galen's gateway into the highest social circles of the Roman ruling class and the recipient of some of his most important works; within the three brief years

---

35 *On the Anatomy of the Veins and Arteries* was also composed as memoranda of "things which you [the addressed, Antisthenes] saw demonstrated on the body of a monkey" (1, 2.779K).

36 "Passionate lover": *Anat. Admin.* 1.1 (2.214–15K). Works dedicated to Boethus: *Anat. Admin.* 1.1 (2.215, 216–17K); *Praecog.* 5 (14.630K); *Libr. Propr.* 1 (19.13, 15–16K). Perished: *Anat. Admin.* 1.1 (2.216K). Possibly they were destroyed by fire, but the reference to fire in Kühn's edition is a Renaissance gloss; Galen did not say how his copy was destroyed. See Boudon-Millot (2007a, CI). On the chronology of *On Anatomical Procedures*, see Bardong (1942, 631–32) for the date of composition (perhaps in three stages over decades) of the fifteen books of this work.

of their acquaintance, and almost immediately from the beginning, Boethus had become the most important person in Galen's life. It is perhaps even possible to speak of—or guess at—something like a close or intimate friendship. Two stories place Galen in the innermost rooms of Boethus's house, treating his wife and child; though both stories also include competition and disputation with other men, too. The patient in the first story is Boethus's son, Cyrillus, who appeared to be suffering from fever, then an ominous symptom in children, or in anyone. After four days, the child had failed to recover and his temperature soared in the night; Boethus went out personally the next day—he did not send a slave or messenger—looking for Galen, his friend and most trusted physician. "Taking hold of me and seizing me, he led me to his house, to the boy." The street was busy, and a crowd collected along the way; among them was Epigenes, the addressee of the work *On Prognosis* in which Galen tells the story ("you were also among them").

Boethus has placed his son in the care of the boy's mother, a silent and shadowy figure in this story. Possibly, but not certainly, this woman was also Boethus's wife, the subject of Galen's next story, but he does not say so unambiguously, identifying her as "the mother of the child." It is not clear whether we here meet Boethus's legitimate wife, an enslaved or freed concubine, or possibly a previous, divorced wife. Galen uses the word *huios* of the boy, the word for a legitimate son, and does not specifically identify him as a *nothos* or illegitimate child, but this is not conclusive.[37] Galen has never met the woman before, and Boethus must introduce him ("This is Galen"). She has been very worried, and Boethus expresses the hope that her fears have been exaggerated—perhaps with some condescension toward feminine weakness, although he had himself fetched Galen to his house.

37　At 14.637K Galen calls the mother "the woman," *gyne*, which could also mean "the wife," but the term is nonspecific (Galen does not write "his [Boethus's] woman"). Roman law would later forbid keeping a (free or freed) concubine concurrently with a wife (*Codex Justinianus* 5.26.1, 7.15.3.2), but it is uncertain when this became illegal or uncustomary. Sex and breeding with one's slaves was normal in all time periods, and slave harems are well attested for the Roman aristocracy. These offspring were not normally openly acknowledged as the master's children, though some were well cared for and well-educated, freed early, and left property, and Roman law recognized that slaves were often the "natural sons" of their masters. See Betzig (1992).

But the moment Galen takes the boy's pulse, the story turns from tense to comic, for Galen foresaw no serious problem. He jokingly promised before the crowd to live up to his own reputation as a prophet. Calling Boethus himself to witness that no one had disclosed any secret knowledge on the way to the house, he declared that the boy had a stash of food hidden in the room, with which he was stuffing himself whenever his mother went to the baths—the *balaneion*, for Boethus had a private bathing suite in his house (which may also have served as the household's latrine). A thorough search of the room and all its furniture (this is described in some detail) revealed nothing, temporarily stumping Galen and jeopardizing his divinatory prowess, until he discovered the food wrapped in the woman's headscarf, to the laughter and cheers of the boy's relieved father and the audience of friends. Galen had guessed at the boy's problem not because the pulse revealed a physiological condition, as he explains; it had told him that the boy was anxious and hiding something (*Praecog.* 7, 14.635–41K).

Galen goes on to relate his next experience in Boethus's household: this time the patient is none other than Boethus's wife (unnamed here perhaps in accordance with the long Greek tradition of reticence about the names of respectable women, although most of Galen's male patients are also anonymous), who has long been suffering from "the so-called female flux." For this she had been under the care of her midwives, too modest to entrust herself to a male physician. In this story as elsewhere, Galen expresses no hostility or condescension toward the midwives with their less educated, more traditional form of medicine, saving all of his contempt for his male colleagues (and some for the woman's hapless female servants, as I shall describe). Boethus's wife's midwives, writes Galen, are "the best in the city," and he writes of her chief caregiver that "I knew her to be very good."

In any case, when his wife's condition showed no improvement under the care of the midwives, Boethus called together all the best doctors, who agreed that the woman should be treated according to Hippocratic principles, with drying remedies to stop the flux by removing the excess fluids that presumably were causing it. Galen himself at first had no better idea, although in the story he is more trusted than the other doctors: Boethus singles him out to work with his wife's female servants, making sure that the remedies are mixed properly. These were applied to the patient's genitals, and Galen seems to have supervised this rather than doing it himself. But the woman's condition deteriorated. She began to swell with edema as though pregnant; the doctors were at a loss, while her midwife prescribed daily baths. One day in the bath the patient was overcome by pains like childbirth, evacuated a large quantity of fluid, and fainted. Her servants, not knowing what to do, shrieked helplessly; Galen happened to be in the house at the time and heard the commotion from outside the bathroom.

He rushed in, presumably found Boethus's wife naked and unconscious on the bathroom floor, and began to massage her abdomen, ordering the women to massage her hands and feet and bring smelling salts. The evacuation had been a positive development, but Galen still worried about the case and lost sleep over it; "the following occurred to me as I was thinking anxiously at night." The patient was being dried by elaborate and exhaustive methods—they were bringing in warm sand from the coast for her to lie down on, and smearing her with pitch and resin—but he determined to treat her with plasters of boiled honey, diuretic drugs, and laxatives. When Boethus called the next collective meeting of doctors, Galen made a point of speaking to him privately, "leading him away from the servants and friends in the house." He took the risky step of asking Boethus to entrust his wife to him entirely—"to do as I like regarding your wife"—for ten days. Boethus consented, and the patient improved steadily under Galen's care, recovering completely in a month. We do not know what condition, in modern terms, afflicted Boethus's wife; the differential diagnosis includes an incomplete miscarriage (but Galen explicitly states that the patient was not pregnant), a hydatid cyst caused by the tapeworm *Echinococcus* in its larval form, which usually however does not infect the uterus, and cancer. If it is true that the patient recovered completely, a pelvic abscess may be the most likely problem.[38]

---

38   For the differential diagnosis, see Nutton (1979, 203).

Boethus was so delighted that he rewarded Galen with four hundred gold coins, a huge sum worth 10,000 *denarii*—not a fee, for Galen insisted that he never accepted these, rather a prize for Galen's successful cure of his beloved wife.[39] But Galen's real triumph in this story occurs at the moment when he wins over Boethus's complete trust. The consul apparently ran a traditional, conservative Greek household, where women were withdrawn as far as possible from the prying eyes of male visitors, and in which he ruled as patriarch over a large female population, including servants, midwives, and perhaps one or more concubines, as well as his wife. When Boethus agrees to allow Galen to "do as I like regarding your wife," he is handing over some of his patriarchal authority, and clearly Galen has privileged access to the women of the house (*Praecog.* 8, 14.641–47K).

In these first few years at Rome Galen was extraordinarily prolific as an author. Besides the anatomical treatises I have mentioned, he also wrote the first six of, eventually, nine books *On the Doctrines of Hippocrates and Plato*, a work in which he strove to show that Plato and Hippocrates agreed on the principles of physiology and that their views were correct, against the intellectual traditions that rejected or questioned them (in particular the Stoics and their belief that the heart is the seat of consciousness). This work he also addressed to Boethus, and when the latter departed for his province, he took these six books of the as yet unfinished work with him. Galen also began to write commentaries on Hippocratic texts, although these would be less erudite and exhaustive than his later efforts—either because, as he writes in *On My Own Books*, he had left his library behind at Pergamum, or perhaps because Hippocratic exegesis did not yet play the fully developed role in his intellectual identity that it would later in his life.[40]

It was also for Boethus that Galen produced the seventeen books *On the Usefulness of the Parts*. Only the first book was complete by the end of Galen's

---

39   On fee vs. prize, see Mattern (2008a, 4 n. 10 and 83). On Galen's claim about fees, see Meyerhof (1929, 84).

40   von Staden (2009); *Libr. Propr.* 9 (19.34–35K). Extant, or mostly extant, treatises dating to this period are Galen's commentaries on the *Aphorisms*, on *Prognostic*, on *On Joints*, on *Fractures*, on *On Regimen in Acute Diseases*, and on book I of the *Epidemics*.

first stay at Rome: he sent it along with Boethus when the latter set out for his province, shortly before Galen's own departure from the city. The whole work took a long time to complete, partly because of the disruption when Galen fled from Rome to Pergamum in 166, and when he was recalled (see chapter 6). He does not seem to have finished all seventeen books until much later, about the year 175, when he sent them to Boethus who was at the time still in his province (on this timeline, Boethus served an exceptionally long term as governor; or perhaps he had stayed on after retirement) and still alive.[41] Although it was addressed to his friend, Galen wrote this treatise with a larger audience in mind and expected it to circulate:

> It does not strive to be clear to one, or two, or three, or four, or some specific number [of readers]; but it aims to teach, in turn, everyone who comes into contact with it.
>
> (*Usu Part.* 7.14, 3.572–73K)

This is a rare statement in Galen, who often claims to be writing for specific friends who asked for his works and refers to many of his treatises as "exercises" or "memoranda," words that suggest a practical and strictly didactic purpose for a relatively narrow audience, though some works circulated more widely than he intended.[42] In *On the Usefulness of the Parts*, however, he spoke broadly to his peers, the intellectual elite, and it is the work most self-consciously addressed to a wider public. Therefore, unlike the first, short version of *On Anatomical Procedures*, which he composed as "memoranda" for Boethus and which perished with the latter's death and the destruction of Galen's own copy, this work circulated right away and was never lost. It was read widely, as Galen claims, by both doctors and Aristotelian philosophers (*Libr. Propr.* 2, 19.20–21K). Indeed, he thought everyone ought to read it: physicians, philosophers, and "whatever people honor the gods," because,

---

41   *Libr. Propr.* 1 (19.15–16K), 2 (19.19–20K); *Anat. Admin.* 1.1 (2.216–17K); Ilberg (1889, 218–19).
42   See von Staden (1997b); Mattern (2008a, 14–21).

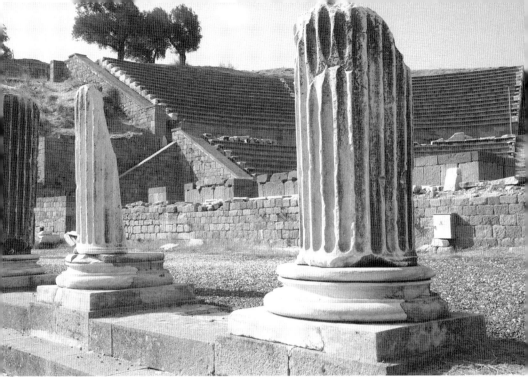

FIG. 1. The ruins of the Asclepieion at Pergamum, with the theater in the background. The precinct of Asclepius was rebuilt in extravagant fashion in the reign of Hadrian, and by Galen's time was the most important of the god's many cult centers around the Mediterranean world. © *Shutterstock.*

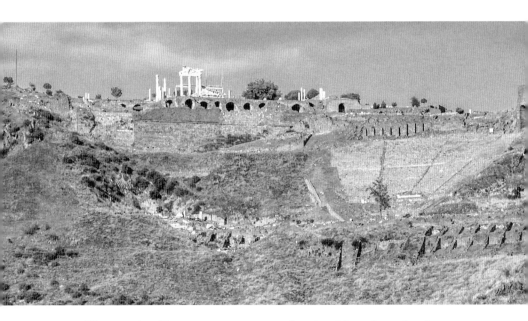

FIG. 2. The acropolis of Pergamum, as it appears today; viewed from the road to the Asclepieion. The most prominent building is the Temple of Zeus and Trajan, center left; to the right is the acropolis' theater. © *Shutterstock.*

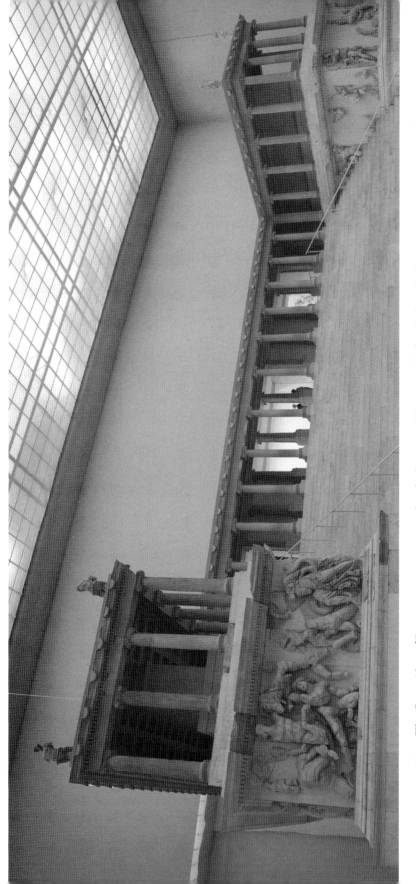

FIG. 3. The Great Altar of Pergamum, as reconstructed in the Pergamon Museum in Berlin. Built under King Eumenes II in the second century B.C.E. Its frieze, 113 meters long, depicts the mythical battle of gods and giants. *Photo courtesy of Album/Art Resource, NY.*

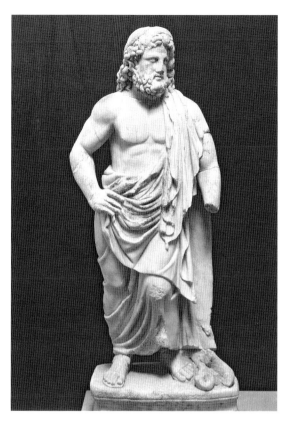

FIG. 4. Small marble statue of Asclepius, 63 cm high, dating to the third or fourth century B.C.E. From the shrine of Asclepius at Epidaurus, and now in the National Archaeological Museum of Athens. Asclepius was usually, but not always, portrayed as a bearded mature man. The snake was one of his attributes, and plays a role in many healing stories. *De Agostini Picture Library/G. Nimatallah.*

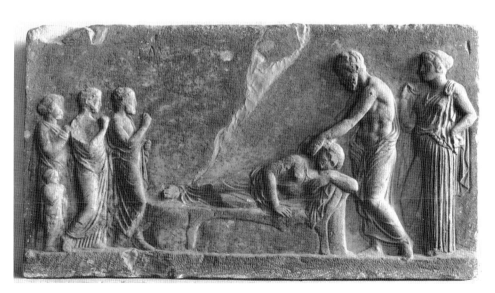

FIG. 5. Asclepius healing a patient in her sleep. Votive relief from the temple of Asclepius at Piraeus, near Athens, Greece; now in the Archaeological Museum of Piraeus. It dates from about 400 B.C.E. Asclepius often healed or gave instructions to patients in dreams; and grateful patients often dedicated votives like this as compensatory offerings. The female figure behind Asclepius is probably his daughter, Hygieia. The figures to the left may be relatives of the patient. *Photo courtesy of Foto Marburg/Art Resource, NY.*

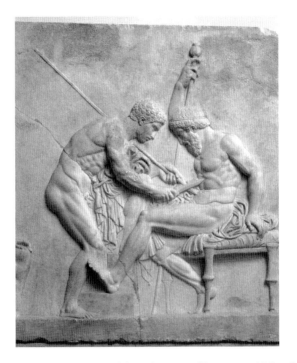

FIG. 6. Two scenes of healing recovered from the ruins of Pompeii and Herculaneum in Italy, buried by Mount Vesuvius in the volcanic eruption of 79 c.e. Both items now at the Museo Archeologico Nazionale di Napoli. (6A), Achilles operates on Telephus. Greek mythology told that in return, Telephus showed the Achaeans the way to Troy. From the House of the Relief of Telephus, Herculaneum. *Photo courtesy Album/Art Resource, NY.*

FIG. 6B. Aeneas, mythic founder of Rome, being attended to by a physician, who removes an arrow head from his thigh. Fresco from the Casa di Sirico in Pompeii. *Photo courtesy of Erich Lessing/Art Resource, NY.*

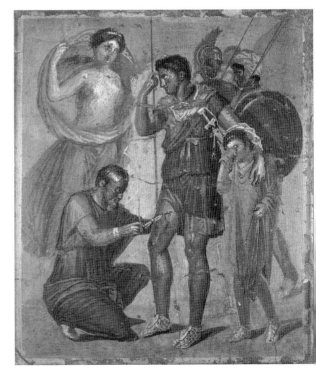

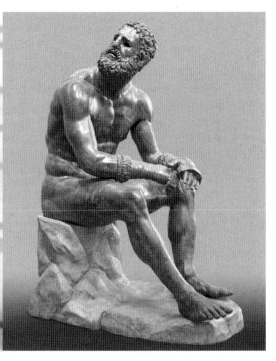

FIG. 7. The Seated Boxer, bronze statue from the first century C.E. (?), wearing leather gloves and a loincloth. His ears are swollen, and blood drips from gashes on his face. At Terme Museum in Rome. *Photo courtesy of Vanni / Art Resource, NY.*

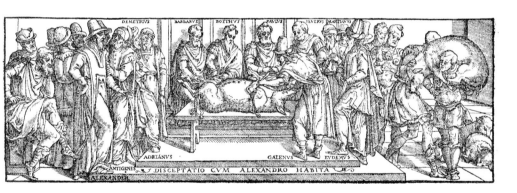

FIG. 8. Detail illustrating the dissection of a pig, from the 1565 edition of Galen's complete works by the Giunta press in Venice. The caption reads "disputation held with Alexander" and refers to Galen's confrontation with Alexander of Damascus at the vivisection he performed for Boethus, described in Chapter Five. Several other scenes from Galen's life were illustrated on the same page. *Photo courtesy of the Wellcome Trust, London © Wellcome Trust.*

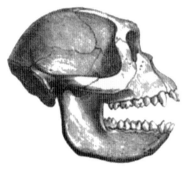
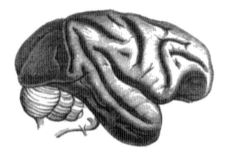

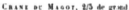
CRANE DU MAGOT, 2/3 de grand.

CERVEAU DU MAGOT, 1/2 de grand

FIG. 9. The skull and brain of the Barbary macaque (*Rhesus sylvanus*), from the *Histoire naturelle des mammifères* by Paul Gervais, L. Curmer 1854. Among the animals with which he was familiar, Galen considered monkeys, and especially macaques, anatomically most similar to humans.

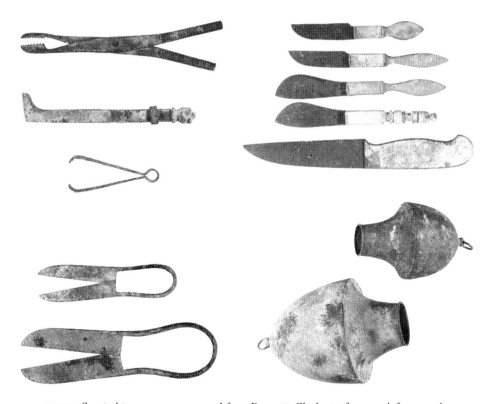

FIG. 10. Surgical instruments recovered from Pompeii. Clockwise from top-left are uvula forceps, scalpels, cups for bloodletting, and surgical scissors. Pompeii, in southern Italy near Naples, was buried in the eruption of Mount Vesuvius in 79 C.E. *Photos courtesy of the Historical Collections & Services of the Health Sciences Library, University of Virginia.*

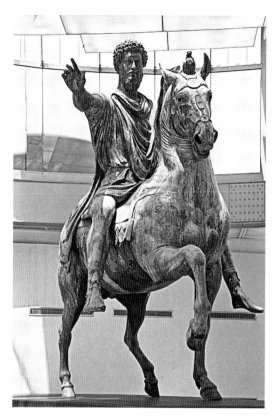

FIG. 11. Bronze statue of Marcus Aurelius, emperor from 161 to 180 c.e., Rome. It was perhaps erected on the occasion of his triumphal visit to the city in 176, and is the only surviving example of many equestrian statues of emperors known to have been produced in antiquity. From 1538 it stood in the Piazza Campidoglio, where it became the centerpiece of Michelangelo's redesigned complex. Badly weathered by pollution in recent years, it is now housed in the nearby Musei Capitolini, while a reproduction stands in its old location. © *Shutterstock.*

FIG. 12. Title page with woodcut from the first volume of the Aldine edition of Galen's complete works, from the press of Aldus Manutius in Venice, 1525. In the text under the illustration, the Pope and the Venetian senate forbid reprinting of these books of Galen anywhere, but they were reprinted many times. *Photo courtesy of the Wellcome Library, London © Wellcome Trust.*

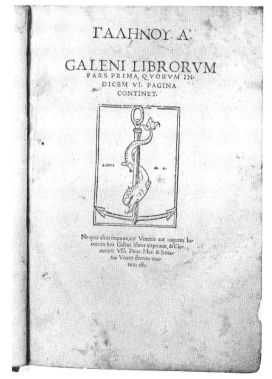

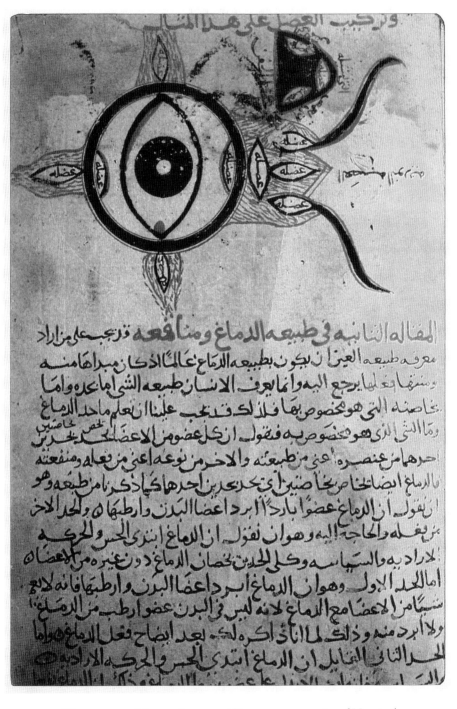

FIG. 13. The anatomy of the eye, from a twelfth-century manuscript of Hunain ibn-Ishaq's "The Book of the Ten Treatises on the Eye." Hunain ibn-Ishaq, who lived in the ninth century, translated most of Galen's known treatises into Syriac and Arabic. "The Book of the Ten Treatises on the Eye" is his best-known original work. *Photo courtesy of SSPL/Science Museum/Art Resource, NY.*

compared to mystery-cults like that of Eleusis with their obscure teachings, "those of Nature are visible in all animals" (*Usu Part.* 17.1, 4.360–61K).

Thus, Galen considered *On the Usefulness of the Parts* a work not just of medicine but of philosophy and also of religious reverence because of its emphasis on "usefulness"—that is, on teleology, and especially ideas of biological teleology tracing back to Aristotle, whom Galen supported against his detractors (especially Erasistratus and Asclepiades) on this point.[43] In this view all living beings and, in particular, all of their anatomical parts were invented by a creator, for a purpose. Some parts might not have a use of their own, arising as by-products of other purposeful parts, but for Galen these examples are rare and he attributes the highest degree of beauty and efficiency to Nature's work. Nature, as he insists repeatedly, following Aristotle, does nothing in vain; he did not acknowledge the restrictions and limitations on this dictum that Aristotle himself seems to have recognized. The providence of the creator, and in particular his or her (Galen calls the creator by the male-gendered word "Demiurge" or Craftsman, and the female-gendered word "Nature" interchangeably) technical skill in designing and modeling the anatomy of the human body, is the unifying theme and message of *On the Usefulness of the Parts*. In the bones and sinews, membranes and fluids of the victims he dissected and vivisected day after day, and lacking an alternate theory to explain the delicately fashioned and finely attuned structures he observed, Galen found cumulative and overpowering evidence of an intelligence at work. I am simplifying here: Galen recognized several types of cause, including some not described by Aristotle, and his philosophy of causation, including creation, is sophisticated. But the point I wish to emphasize here is his metaphysical belief in an intelligence behind creation; for Galen was in many ways, and not only in this one, a surprisingly pious man.

---

43 On the intended audience for *Usu Part.* (doctors and philosophers), *Anat. Admin.* 2.3 (2.291K); *Usu Part.* 17.1 (4.360–61K). On teleology and Aristotle, see Hankinson (2008b, 225–36; 1994a, b; 1989). On Galenic theology and religious views more generally, see Frede (2003). On Galen's Demiurge (below), see Flemming (2008). For an interesting discussion of the relationship between teleology and anatomy in Greek culture, see Kuriyama (1999, 116–29).

Galen revered this intelligence without being able to imagine its form, a point to which I return below. One theme is clear however: in Galen's mind the creator is an engineer or artisan, whom he compares to Prometheus, the mythical Titan who molded the first man out of potter's clay, or to the famous sculptor Phidias, who made the cult statue of Zeus at Olympia out of ivory and gold; or the anonymous artisan who carved a signet ring depicting Phaethon's disastrous attempt to drive the chariot of the sun, in such fine detail that Galen could scarcely make out all sixteen limbs of the horses, except by close scrutiny in the brightest light; but each of the limbs seemed perfect on inspection.[44] This was surely amazing, but how much more amazing the perfect leg of a flea, created by Nature? The artistry that Galen attributes to the creator is also, in his view, the most characteristic quality of humans; and he begins *On the Usefulness of the Parts* with a description of the hand, the anatomical part that, together with reason, enables it.

Galen's creator was limited by the humble nature of the materials available (semen and menstrual blood), which explained any imperfections in the results of his or her design. Judeo-Christian ideas of the creator as an omnipotent being who called creatures into existence by fiat struck Galen as irrational and wrong. Passionately committed to logical demonstration, he criticized Jewish religion for what seemed to him an unsophisticated reliance on God's directives to Moses as the source of law. He refers three times in surviving passages to the "followers of Moses and Christ" as doctrinaire schools that insist that their adherents accept their tenets on faith, without logical demonstration: "One might sooner teach something new to the followers of Moses and Christ than to those doctors and philosophers who cling to their *haireseis*" (*Diff. Puls.* 3.3, 8.657K). Comparing the creator-god of Moses (whom he always cites as the originator of Jewish ideas, seeing him as similar to the founders of the Greek philosophical schools) to the Craftsman of Plato and of his own *On the Usefulness of the Parts*, he argues that Moses ought to have recognized the material cause of creation; no god could simply will

---

44   Phidias: *Usu Part.* 3.10 (3.239K). Prometheus: *Usu Part.* 10.9 (3.801–2K), 12.11 (4.45K). Phaethon: *Usu Part.* 17.1 (4.361K).

creatures into existence out of any material whatsoever, as though humans could be made of stone or a bull from ashes (*Usu Part.* 11.14, 3.905–7K). The thought that a good and omnipotent creator would have seen fit to invent scorpions, mosquitoes, and the like repelled him; he does not associate this idea with Judaism, but it troubled his thoughts on the nature of the Platonic creator (*Foet. Form.* 6, 4.700K).

Some of Galen's references to Jews and Christians survive only in Arabic excerpts from lost treatises and were collected and studied in a classic book by Richard Walzer (himself a Jewish refugee and émigré to Oxford from Germany) published in 1949. Walzer demonstrates that Galen's views, with perhaps one exception (on Christian virtue; see below) were typical of the Greek tradition and that the first chapters of Genesis, for example, may have been well known to pagan intellectuals. It is therefore not necessary to postulate that Galen had an unusually intimate knowledge of Judeo-Christian religion or direct contact with Jews or Christians in Rome, although both communities were large and this is not excluded.[45] Galen's close friend Boethus was from Palestine and may well have had Jewish friends or connections.

In one passage, Galen excuses Christians for using parables in place of logical demonstration, given that most people cannot follow rigorous arguments anyway (this passage occurs in Galen's lost commentary on Plato's *Republic* and assimilates Christian parables to Plato's "myths"). He also lauds their contempt for death, their lifestyle of celibacy and restraint in food and drink, and—rather vaguely—their passion for "justice." This praise of Christianity is unique among pagan philosophers and, if it does not reflect a lost literary tradition, may be based on personal interaction with Christians in Alexandria or Rome, or possibly Galen witnessed one or more Christian martyrdoms in Pergamum or Smyrna during his sojourn there (see chapter 6), or in Rome before or after his return. Many such martyrdoms are attested, including that of Justin, beheaded in Rome some time during Galen's first stay there; but it is impossible to speculate based on his vague comment. As with Jews, Galen does not mention having Christian friends,

---

45   On the Jewish community at Rome, see Cappelletti (2006); Gruen (2002, chapter 1).

hearing Christian speakers debating in public, or reading Christian writings, although all are possible.[46]

We should also note that Galen's polemics against Jews and Christians are few (five passages in all, plus the praise of the Christian lifestyle just mentioned) and they betray no special hostility toward those religions; they pale in number, length, and vitriol by comparison with his polemics against Methodists, Erasistrateans, Pneumatists, and other medical or philosophical schools with which he disagreed, which is to say nearly all of them. He treats Judaism and Christianity like two (or one, for he sometimes seems to conflate them) of these sects and not as unusually alien or contemptible cults, and in general does not seem especially interested in either one of these religions. On the other hand, the reverse is not true. As early as 210—Galen was still alive— an anonymous theologian denounced a heretical group in Rome, led by one Theophrastus, a shoemaker, that had forsaken orthodox Christian doctrine for geometry and the tenets of certain Greek philosophers, including Euclid, Aristotle, and Galen. The heretics were, perhaps, responding to Galen's criticism of Christian irrationality; and perhaps even to *On the Usefulness of the Parts* in particular, which Origen, for example, may have read.[47]

In a famous passage from book 10 of *On the Usefulness of the Parts*, which describes the eye, Galen expounds certain geometric arguments on optics in obedience to a dream. He had been inclined to leave this passage out for fear of boring or offending his audience, of whose patience for this level of erudition he had a low opinion.[48] Galen states many times his belief that the dream came from a divinity, which he calls here a *daimon*. Following Plato and a long philosophical tradition, especially that of the Stoics, Galen believed that a human's highest, rational soul was a divine entity that resides within us, guides us, and speaks to us, in this case through a dream.[49]

---

46 Martyrdoms: Schlange-Schöningen (2003, 251). On the Christian community in Rome in Galen's time, see Lane Fox (1986, 268–69); Frend (1965, 121–26, 234–38).

47 Walzer (1949, 77); Nutton (1984b, 316–17); Eusebius, *Ecclesiastical History* 5.28.13–14; Epiphanius, *Adversos Haereses* 54.3.1.

48 *Usu Part.* 10.12 (3.812, 814K), 10.14 (3.835–36K).

49 See von Staden (2003, 31–43).

Galen took dreams very seriously, as most people in his culture also did. He often comments on this in passing: Empiricists, as I have mentioned, relied on dreams for many of the remedies they tested, probably including Aeschrion's mystical remedy for rabies, which Galen praised.[50] While Galen is critical of this sect's excessive use of dreams for pharmacological inspiration, he does not dispute the usefulness of dreams in many contexts and he trusts in them himself. Two pivotal events in his life had been triggered by dreams, as we have already seen: as a teenager, his father's decision to educate him in medicine; and his own recovery of health after self-treatment for a chronic illness at age twenty-seven (see chapter 2). A work *On Diagnosis from Dreams* survives under Galen's name; this brief text may be a summary or extract of a longer work,[51] perhaps his lost treatise on the subject of "dreams, birds, omens, and all of astrology" that he mentions having composed in *On the Natural Faculties* (*Nat. Fac.* 1.2, 2.29K).

When a patient, a sixty-year-old man, suffered from a tongue so badly swollen that it did not fit in his mouth, Galen and another physician disagreed on the remedy until the other doctor had "a very vivid dream in the night, and assented to my advice"; Galen washed out the patient's mouth with lettuce juice, and he was cured (*Meth. Med.* 14.8, 10.971–72K). At Alexandria Galen watched the sick plaster themselves in mud, "many spontaneously and using their own judgment, and many who had been advised by dreams" (*Simp. Med.* 9.1.2, 12.177K); he makes this observation without apparent comment or criticism. He also believed in the healing power of the god Asclepius, who often worked through dreams, and relates examples of this: a Thracian suffering from elephantiasis (leprosy) went to Pergamum on the advice of a dream, whereupon the god there (certainly Galen means Asclepius) advised him in another dream to cure his condition with medicine made from viper flesh.[52] Another worshipper of Asclepius at Pergamum dreamed that he might relieve a chronic pain in the side by arteriotomy of the

---

50　*Sect. Intro.* (1.66–67K); *Comp. Med. Gen.* 1.1 (13.366K); *Simp. Med.* 11.1.34 (12.356–57K).
51　See Harris (2009, 210 n. 520).
52　*Simp. Med.* 11.1.1 (12.315K); *Subfig. Emp.* 10 (78–79 Deichgräber).

hand, a case Galen considers similar to the chronic illness of his own youth, also cured by a dream (*Cur. Ven. Sect.* 23, 11.315K).[53]

Following Hippocrates and other predecessors, Galen recognized several sources of dreams, including some that might make sense to modern readers. A dream could reflect an imbalance of the humors, and a wrestler suffering from an excess of blood, for example, dreamed of standing in a cistern of blood; snow or ice would represent the cold, wet humor of phlegm, and so on. Thus, it was important to pay attention to the dreams of patients, though they might not always be interpreted correctly, as in the case of a man who dreamed his leg had turned to wood. Galen and the others treating him assumed that this symbolized something to do with slaves (an interpretation attested independently in an ancient dream book), but later the leg became paralyzed. But although some dreams arose from physiological imbalances, Galen also attributed a divine prophetic power to the soul, which could be the source of dreams, and clearly believed that some dreams were direct messages from a god.[54] In old age, pessimistically expressing agnosticism about the nature of the gods, he nevertheless insists that they must exist: "I say … that I know they exist from their deeds; for the equipment of animals is their deed, and also the things that they proclaim through omens and auguries and dreams" (*Plac. Propr.* 2, 173 Boudon-Millot and Pietrobelli).

Galen many times contrasts medical prognosis with divination by birds, omens, or astrology, always insisting that the two procedures are completely distinct from one another, however much his rivals might accuse him of divination when they did not understand one of his (preternaturally accurate) predictions. He sometimes associates divination with lowlife characters, magicians or sorcerers.[55] However, Galen did not reject divination nor disbelieve in its efficacy; on the contrary, besides the passage just quoted from

---

53 On Galen's relationship to Asclepius, see especially Schlange-Schöningen (2003, 223–35).

54 Examples come from *Dign. Insomn.* (6.832–35K). For translation and discussion, Oberhelman (1983). Further on dreams in Galen: Harris (2009, 64, 209–12); von Staden (2003, 21–28); Oberhelman (1993).

55 Divination vs. prognosis, and accusations of divination: e.g., *Febr. Diff.* 2.7 (7.354K); *Syn. Puls.* 6 (9.446–47K); *Loc. Affect.* 3.7 (8.168K), 5.8 (8.362K); *Praecog.* 1 (14.601–2K), 5 (14.625K). Lowlifes: e.g., *Opt. Med. Philosoph.* 1 (1.54–55K); *Simp. Med.* 10.2.6 (12.263K).

On My Own Opinions, another, for example, criticizes the Epicureans' belief that the gods do not intervene in the world, also accusing them of the view that the soul has no reasoning power, two opinions with which he clearly disagreed. He adds that "they also despise dreams and [divination from] birds and omens and all of astrology," as though this were part of his criticism, and mentions that he himself has produced a treatise, now lost, on these subjects (*Nat. Fac.* 1.12, 2.29K). In a passage from *On Prognosis*, Galen makes Eudemus deplore the degenerate education of the aristocrats of his time, who seek only the practical benefits from knowledge of geometry, arithmetic, philosophy, astronomy, *and divination* (*Praecog.* 1, 14.604–5K). He attributes a respect for augury to Hippocrates and also recounts at length how he himself witnessed a contest between a Greek augur and an Arab, praising the Greek as more "discriminating and skilled" (*technikos*; *Hipp. Acut. Vict.* 1.15, 15.441–42K). One of Galen's patients, after consulting a friend who was "amazingly successful" at augury, agreed to try Galen's remedy for elephantiasis, although he was in despair.[56] It is undeniable that Galen considered divination not only a skill at which one might be more or less adept but also an element of piety.[57]

Galen rejects as nonsense many magical practices, especially in a few passages from his treatise *On the Mixtures and Powers of Simple Drugs*—pharmacology being a discipline on the shadowy boundary of medicine and magic.[58] The incantations, libations, and offerings of incense that crept into some drug recipes he calls "stories not even useful for young boys" and dismisses love potions, spells for manipulating the dreams or thoughts of others, and so on as "ridiculous," as also amulets—very popular in antiquity for everything from protection against worms to help in childbirth. However, an intriguing reference in a much later source, Alexander of Tralles, writing in the sixth century C.E., tells us that in a lost work *On Homeric Medicine* Galen changed his mind about incantations after witnessing their efficacy in patients

---

56   *Simp. Med.* 11.1.1 (12.314–15K); *Subfig. Emp.* 10 (77–78 Deichgräber).

57   On Galen's views on divination, see von Staden (2003, 26).

58   *Simp. Med.* 6 *proem* (11.792–97K), 10.1 (12.251K), 10.2.16 (12.289–90K). See von Staden (2003, 19) for this and what follows.

suffering from scorpion stings or choking on chicken bones (*Therapeutica*, 2.475 Puschmann).

This is all the more plausible because in the same work *On…Simple Drugs* in which Galen ridicules incantations and amulets, he also tells the story of one young patient, a child, protected from epilepsy by a *periapton*—the word for "amulet," literally something "hanging round [the neck]," in this case a piece of peony root. Galen was dubious at first, but experiment revealed that the amulet worked:

> I know a child [*paidion*] who had no epileptic seizures at all for eight months, while he was carrying around this root, and when once the amulet [*periapton*] fell off from around his neck, straightaway he suffered an attack, and when another was hung around it he was fine again. I thought it best to remove it once more for the sake of experiment, and having done this, when again he suffered a seizure, we suspended a large and fresh portion of the root from his neck, and from then on the boy was completely healthy and never suffered an epileptic seizure.
>
> (*Simp. Med.* 6.3.10, 11.859–60K)

Galen adds a rationalizing explanation for the remedy: the patient inhaled particles of the root, or the root altered the air he breathed in some way—but my point is that his attitude to some magical practices is complicated and not simply dismissive.[59]

On many metaphysical questions he expressed agnosticism and doubt. He did not know the substance of the soul (despite having very specific views on its tripartite nature and its location in the body, as I have mentioned), nor whether it was or was not immortal, both points much debated in antiquity, and on which the major philosophical schools took differing stances. He professed a lack of curiosity on these questions, declaring them irrelevant to medical science. Similarly he confessed doubt on other great unknowns,

---

59 For similar examples of the rationalizing of magical practices and of the semi-magical idea of sympathy in Galen's pharmacology, see Keyser (1997).

the form and substance of the gods and of the creator whose providence and skill he believed was so amply attested in anatomy, and the mechanisms by which complex beings develop and grow. The theme of agnosticism is especially prominent in Galen's later works—*On the Formation of the Fetus, On My Own Opinions*. A lifetime of reflection produced no insight into the nature of the intelligence he had so long studied and revered, and it is possible that, although he does not say so, he found this discouraging:[60]

> Whether the universe is uncreated or created, and whether there is something outside it or not, I say that I don't know; and since I say that I don't know these things, it is obvious that I also do not know what kind of being is the creator of all things in the universe, and whether he is incorporeal or corporeal, and even more, where he lives.
>
> (*Plac. Propr.* 2, 172 Boudon-Millot and Pietrobelli)

> I confess that I am at a loss about the substance of the soul … and so I confess that I am in doubt about the formative cause of the fetus. For I see the highest wisdom and power in its construction, and I cannot admit that the soul in the seed, which is called vegetative by Aristotle and desiderative by Plato, and which the Stoics do not consider the soul at all, but nature, forms the embryo; for not only is it not wise, but it is wholly irrational; and on the other hand I am not entirely able to stand aloof from this, because of the similarity of offspring to their parents.
>
> (*Foet. Form.* 6, 4.700K)

---

60   Galen, *Plac. Propr.* 2–3 (172–74 Bouton-Millot and Pietrobelli), 7 (178 Boudon-Millot and Pietrobelli), 11 (182 Boudon-Millot and Pietrobelli); *Foet. Form.* 6 (4.699–702K); Nutton (1999, 142–44). On Galen's agnosticism about the soul in the context of debates on its mortality and substance in the ancient philosophical tradition, see von Staden (2000). Nutton's edition of *On My Own Opinions* is based mainly on a medieval Latin translation of an Arabic translation, supplemented by fragments and extracts in the original Greek and in Hebrew. It was only very recently that a complete Greek text of *On My Own Opinions* was discovered in a collection of thirteen Galenic treatises in a monastery in Thessaloniki (see Boudon-Millot and Pietrobelli 2005). It is important to note that the Arabic translation that was the basis for the Latin text censored Galen's references to the gods in order to downplay his polytheism (Boudon-Millot and Pietrobelli 2005, 192 n. 10).

Regarding, then, the role of religion in Galen's life: It is no exaggeration to say that Galen had a personal, spiritual relationship to Asclepius, whose power and efficacy he did not question, who had (most likely, if he was the god who sent dreams to Galen's father) chosen his career for him, and who had spoken to him personally in dreams and saved his life. Galen calls himself a *therapeutes*, or devotee, of the god, tracing this relationship to his miraculous cure at age twenty-seven, and reaffirms this in old age in *On My Own Opinions*. Here he claims to have no doubt that Asclepius exists, for "he showed me his power and providence in many other ways and also when he healed me" (*Plac. Propr.* 2, 173 Boudon-Millot and Pietrobelli).[61] He did not question Asclepius's medical prowess and was particularly impressed by the god's ability to command the obedience of his patients, always a challenge and potential source of frustration for himself and his colleagues. Patients would go fifteen days without drinking, for example, "which they would never do if a doctor had ordered it. For he [Asclepius] has a great influence to make the patient obey all of his commands."[62]

But his reverence for Asclepius is not the only way in which Galen could be described as pious; his piety was complex and many-faceted. It included some elements that may strike modern readers as irrational: Galen believed in direct and indirect communication between humans and external, supernatural forces, through dreams, omens, and astrology. That these supernatural forces moved in the world, cryptically and sometimes powerfully, he did not question, and in this he was a creature of his cultural environment. But Galen's piety also encompassed his highly philosophical reverence for the artistry of the creator, whose design he found inscribed so intricately in the anatomy of animals; and also his sense of the creator's mystery and inaccessibility. Galen studied and anatomized animals all his life without ever coming closer to understanding the factors explaining the complexity of nature,

---

61   He goes on in this passage to write that he has experienced the "power and providence" of the Dioscuri, the twins Castor and Pollux, at sea. Salvation from shipwreck is a frequently attested intervention of the gods, though healing is by far the most common. See MacMullen (1981, 50 with n. 7).

62   *Hipp. 6 Epid.* 4.8 (17B.137K). On the obedience of patients, see Mattern (2008a, 145–49).

a limitation he acknowledged repeatedly. It is difficult not to wish one could grant him a glimpse into the future so that he could see the answers in modern evolutionary biology, a field to which I have no doubt that Galen, if born today, would be a most eminent and enthusiastic contributor.

Galen wrote profusely during his first stay at Rome and dedicated most of what he produced to Boethus, his friend and—although Galen would never acknowledge this, excoriating rivals who enslaved themselves to dependency on the rich and powerful—his patron.[63] All the anatomical works he wrote in this period, mostly lost today—his four books on the voice, the lost original of *On Anatomical Procedures*, his two books *On the Causes of Respiration*, his works *On the Anatomy of Hippocrates* in five books and *On the Anatomy of Erasistratus* in three books, his treatises on the anatomy of living and of dead animals; as well as his major works *On the Doctrines of Hippocrates and Plato* and the first book of *On the Usefulness of the Parts*, composed before his departure from Rome—all these were for Boethus, although Galen also composed minor anatomical works for others, early Hippocratic commentaries, and, as I have mentioned, works "for beginners" as he began to take on the role of teacher in earnest. But Boethus departed Rome before Galen— shortly before, as Galen implies—as governor of Syria Palestina.[64] He never returned, although Galen kept in touch with him, sending him the seventeen books of *On the Usefulness of the Parts* when it was complete many years later; it is not impossible that Galen saw his friend again, when Galen returned home to Pergamum in 166, especially if the pharmacological journeys described in chapter 4 date to that period and not earlier, a contingency the evidence does not exclude. When Boethus died, Galen knew about it, although no expressions of grief survive in his works; this is also true of the death of his father, as I have mentioned, and of his childhood friend Teuthras, who will die of the "Great Plague" in 166.

It is only through a casual reference in Galen's commentary on a well-known passage from the Hippocratic treatise *On Joints* that we learn of

---

63 On patronage, see Mattern (2008a, 21–27 and 1999).
64 *Anat. Admin.* 1.1 (2.215, 217–18K); *Libr. Propr.* 1 (19.15–16K).

a major injury he suffered "in my thirty-fifth year" (that is in 164, for it happened in summer), while wrestling. It took place after the cure of Eudemus in the winter of 162/163, and after he wrote the treatise on venesection for Teuthras, in his thirty-fourth year; it is not clear where to place the injury in relation to the demonstration at Boethus's house or the treatment of the ex-consul's wife and child.

There can be no doubt that wrestling and other (as he would have called them) "gymnastic" exercises were part of his daily, or at least regular, routine. Galen's criticisms of heavy athletes are well known; these are men who (as he writes) spend most of their time working out at the gymnasium with trainers and are obsessed with victory and competition. The pensions they earned at major festivals could be lucrative, even for a single victory, and were heritable. But in Galen's view their lifestyle is a perverse extreme, their constitutions unbalanced; and they are not only ugly but useless as citizens and friends, as well as sexually impotent, having unusually small or shrivelled genitals. Even as he is merciless in his criticism of this group, it is also abundantly clear from his work that Galen considered gymnastic exercise in moderation a normal part of a healthy lifestyle. He prescribed daily visits to the gymnasium in his treatise *On Healthfulness* and was proud of his physical condition, boasting that he was stronger than many athletes.[65]

Galen dislocated his collarbone, an injury that today would be called an acromioclavicular joint separation. He writes:

> It is clear that the acromion, where it lies at the juncture of the collarbone (*kleis,* clavicle) and the shoulder blade (*omoplate,* scapula), is of cartilaginous bone, having ligaments originating in it, with which it binds together the ends of the bones …

---

65   Athletes ugly: *San. Tuend.* 5.3 (6.327K = 5.10, 157 Koch); *Adhort. Art.* 12 (131–32K). Useless: *Bon. Hab.* (4.753K, commenting on Plato's *Republic*); *Thras. Med. Gymn.* 45–46 (5.893–94K). Their unbalanced constitution: *Adhort. Art.* 9–10 (1.20–39K); *Bon. Hab.* (4.750–56K); *Thras. Med. Gymn.* (5.806–98K). Athletes and sex: *San. Tuend.* 6.14 (6.446K); *Simp. Med.* 9.3.23 (12.232K); *Hipp. 3 Epid.* 1.4 (17A.520–21K); *Loc. Affec.* 6.5 (8.451K); *Sem.* 1.15 (4.571K). Galen's boast: *Thras. Med. Gymn.* 46 (5.893–94K). On pensions, see Potter (2012, 279–86). See further discussion in Mattern (2008a, 128–30; 2008b); König (2005, 274–300).

an accurate description of the acromioclavicular joint, whose anatomy was already reasonably well known to the original, Hippocratic author (*Hipp. Artic.* 1.61, 18A.400K).

> And when this is displaced the collarbone is usually displaced as well [? some unclarity here], and for this reason the correction is to force the collarbone downward.

Galen's injury was severe and probably involved the muscle attachments, as well as the ligaments, which were totally separated. Three fingers' worth of space could be felt between the clavicle and the tip of the shoulder. The gymnasium's professional trainer—the *paidotribes*—apparently believed the injury to be a dislocation of the humerus, a common mistake, according to Hippocrates (*Artic.* 13, 3.313 Loeb); Galen himself believed the same thing. The trainer pulled down on the arm while pushing the head of the humerus, as he thought, from the armpit up toward its correct position, "and he did this skillfully" (Galen, *Hipp. Artic.* 1.61, 18A.402K).

By this time a crowd seems to have gathered; perhaps these injuries, and the commotion they caused as trainers and bystanders rushed to treat them, each with his own opinion about the problem and what should be done, were a common source of entertainment in the gymnasium. On Galen's orders they tried pulling on the arm and, in opposition, on the shoulder from above, while Galen himself placed his good hand in the armpit of the injured shoulder and tried to push the joint back into place. But at this point, "finding nothing in the armpit contrary to nature," he realized that the humerus was not, in fact, dislocated. "I ordered those who were stretching [the arm] together with the trainer to stop stretching and counter-stretching, for the joint had not fallen out." Galen's helpers thought he was backing off because of the pain and chided him as soft while continuing to pull mercilessly on the arm, until someone more knowledgeable happened along—Galen does not say who, but perhaps this was an educated, well-informed layman of the type he idealized—and Galen was able to explain that the problem was a displaced acromion, not the humerus. This required, according to

Hippocrates, conservative therapy with bandaging (and modern physicians agree, though today an injury of the severity Galen describes might be corrected with surgery). Galen asked for wool and oil and proceeded to the baths, where he soaked for a long time while he waited for his servants to bring the supplies.

In a child or adolescent the injury would have been easier to treat; but Galen was thirty-four, and the stretching had done extra damage. He resorted to a very tight bandage, more painful than most could have borne; most of his own patients, as he writes, "choose to suffer disability in the future," rather than endure the remedy. The bone "throbbed deeply"; the muscles of his arm and forearm atrophied; the shoulder felt so cold that he was forced to lie naked on a skin (it was summer, and very hot) while his servants poured warm oil over it night and day, collecting the runoff in a bowl by his feet and reheating it. This treatment he endured for forty days, and in the end the joint healed so well that no one could believe it had ever been injured (*Hipp. Artic.* 1.61, 401–4K).

Where did Galen live in Rome during this time, the four-year duration of his first stay? We know that he bought a house because his steward will later sell it at auction when he flees the city (see chapter 6). Galen also bought a country estate in Campania, the area around Naples, a location very popular among the Roman aristocracy—who often built luxurious villas on some of the farms they owned, viewing them as idyllic retreats from the demands of the city, where they could study and write in peace. These estates were working, income-producing farms with storerooms and presses for grapes and olives, and required a permanent staff of slaves and tenants; but they were also designed to entertain hordes of guests, with multiple bedrooms and dining rooms. We know nothing about Galen's estate in Campania except for one reference in the recently recovered treatise *Avoiding Distress* (*Peri Alupias* or, in Latin, *De Indolentia*), composed after the fire of 192 c.e., in which he mentions that he stored backup copies of his manuscripts in Campania against the contingency of fire in Rome, without complete success (*Ind.* 22–23, and see chapter 8). It is likely that Galen bought the estate during his first stay in Rome and did not sell it when he left; fleeing the city, he will tell his friends that he is going to Campania to avert their suspicions, as though this were a normal thing for him to do (see chapter 6).[66]

As for his house in Rome, I suspect, admittedly on little evidence, that in this period Galen lived in or near the district he calls the "Sandaliarion," which was the *vicus Sandaliarius* in Latin. He tells us that he lived close to his patient Eudemus (*Praecog.* 3, 14.613K), and that one day as he was leaving Eudemus's house he ran into his arch-rival Martianus in the Sandaliarion. Maritanus was himself on his way to visit Eudemus, suggesting that they crossed paths close to the latter's house (*Praecog.* 4, 14.620–21K). Although the street's name may reflect a history as the traditional locale for shoemakers, in Galen's time booksellers congregated there; he even describes a heated debate that broke out in this neighborhood between two of his readers over the authenticity of one of his own books, and there is some other evidence that it was a popular venue for intellectual contests and debates.[67] The Sandaliarion was in one of Rome's busiest and most central sectors (Region IV), and probably bordered on the northeast side of the Temple of Peace—another location Galen mentions as the site of public orations and debates, and which also housed one of Rome's largest libraries. Galen kept his most precious books and possessions in a supposedly fireproof storage room near the Temple of Peace, with tragic results when the area later burned; but by that time he had sold his original house in Rome and may have been living in another part of the city.

One final story must be told before we move on to the dark year 166, when Galen departed Rome amid terrifying rumors of a plague making its way to Italy from the east. The story of the slave of Maryllus must belong to this period, provided the venue is Rome and not Pergamum—certainly the event happened before Galen's departure, for he relates one version of the story (two survive) in the first book of *On the Doctrines of Hippocrates and Plato*, which Boethus took with him to his province. The first section of this work is lost in Greek and the story survives mainly in Arabic translation, although the Greek text picks up at the very end; Galen also told it again

---

66   On Galen's house in Campania, see Boudon-Millot and Jouana (2010, xxviii–xxxi).
67   See Mattern (2008a, 52–53); also Richardson (1992), s.v. "Vicus Sandalarius"; and Peter White (2009).

much later, in the seventh book of the surviving version of *On Anatomical Procedures*. It must have been one of his most famous cases, and perfectly epitomizes the anatomical virtuosity for which he became renowned in these early years of his career in Rome, when he burst so swiftly and astonishingly onto the scene of medicine, and quickly unseated all the ranking physicians in that cutthroat atmosphere.

The patient was a boy—Galen calls him *pais* and *paidarion*, terms he uses for children under the age of 15 or so; he does not seem to use the term of adult slaves, as some other ancient sources do.[68] The boy was, in any case, the slave of Maryllus "the mime-writer"; the latter apparently made his living composing the immensely popular theatrical performances to which the Roman populace flocked at festivals. The slave was much beloved, either as a sex object or, equally plausibly, he was Maryllus's natural son. In any case Maryllus spared no effort or expense to save his life.

The boy had been injured wrestling. The wound, an injury to the sternum, had formed an abscess; other physicians had twice tried to drain the pus, but the abscess would not close or cicatrize. One version of Galen's story says that a fistula had formed; and he appears to say that the patient's heart had been displaced to the left. Thus, several months after the injury, it was obvious that the boy was seriously or fatally ill. He had developed osteomyelitis of the sternum following the trauma.

Maryllus called together several physicians, including Galen, to consult on the case. They all agreed that the affected part of the sternum needed to be cut out; no one, however, dared to perform the operation, knowing that the slightest error would result in a catastrophic perforation of the pleural membrane. But Galen had vivisected hundreds of animals. He had held their beating hearts in his fingers. Still, I imagine an awkward silence in which he took a deep breath to steady himself before he spoke up. "I said that I would excise the sternum without creating what the physicians, for their part, were calling a 'perforation.'"

---

68   On Galen's terms for children and also on the relationship between *pais* and "slave," see Mattern (2008a, 108–9).

Galen is silent on most of the details of the operation—perhaps he strapped the young patient to one of the boards he used to vivisect animals, or perhaps assistants held him down, as Celsus advises when describing surgery to remove kidney stones. Galen may have performed the surgery in a bath house, which is the setting he recommends for vivisection of an animal's heart, because it is warm there; if so he would have needed to be near the door, or else not indoors at all but outside, in a courtyard, for no artificial light was, of course, available.

He probably used no anesthesia. Two or three brief references from the Roman period mention giving mandrake to those about to be cut or cauterized, so that they will not feel pain—a passage in Pliny the Elder's *Natural History* of the first century C.E., and another in Dioscorides' famous drug encyclopedia, which was probably Pliny's source for this item. But surgical texts, notably Celsus and Soranus, the most substantial discussions of surgery to survive from antiquity, mention no form of anesthesia; and Celsus clearly thought the patient's suffering was a problem to be managed with force and fortitude. It is unclear whether anesthesia was commonly or ever used, perhaps because the dangers of overdose were well known. Galen mentions mandrake many times as a drug with wet, cooling properties, causing deep sleep and numbing the senses, but does not describe using this or any other anesthesia for surgery.[69]

The operation went well at first—the infection had spared the veins and arteries around the wound—but when Galen removed the affected bone, he saw, to his despair, that part of the pericardium beneath had putrefied and disintegrated, forcing him to excise it. Then, "we saw the heart as clearly as we see it when we deliberately lay it bare during [animal] dissection."

---

69   Pliny, *Naturalis historia*, 25.150; Dioscorides, *Materia medica* 4.75. On mandrake as anesthetic, see Ramoutsaki, Askitopoulou, and Konsolaki (2002) and von Hintzenstern (1989); the former article should be used with caution as many of the references to ancient sources are problematic. For a review of the exiguous evidence for anesthesia in Mediterranean antiquity, Nunn (1989). Mandragora in Galen: *Temp.* 2.2 (1.585K); *Meth. Med.* 3.2 (10.171K); *Simp. Med.* 7.12.4 (12.67K); *Comp. Med. Loc.* 3.1 (12.644K); and many other references. On the dangers of overdose of mandragora (and opium): *Comp. Med. Loc.* 8.3 (13.157K); also *Hipp. Aph.* 2.17 (17B.477–78K). Besides Pliny and Dioscorides, the third possible reference to mandrake as surgical anesthesia is in the obscure *Herbarium* of Apuleius or Pseudo-Apuleius.

Galen was pessimistic about the boy's recovery, but against all odds he survived, and was still alive many years later when Galen wrote the seventh book of *On Anatomical Procedures*. The wound closed, and scar tissue replaced the excised tissue and bone, protecting the heart. I have no doubt that this story is true. Galen's audience for both of the versions he recounts would have included witnesses to the event itself, or people who heard about it at the time. Even today, it is difficult not to be impressed by the surgical skill and speed implied here, given the primitive conditions under which Galen was working; and by the luck of both patient and doctor, for without antisepsis this operation should have been fatal almost always. But imagine, in that day and age, being the patient, who had suffered an experience perhaps unique in human history at the time: his heart had been exposed, and he had lived! He had been saved by surely the world's greatest and most skilled—surely its most celebrated—physician. The story rivaled the most bizarre and fantastical of Asclepius's miracles, and put the healing powers of Jesus and the early Christian saints, relatively mundane by comparison, to shame. I cannot explain why Galen does not include it in *On Prognosis*, which narrates his rise to fame in Rome; perhaps because Maryllus's social status, as part of the entertainment industry, was marginal, and he was thus not part of the aristocratic circle whose stories mostly occupy that treatise. But it seems likely that this event, unparalleled in any surviving ancient source, sealed Galen's reputation as Rome's most brilliant physician.[70]

---

70   The story of Maryllus's slave is told in *Plac. Hipp. Plat.*, Testimonies and Fragments 7 (72–76 de Lacy and 5.181K) and *Anat. Admin.* 7.12–13 (2.631, 632–33K). The first quotation ("I said that I ... ") is *Anat. Admin.* 7.13 (2.633K); the second quotation ("We saw the heart ... ") is *Plac. Hipp. Plat.*, Testimonies and Fragments 7 (74 de Lacy, tr. de Lacy). For slaves as the natural children of their masters, see Betzig (1992).

Chapter Six

MARCUS AURELIUS AND THE PLAGUE

alen had been in Rome for about four years when he departed suddenly and in a hurry. This was probably in the summer in 166.[1] Ordering one of his slaves to stay behind and put his house up for auction, he headed south—"pretending," he writes, "to depart for Campania," where he owned other property.

> Leaving one servant behind to guard the property [at Rome], I instructed him to wait for one of the ships departing for Asia, and then in a single day to hire one of the hustlers from the Subura to sell the property, depart immediately, embark on a boat and arrive at the homeland by way of Sicily. This was done a little later—I was at Campania, and then from there I hurried to Brundisium; once there, I decided to cross [the Adriatic] on the first boat that was putting out, whether it was sailing for Dyrrhachium [in modern Albania] or for Greece.
>
> (*Praecog.* 9, 14.648K)

What explains the haste and secrecy with which Galen left for Pergamum? Before this passage from his autobiographical work *On Prognosis*, he names

---

1   Schlange-Schöningen (2003, 141–42).

two anxieties behind his departure: first, the jealousy of his rivals had inten-sified; second, he was afraid of being dragged back to Rome and detained by a powerful person or by the emperors, and worried that they might send sol-diers after him to fetch him back. For his reputation had grown to the point where he might well find himself pressed into service by those in a position to command him.

And so, Galen departed "like a runaway slave." His friends looked for him, only to be told by his sole remaining servant that he had departed for Campania, with the truth dawning on them only gradually. It is with some satisfaction that Galen imagines their chagrin—for he had long threatened to leave what he describes as the corrupt and competitive atmosphere of the city, and his resolve had apparently been doubted.

But what specific circumstance might have precipitated Galen's decision to leave so abruptly? It is, frankly, difficult to make sense of his account. The event he refers to at this point in *On Prognosis*—the stunning cure of Boethus's wife (see chapter 5), and in particular the extravagant reward of 400 gold pieces, which provoked new heights of envy and hostility in his rivals— almost certainly occurred much earlier, a year or even two years before his departure.[2] Writing years after the events he describes, Galen may have trans-posed episodes in his mind. Furthermore, he makes it clear that he did not leave as soon as his concerns first arose, but had to wait for a better political situation in Pergamum.

That Galen was unsettled by ramped-up hostility from his enemies is hardly implausible; enemies could be dangerous. In the beginning of this treatise Galen's friend Eudemus warns him that disgruntled rivals might plot to poison him (*Praecog.* 1,14.601K; 4, 624K). To a modern reader this, of course, sounds paranoid and hyperbolic; it would not have to Eudemus's contemporaries. Poison was a widely feared hazard and a common criminal charge among the Roman aristocracy: both professional poisoners and pro-fessional food-tasters (the latter had their own trade organization) are well

---

2   Nutton (1979, 202–3); see also Hankinson (2008, 14). For fuller discussion of the date of Galen's departure, see Boudon-Millot (2007a, lxiii–lxvii); Schlange-Schöningen (2003, 142–45).

attested. Eudemus offers as example the story of another doctor who had been poisoned along with two servants after a successful public demonstration of his skill (*Praecog.* 4, 14.624K). Even more plausible is Eudemus's claim that the renowned doctor Quintus—who had practiced in Rome a generation before Galen—fled charges of murdering his patients (*Praecog.* 1, 14.602K). Spurious denunciations were a time-honored weapon against one's enemies in the upper echelons of Roman society. In the same treatise, Galen mentions being called a sorcerer or a diviner by rivals jealous of the accuracy of his prognoses. Some kinds of divination were a respectable part of mainstream culture, as I have mentioned, and Galen does not seem to mind when Eudemus compares him to Apollo, the god of prophecy. But such a reputation also created a gray area that enemies might exploit; divination could be practiced by marginal characters for treasonous purposes, and sorcery was a capital crime in Roman law. Galen may have feared prosecution, however baseless. Living a life of relentless and continuous public conflict, it is hardly unreasonable that he came to fear for his social standing or even for his life.[3]

As Galen's reputation grew and friends began to speak of praising him to the emperor, Galen asked them to wait for his signal to do so, or so he tells us (*Praecog.* 9, 14.648K). But his claim to be afraid of a summons from the emperor—and to prefer the friendly values and homegrown atmosphere of Pergamum to the corruption of the capital city—strikes one as possibly disingenuous; at the very least, Galen's feelings were probably mixed. On the one hand, his fear of being summoned by a soldier—a sudden knock on the door that would change his life forever, in ways he would be powerless to resist—rings true enough. In that time, place, and situation, one could not assert liberties or rights. Galen will later express his resentment at the duties imposed on him by his service at court and will narrowly avoid a prolonged stint on military campaign with the emperor. On the other hand, for many

---

3   On poisoning among the Roman aristocracy, see Gilbert Watson (1966, 82–91). On sorcery: *Praecog.* 1 (14.601–3K). On Galen's reputation for divination: Tamsyn S. Barton (1994, 140–43). For an illuminating discussion of the trial of Galen's contemporary Apuleius for magical seduction, see Bradley (1997). For a recent discussion of Roman laws against magic, which by the early third century included some types of divination, see Rives (2003).

Greek intellectuals, an invitation to join the imperial staff or entourage was the pinnacle of a career and most doctors would have considered the position of "physician to the emperor"—*archiatros*—the highest social standing that they could hope to achieve.[4] The *fons et origo* of all patronage in the empire, the monarch's power was more social than strictly political. Being talked about and praised to the emperor, as Galen says he began to be after he cured Boethus's wife, was a development that many among the Greco-Roman elite desired fervently, and there is an element of braggadocio in Galen's mention of it here. Galen's contemporary, the sophist Aelius Aristides, met the emperors just once; and yet his writings recount how they haunted his dreams, where he hangs on their praise.[5]

It is at this point, then, that the Emperor Marcus Aurelius begins to cast his shadow over Galen's life. Marcus was a hard man, with a lifelong reputation for austerity. Renowned for his philosophical education, he also lived up to the Stoic precepts upon which he expounded. Tradition held that it was his studious and frugal lifestyle as a youth that inspired the emperor Hadrian to single out Marcus at the age of seventeen. When, in 138 C.E., the dying emperor adopted Antoninus Pius as his successor (the adoption of adult heirs being common among the Roman aristocracy), he also insisted that Pius adopt Marcus, then called Marcus Annius Verus, as well as Marcus's future co-ruler, Lucius Ceionius Commodus (known to historiography as Lucius Verus, and not identical with Marcus Aurelius's son and heir, later to be known as Commodus), as yet a child only seven years old. Thus, Hadrian established the imperial succession for the next two generations.

Marcus would be remembered as a monarch who remained impassive in joy and in grief, who lived soberly and unpretentiously, who sold treasures from the imperial household rather than raise taxes to finance his wars, and

---

4   On Galen's position under Marcus Aurelius, see Schlange-Schöningen (2003, 187–98). On *archiatroi* more generally, see Mattern (2008a, 7–8 with note 16; 1999a, 6–7); Nutton (1977, 193–98).

5   Reputation with the emperor: Mattern (1999a, 12–14). Aristides: e.g., *Sacred Tales* 1.23, 33, 36, and 46–49 (praise). On the emperor's role in Roman politics and society, Millar (1992) is the most important reference.

heard cases until late in the day instead of relaxing and enjoying the usual evening entertainments. The historians who later wrote of his reign extolled him as a model of the philosophical life and of the Stoic ethics long fashionable among the Roman ruling class. Their only major criticism was his perhaps excessive tolerance of his wife's rumored infidelities with ballet dancers and gladiators. The people of Rome, however, resented his austerity and his distaste for the bloody gladiatorial games and mime performances that they loved—all the more so when Marcus curtailed the number of dance performances permitted and conscripted gladiators into the army.[6]

He spent most of the second half of his reign on campaign in central Europe, fighting Rome's most-feared tribal enemies. And it was in the course of this continual series of wars that he wrote his *Meditations* in Greek—a work in twelve books on Stoic philosophy. Today Marcus is one of the most important Stoic writers whose work survives. Stoic ethics, which arose in a world much more difficult to bear than the modern one, dictated that virtue itself was the only good, and its pursuit the only purpose of life; they emphasized sober and frugal living, duty to society, control of the passions or emotions, and living in harmony with the providential universe, which often translated into impassive acceptance of fate. Ancient sources praise Marcus as having lived their tenets (even if, understandably, he found it difficult to achieve a materially simple life amidst the pomp of the palace and court). Marcus's father died when he was three years old. Eight of his fourteen known children by his wife Faustina predeceased him, most of them dying in the first five years of life; and Faustina herself died in 170, after thirty years of marriage. Marcus never remarried, instead taking a former slave as concubine.[7]

Lucius Verus, born Lucius Ceionius Commodus, ten years Marcus's junior, was known as more the pleasure-loving and frivolous of Antoninus Pius's two heirs. When Pius died, he and Marcus ruled together for seven years until Lucius died, probably of the plague, early in 169 (see below). Galen mentions his death but does not discuss Lucius in any other context

---

6   On Marcus's life, see Birley (1987); on the imperial court in his reign also Champlin (1980, chapter 7).

7   On Marcus's children: Birley (1987, Appendix 2).

and may not have known him well or at all. This was the empire's first experience with joint rule. But from the beginning of their reign, Marcus clearly outranked his younger brother-by-adoption and held most of the imperial authority.

Marcus's own health was notoriously frail, abdominal and chest pain being his main complaints (Cass. Dio 72[71].6.3). The Stoic emperor's preoccupation with his health—evident in his surviving correspondence with his former tutor and friend, Cornelius Fronto—surprises some modern readers, but he may be forgiven this quality in an environment where infectious disease killed rich and poor indiscriminately, and any symptom might herald serious illness or even death. As we saw in chapter 5, an amateur knowledge of medicine was essential to the intellectual image of many aristocrats. And it is in this context—rather than just because Marcus needed to stay healthy—that the emperor included physicians in his entourage.[8]

Galen writes with scorn of doctors who advance their careers by flattering and fawning on aristocrats, joining them at dinner and accompanying them on trips—practices he perceives as all too typical. He himself, as he claims, succeeded by virtue of public displays of excellence that won him reputation, followers, and respect. Still, social connections and favors were the standard currency in Roman society, and later in his very same treatise, *On Prognosis*, which opens with a denunciation of sycophantic doctors, Galen boasts about his cure of the emperor's digestive problem (*Praecog.* 11, 14.657–61K). Indeed, he records the exact words of the emperor's praise on this occasion. In his scorn for those who court the aristocracy, he perhaps "protests too much," defensive about his dependence on their favor.[9]

It was hardly unreasonable, then, if Galen's friends doubted his professed resolve to leave Rome at the earliest opportunity. It is a common theme in

---

8   On Marcus's "hypochondria," see Bowersock (1969, 72–73). Whether people in the second century generally suffered more anxiety about their health than those in other eras, as he asserts, is difficult to prove, but it is possible that the high prestige of medicine among elites at this time encouraged more talk about health and sickness.

9   On doctors and patronage, see Mattern (1999a) for references. On the idea of patronage in general, the classic work is Saller (1982).

Galen, after all, as in any number of other Greco-Roman writers, that they do only reluctantly and under coercion the things that advance their reputation and standing in society. Galen often makes this claim about writing books, for example.[10]

In any case, despite his concerns that the emperor's attention might be drawn to him at any minute, Galen was unable to depart before receiving news of the end of what he calls *stasis* back at Pergamum. As discussed above in chapter 3, *stasis* was a loaded term, most likely referring here to heightened tensions and outbreaks of violence in the city. In any event, dire conditions now prevented his immediate return.[11]

In another work, his treatise *On My Own Books*, Galen mentions an entirely different motive for his departure, namely the outbreak of the deadly disease he refers to only as "the plague": "When the great plague began, I immediately left the city and traveled to my homeland" (*Libr. Propr.* 1, 19.15K). If the plague came to Rome with the army of Lucius Verus, which had been fighting the kingdom of Parthia in the East (as attested in one late and not especially reliable source claiming that a "pestilential vapor" had escaped its container, a golden casket housed in a temple of Apollo, when one of Lucius's soldiers accidentally pierced it with his sword), then in Rome itself the epidemic was as yet only a shadow on the horizon, a rumor of a calamity ravaging the army. For Galen is specific that he left Rome before the army returned.[12]

Galen's recollections in *On My Own Books*, produced late in life, may be clouded, and it is hard to understand why he does not mention the plague in the more detailed discussion of his flight from Rome in *On Prognosis*, composed at least fifteen years earlier, in 178. Yet if his memory is accurate on this point, then in 166 Galen fled not from the plague, but toward it—motivated, perhaps, by worry about his hometown and a desire to be there for his people. Galen had relatives, a house, and childhood friends

---

10   Mattern (2008a, 14–15).

11   *Stasis* at Pergamum: *Praecog.* 9 (14.648K); see also 4 (14.622K).

12   *Praecog.* 9 (14.649–50K). Vapor: SHA *Verus* 8.1–2.

at Pergamum, the city that, even in old age, he continued to refer to as his home. It is possible that horrific rumors reached him at about this time. The plague struck the city of Smyrna, about 66 miles from Pergamum, in 165, where it infected the household of Aelius Aristides, who barely survived it. This would perhaps explain Galen's urgency and the extraordinary precautions he took not to be recalled or detained at Rome. In the end, though, Pergamum may have escaped the plague's ravages—Galen seems to describe his first major confrontation with the terrible disease at Aquileia in Italy, as I shall discuss below.[13]

In the event, Galen and his household embarked not for Dyrrhachium or for the Greek mainland, but for Cassiope, on the island of Corcyra (*Praecog.* 9, 14.649K). From there he sailed to Corinth, and proceeded on foot to Athens, where he could embark to cross the Aegean.[14] Between Corinth and Athens—as he writes in an anecdote illustrating the dangers of the passion of anger—he fell in with a friend, a man from Gortyn, on Crete, who was traveling with his own coterie of slaves. The man's weakness, as Galen writes, was a savage temper—and as with many of his contemporaries, the paradigmatic manifestation of anger was violence against slaves. This man, Galen writes, would habitually hit and kick his servants and beat them with leather straps or blunt objects. Near Athens the man met up with two of his young slaves, who failed to produce a certain item of luggage he had apparently asked them to bring; whereupon he assaulted them with a knife, bringing it crashing down on their heads. As Galen writes,

> He used not the flat part (which would have produced no serious result), but the edge of the knife. The knife cut straight through the sheath, and inflicted two very major injuries on each of their heads—for he hit each of them twice.
>
> (*Anim. Affect. Dign.* 4, 5.18–20K)

---

13   On Galen's departure and the plague, see Schlange-Schöningen (2003, 145). Aristides: *Sacred Tales* 2.38–44 with Duncan-Jones (1996, 118) and Behr (1968, 96 n. 9).
14   See Nutton (1973, 168).

As blood spurted from these wounds, the master fled in panic, perhaps fearing prosecution if the slaves died. Quickly stepping in to treat the victims, Galen saved their lives, following which his contrite and distraught friend begged Galen to beat him as punishment. Galen only laughed at him and delivered a moral lecture; which seems to have had some effect, as the man's behavior, he writes, improved greatly afterward.

Galen spent the following two years at Pergamum.[15] Of his time there he tells us only that he edited a few books he had written before his departure for Rome and that were now brought back to him. He mentions in particular one work, *On the Motion of the Chest and Lungs*, written in his youth at Smyrna for a friend who had since died. Someone else had, apparently, tried to circulate the book under his own name, but without success. Here as elsewhere, Galen is proud of having a discerning and loyal audience that can recognize his work. He was, however, embarrassed by the contents of the treatise, which did not contain his more recent discoveries on the intercostal muscles—some of his most important contributions to anatomy—and which, as he writes, he had never intended for a public audience. Galen updated the treatise and later wrote a fuller exposition of the same subject in *On the Causes of Respiration*.[16] Aside from this, he tells us, "I went about my usual business." If he had been concerned about a visitation of plague on his homeland, that contingency never materialized (*Libr. Propr.* 2, 19.16–17K).

Late in the year 168 Galen received the message he so dreaded—"a letter from the emperors, summoning me" (*Libr. Propr.* 2, 19.17K). The emperors were preparing a military campaign and required his presence. It is unclear whether Marcus and Lucius wanted him in attendance as a personal physician, or whether he was simply to treat soldiers wounded in battle; the army

---

15　On the chronology, see Schlange-Schöningen (2003, 146–47). In *On My Own Books* Galen writes that his summons to Aquileia came "immediately" after his return to Pergamum, but this must be inaccurate.

16　*On the Motion of the Chest and Lungs*: *Anat. Admin.* 1.1 (2.217–18K), 8.2 (2.659–60K). An English translation of the short extant treatise *On the Causes of Respiration* is available in Furley and Wilkie (1984), but this is probably not identical with the work Galen refers to here and elsewhere; that work ran to two books. What survives is probably a summary by a later editor. See ibid., 231–32.

employed many doctors.[17] The former explanation seems more probable, though, for Galen tells us that "a discussion had arisen about those who demonstrated both medicine and philosophy with deeds rather than words; and not a few of those around them [the emperors] named me in this category"; these seem better qualifications for a personal physician than for a military doctor (*Praecog.* 9, 24.649K).

With Lucius's war against the Parthians concluded, the co-rulers were gathering an army at Aquileia, in northern Italy, for a planned assault on "the Germans"—tribes in the area later known as Bohemia. We have only fragmentary information about the complex events of this war, depicted on the relief that winds around the Column of Marcus Aurelius in Rome and mentioned in a few historical sources. Its most famous episode was a rain miracle that saved Marcus's army from sure defeat, and for which the Christians eventually took credit, claiming that the faithful of the Twelfth Legion had prayed successfully for rain. Early in the conflict, in 170, the tribes known to the Romans as the Quadi and the Marcomanni invaded Italy and besieged Aquileia. Over the next years Marcus subjugated them and occupied their territory, intending to add two new provinces to the empire (abandoned after his death by his son and successor, Commodus).[18] He spent the rest of his life on the northern frontier, save for two years from 175 to 177, when he toured the East in the wake of the rebellion of Avidius Cassius, governor of Syria, and then visited Rome to establish Commodus as co-emperor.

Galen is justly proud of his reputation "for both medicine and philosophy"—won not just through talk, as he insisted all his life, but through practical demonstrations. And he is proud to be recognized as a doctor and philosopher by the emperors themselves. Still, we need not doubt that he obeyed the summons with reluctance or, at the very least, deep ambivalence. The prospect of a potentially long campaign—in the event, Marcus Aurelius's German war dragged on for nine years—in what Galen and other educated people

---

17   See Patricia Ann Baker (2004); Cruse (2004, 93–100); Davies (1989, chapter 10).

18   On the campaigns, see Birley (1987, chapter 8). On Marcus's temporary occupation of territory in Bohemia, see Cass. Dio 71[72].20.2.

thought of as barbaric, barely habitable territory cannot have been appealing. "Germans" were, in Greco-Roman ethnography, fierce, uncouth, aggressive, drunken, nomadic, and totally uncivilized—in extreme descriptions, they are said to dress in skins or leaves and eat raw meat, utterly insensible to the rule of law—while "free Germany" itself was a damp, frostbitten land of dense woods, swamps, and bizarre animals. Galen's own work shows evidence that he bought into the prevailing stereotypes of northern tribal peoples.[19] Certainly, compared to the more developed urban environment he was accustomed to, life in the frontier provinces was rough and isolated; not to speak of the hardships associated with accompanying an army on campaign in enemy territory. But Galen had no choice. "By necessity, I went" (*Libr. Propr.* 2, 19.18K).

To reach Aquileia Galen made his way first to Alexandria Troas, on the far north of Turkey's western coast. From there he sailed to Thessalonike via the island of Lemnos, where he hoped to buy some of its most famous product, the stamped signets of sacred earth discussed in chapter 4. As I have described, he was intent on finding a hill sacred to the god Hephaestus and its temple of Philoctetes, but to his dismay, Galen learned that the ship had put in at the wrong city; his purchase would have to wait until he made a return trip to Asia.

On his arrival in Aquileia, Galen encountered the plague full-force:

> When I reached Aquileia, the plague descended as never before; so that the emperors immediately fled to Rome with a few soldiers, while most of us struggled for a long time to stay alive, and a great many died—not only because of the plague, but also because these things were happening in the middle of winter.
>
> (*Libr. Propr.* 2, 19.18K)

The younger co-emperor, Lucius Verus, himself died on the road to Rome. It seems that Galen met the emperors in person at Aquileia—most likely

---

19   On the ethnography of Germany, see Isaac (2004, chapter 12); Mattern (1999b, 70–78). Barbarians in Galen: *Plac. Hipp. Plat.* 3.3 (5.303K); *Simp. Med.* 2.20 (11.513–14K).

for the first time, for he writes as though they knew him by reputation only before that juncture. The passage above strongly suggests that he did not follow the emperors to Rome and—although he had another conversation with Marcus in 169, in which he convinced the emperor to let him stay in Italy (see below)—that conversation happened in Aquileia on Marcus's return to the front, not at the capital. Marcus and Galen were not together in Rome, then, until the former returned after many years, in 176.[20]

What exactly was the disease that Galen faced in Aquileia? He calls it only "the plague" or "the great plague," and in later years "the long plague" or "the very long plague." Lethal outbreaks of epidemic disease were common in antiquity; the historical record is full of casual references to episodes of this kind, always using the general term "plague" or "pestilence" with no attempt to distinguish one visitation clinically from another. The most common epidemic diseases were probably typhoid, typhus, malaria, possibly cholera, and various diarrheal diseases; tuberculosis was also endemic in Rome and other areas, and bubonic plague is attested beginning in the sixth century C.E.[21] Recall that Galen himself described a gruesome epidemic that he witnessed in 152 C.E., while still a young man studying at Pergamum, that consumed the skin and even the flesh from its victims' bodies. As for the "great plague"— Galen never names the disease that he battled for years, distinguishing it from other epidemics only by its magnitude and duration, in which it stood alone.

Galen is not the only author of the Antonine period to record his experiences with the plague. Aelius Aristides recounts horrific details from its assault on the city of Smyrna. He was in the suburbs at the time; nevertheless, all his neighbors and his entire household fell ill. His beloved foster son Hermias died, and so intense was the misery and suffering in his household at its worst stage, that it seemed anyone who so much as tried to move died on the spot. Aristides himself fell ill, and the doctors attending him predicted his death, but he recovered following a diet prescribed in his dreams by the god Asclepius (*Sacred Tales* 2.38–44, 5.25). Most other contemporary descriptions

---

20   Schlange-Schöningen (2003, 175).
21   On plagues in ancient historiography, Duncan-Jones (1996).

have been lost, though many sources from the later imperial period mention the Antonine plague.[22]

Once established, the plague returned in a series of epidemic outbreaks over several years. Galen frequently describes it as "the very long plague." Although most of the evidence for the plague's demographic effects is indirect, what survives suggests a catastrophe of the highest magnitude. In Egypt, whole villages practically disappear from the tax rolls, wiped out by a combination of mortality and the flight of whatever inhabitants managed to survive. Huge gaps or dramatic reductions in the documentary record, too—papyri from Egypt, inscriptions on stone from the city of Rome, the military diplomas issued to discharged soldiers, which mainly survive from the Balkan region—occur in the decade after 166 or so. Public building in Italy dropped by more than one-half.[23]

About 25 percent of the Roman Empire's population—perhaps fifteen million people—may have died in the Antonine pandemic, if it was the first visitation of smallpox on a virgin population (see below). Areas directly affected probably suffered much heavier losses, mortality being very high among those infected, but communications in the empire were not everywhere easy and efficient, and some areas escaped the plague.[24] The city of Rome, however, did not. Like Aelius Aristides, whose household in Smyrna was decimated, Galen lost almost all of his slaves at Rome, as well as his good friend and compatriot Teuthras (*Ind.* 35).

Among ancient sources on the plague, Galen is the only one who describes its symptoms, but no detailed discussion of these survives in his work and we have only scattered and passing references. It is difficult to make diagnoses based on ancient descriptions of diseases even when they are very specific, but modern scholars have most often identified the plague Galen describes

---

22   See Duncan-Jones (1996, 118–20).

23   For the demographic and economic effects of the plague, Scheidel (2010b, 2002); Duncan-Jones (1996). Contemporary literary and historical sources on the plague are collected in Duncan-Jones (1996, 118–20).

24   Twenty-five percent: Scheidel (2002, 100–101). On the regionality of the plague, see Duncan-Jones (1996, 134–36).

as smallpox.[25] Few physicians practicing today have seen a case of smallpox, which was eradicated in 1977, but after 168 this scourge may have been a major factor shaping Galen's life and practice. If so, it was probably the first visitation of smallpox in the Mediterranean region, or possibly the first such visitation in over a millennium. No disease like smallpox appears in Greek literature before Galen. The best candidate, the plague that struck Athens in 429 B.C.E. and was described by the historian Thucydides in his most famous passage, is now thought to be typhoid fever.[26] The weight of literary tradition led Galen himself to identify disease he battled with the one described by Thucydides (*Simp. Med.* 9.1.4, 12.189K), but he writes as though it were new to his experience, rather than something he had seen before.

Most clinical descriptions of smallpox in modern times have emphasized the disease's virulent rash as its most pronounced and characteristic symptom, the high fever that strikes patients in the first few days of its onset not being

---

25   See Littman and Littman (1973).

26   Leading candidates for the plague of Athens have been smallpox, measles, typhus, and typhoid fever; typhoid fever is implicated in recent DNA testing of dental pulp from a mass grave in the Kerameikos district, but these results are still being debated and are not conclusive. See Papagrigorakis et al. (2006). The phylogenetic study of Li et al. (2007) suggests that virulent smallpox diverged from its less aggressive modern clades some 6,300 years ago in East Asia and assumes that its radiation began around 400 C.E., the date it assigns to the first appearance of a good description of smallpox (in the work of Ge Hong or Ko Hung, who however wrote in the first half of the fourth century C.E. and describes it as a disease imported from the west or from tribal peoples, perhaps in the first century C.E.). The authors use this event to calibrate the molecular clock timing the virus's evolution. In this view, smallpox would not have reached the Mediterranean until much later, but the accuracy of the timeline depends on what seems like an arbitrary use of historical evidence. Shchelkunov (2011) proposes a different scenario using different molecular dates, speculating that smallpox may have been responsible for the fall of Bronze Age civilization in the Mediterranean region around 1100 B.C.E., an intriguing suggestion that would account for the possible findings of smallpox virus and antibody in the mummy of the pharaoh Rameses V, who died in the twelfth century B.C.E. (Hopkins 2002, 14–16; Sandison and Tapp 1998, 44; Fenner et al. 1988, 210–11). However, he also suggests that the disease died out with the collapse of the population and that the virus re-emerged in India after 500 B.C.E. The study of Hopkins (2002), originally published in 1983, and the classic essay of Fenner et al. (1988, chapter 5, "The History of Smallpox and Its Spread around the World"; see p. 216 on Ko Hung) are still the best treatments of smallpox in the ancient historical record. The online collection of information by the Center for Infectious Disease Research and Policy at the University of Minnesota is especially helpful: http://www.cidrap.umn.edu/cidrap/content/bt/smallpox/index.html.

nearly as specific to smallpox. Galen describes a black, often ulcerated rash, with eruptions "close together" over the whole body; these eventually formed scabs that fell away. He considered the rash a hopeful sign, as also the excretion of black diarrhea.[27] This is because he viewed the plague as one of many diseases caused by an excessive accumulation of black bile. His description of the rash as black and resembling a deposit of ashes on the skin (*Meth. Med.* 5.12, 10.367K) suggests the late-forming variety of hemorrhagic smallpox, a presentation rare in modern times, and almost always fatal; it is possible that the disease he faced took a different, more virulent form than that described by modern physicians in populations long exposed to it.

Galen's view and experience of the disease reflect the medical knowledge and predispositions of his times, as, for example, in the story he tells of one patient with the plague:

> In the beginning of this great plague—if only it would end!—a certain youth, who had been ill for nine days, suffered from ulcers erupting on his whole body, just like almost everyone else who survived. On that day he coughed a little. On the next day when he bathed, he coughed more strongly and he expelled with the cough what they call an *ephelkis* [scab of a sore or wound]. The sensation for him was in the rough artery in the neck [the trachea] near the throat, as this was the ulcerated part. We [sc. I] opened his mouth and inspected his pharynx, in case there was an ulceration there; he did not seem to us, inspecting him, to be thus affected [ulcerated]; and anyway the patient would have perceived the sensation as arising from the passage of food and drink, if an ulceration had been present there. Nevertheless we gave him vinegar and mustard to eat, in order to achieve a clearer understanding of the cause. None of these things hurt him, but there was clearly a sensation in his neck; he was so irritated in that place that he was compelled to cough; we

---

27   *Atra bile* 4 (5.115K); *Meth. Med.* 5.12 (10.367K, "black *exanthemata* appeared close together over the whole body"). I am not sure why Johnston and Horsley (2011) do not translate the word "black" (*melana*) in the latter passage, which is his best description of the rash.

encouraged him to resist as much as he could and not to cough, which he did. For the irritation was small, and we made efforts of all kinds to bring the ulceration to scarring, applying a drying medicine externally as he was lying on his back.

(Meth. Med. 5.12, 10.360–63K)

Ulceration of the larynx, trachea, and esophagus are symptoms of smallpox, and in modern times the rash usually began in the mouth. But it is interesting that, while Galen mentions this patient's full-body rash, he has little to say about it, focusing his entire attention on the patient's perception of an internal ulceration (granted, in this section of *On the Method of Healing* he is discussing ulcerations of the trachea, so his focus on this symptom is logical). Similarly, if this patient suffered from a high temperature, Galen does not mention it—although in another treatise he describes the intense heat of the first few days of the disease, and a characteristic pulse that, as he believed, accompanied this symptom (*Praes. Puls*. 3.3, 9.341, 358K). Galen makes only one dubious reference to the disfiguring scarring that affected about 65 to 80 percent of survivors of smallpox in modern times and has contributed so much to the disease's gruesome reputation. Cultural differences might explain this (the scars may not have been very interesting to Galen); we might also note that hemorrhagic smallpox sometimes caused less scarring in the survivors than the ordinary form of the disease.[28]

One can scarcely imagine the horror and suffering that the "great plague" must have caused when it struck the overcrowded, squalid city of Rome itself. The detached tone with which Galen recounts his treatment of the patient above is, however, typical of him. Even when describing intensely painful or visually repellent conditions or victims of tender years, Galen practically never expresses sympathy, revulsion, weariness, sadness, or any emotion other than outrage at the poor performance of his rivals or pride in accomplishing

---

28 For an intriguing discussion of modern views of smallpox, see Shuttleton (2007, part III, "Disfigurement"). On late hemorrhagic smallpox, see Fenner et al. (1988, 38). Galen's word *epoulouto* at *Meth. Med*. 5.13 (10.367K) probably implies that the skin lesions "scarred over" after the scabs fell off.

a cure. These last sentiments he expresses very frequently. But they were socially condoned, even required, in Galen's competitive and hypermasculine world. If Galen is reticent about his other feelings, this is most likely because he did not wish to appear weak, and not because he felt no empathy for the plague victims, or no sense of overwhelming horror in confronting the plague. On the contrary—his exclamations about the duration of the plague ("If only it would end!") or commentary on the desperation of a situation ("most of us struggled ... to stay alive") are so rare in the rest of his work that they stand out strikingly here. The plague was a central and traumatic event in his life. Although hardened by years of treating deadly infectious diseases in the city of Rome, what Galen encountered and endured at Aquileia nevertheless shook him to the core.

The "great plague" was obviously highly contagious, as its clustering in the households of Galen and Aristides suggests.[29] Smallpox spreads through the air in atomized droplets breathed out by an infected person; face-to-face contact within a range of six feet or so is the normal method of transmission. The idea of contagion is not unattested in antiquity, for example, when Thucydides writes of the Athenian plague that those who nursed the sick were the most likely to catch it (2.51); and Pliny the Elder described the transmission of the disease he called *mentagra* by kissing, as I have mentioned. Galen is mostly silent on the question of plague's transmission, save one passage that attributes this, following Hippocratic ideas, to breathing corrupted air (*Praes. Puls.* 3.3, 9.342K). Thus, Hippocrates, as Galen (or the anonymous author of the possibly spurious treatise *On Theriac to Piso*) writes, treated the plague that attacked classical Greece in 429 by purifying the air with fires (*Ther. Pis.* 16, 14.280–81K). In the case of plague victims like the one whose treatment Galen describes above, he clearly did nothing to limit the touching and close examination of the patient that was typical of his practice. It is unclear why Galen did not contract the disease, for he never mentions having done so; and while I am skeptical of arguments from silence in general, I find it hard to believe that in this case some evidence of the event

---

29   Also see Lucian, *Alexander* 36.

would not have survived. If the "great plague" was smallpox, it is not clear whether or how often subclinical forms, with few or no symptoms, occurred in unvaccinated people in modern times, but perhaps this is a possibility.[30] It is also possible that in his long history of dissecting and vivisecting domestic animals and monkeys he had acquired a similar virus causing only mild symptoms, if a zoonotic relative of smallpox was endemic to the region in his day, like the cowpox virus that in the eighteenth century became the first vaccine used in history, or the monkeypox virus now found in parts of Africa. (Monkeypox is, however, today a serious disease when it infects humans, and like all orthopoxviruses may be the source of a new human smallpox virus if it adapts to human hosts sometime in the future.)[31]

Galen himself treated hundreds of victims of the great plague (*Praes. Puls.* 3.4, 9.357K). He considers certain unusual remedies efficacious: milk from Stabiae, near Pompeii, is supposed to have cured the patient described in the passage quoted above and others similarly afflicted; while earth from Armenia miraculously cured others, but those who received no benefit from it all died (*Simp. Med.* 9.1.4, 12.191K). In Syria a popular remedy was the urine of a boy, and Galen acknowledges that, although repulsive, it could work (*Simp. Med.* 10.1.15, 12.285K). Of the complex antidote described in *On Theriac to Piso*, he or its author writes,

> In plague-ridden conditions, this antidote seemed to us to be the only one capable of helping those who had been attacked…. For that plague, like some beast, foully destroyed not a few people, but even rampaged over whole cities and destroyed them.
>
> (*Ther. Pis.* 16, 14.280–81K)

The onset of the plague did not prompt Marcus to back down from his plans for European conquest. Returning to the front in 169 in sole command of the

---

30   Fenner et al. (1988, 30–31) on subclinical smallpox in the vaccinated contacts of smallpox patients.
31   Cf. Shchelkunov (2011) on the periodic emergence of smallpox from zoonotic ancestor viruses.

army, he would remain occupied with the German wars until 175. Galen, desperate to avoid being forced to accompany the emperor to the front, invented an excuse not to go: Asclepius, he said, had spoken to him in a dream and forbidden it (*Libr. Propr.* 2, 19.18–19K). Instead, he spent the next several years treating the imperial heir, Commodus. Marcus's anxiety for the health of his only living son, then eight years old, was very obvious; Galen writes that the emperor "enjoined those who took care of [Commodus] to make every effort to preserve his health, and if they should ever judge it necessary, to call on me for his therapy" (*Lib. Propr.* 2, 19.19K).

Galen introduces this period in *On Prognosis* as a break from public life: "Remembering the customary malice of the doctors and philosophers in the city," he writes, "I decided to withdraw from it, at different times to the different places in the country, wherever [Marcus's] son Commodus might be" (*Praecog.* 9, 14.650K). The emperor owned villas all over Italy, and here Galen implies a rural interval away from the intensity and competitiveness of the city. Galen would soon be drawn back into that arena, but seems to have experienced relative peace in the years between Marcus's departure in 169 and his return visit to Rome in 176.

During these seven years, Galen was extraordinarily productive as a writer, a circumstance he seems to attribute to his greater time for leisure. "Antoninus [i.e., Marcus] was away for much longer than could have been hoped," he writes, making no attempt at flattery in this passage written long after Marcus's death (*Libr. Propr.* 2, 19.19K). "This whole time," he goes on, "provided me with the most noteworthy discipline" (*askesis*, which meant exercise or training but could also refer to a rigorous way of life). Thus, Galen looked back on the years 169–176 as a time of unusual focus on his research and writing, though he complains in this same passage that much of what resulted burned in the fire of 192 C.E.[32]

To name only the best-known of Galen's works dating from this period: he completed books two through seventeen of *On the Usefulness of the Parts*, as well as the last three books of his medical-philosophical treatise *On the*

---

32   See also *Praecog.* 9 (14.650K).

Doctrines of Hippocrates and Plato, and the first five books of his other great anatomical treatise, *On Anatomical Procedures*. (These works, dedicated to Galen's friend Boethus or—in the case of *On Anatomical Procedures*—replacing lost works dedicated to him, are discussed in the previous chapter.) He wrote sixteen books on pulses: namely, the treatises *On the Differences in Pulses*, *On the Diagnosis of Pulses*, *On the Causes of Pulses*, and *On Prognosis from Pulses*, in four books each. He wrote a series of diagnostic and prognostic treatises: *On Critical Days*, *On the Differences in Fevers*, and *On Crises*; and nosological treatises *On the Differences in Diseases*, *On the Causes of Diseases*, *On the Differences in Symptoms*, and *On the Causes of Symptoms*. He wrote the three books *On Mixtures*, which address the canonical humors and qualities associated with them, and the physiological treatise *On the Natural Faculties* in three books. He wrote the first six books of his massive therapeutic work *On the Method of Healing*, and his shorter and more user-friendly *On the Method of Healing to Glaucon* in one book; the first eight books of his pharmacological work *On the Mixtures and Powers of Simple Drugs*, almost entirely a collection of recipes (some very ancient or obscure), like all his works on drugs; and the first five books of his manual on the healthy lifestyle, *On Healthfulness*, a work *sui generis* in which he discusses the proper diet and exercise for a hypothetical patient across the human lifespan.[33]

Commodus, whose health was now partly Galen's responsibility, was under the care of Peitholaus, the imperial chamberlain (*koitonites*) or head of domestic staff; Galen describes the latter as Commodus's *tropheus*, or what we might call a primary caregiver. It is unclear whether Peitholaus was a slave or freedman, but certainly he belonged to one of those categories. As the story of Sextus (below) indicates, he was assumed to be on intimate terms with the emperor and to be influential with him. Galen seems proud of his

---

33   For an English translation of the nosological treatises on diseases and symptoms, see Johnston (2006). A translation of *On Mixtures* is available in Singer (1997) and of *On the Natural Faculties* in Brock (1916). A modern translation of *Meth. Med.* is now available; see Johnston and Horsley (2011). Books 1 and 2 are edited with an English translation by Hankinson (1991a). An English translation of *On Healthfulness* exists (Green 1951) but should be used with caution. On the chronology of Galen's works in this period, see Bardong (1942) and Peterson (1977), updating and correcting the original work of Ilberg (1889).

relationship with Peitholaus and boasts of giving him orders in the course of a cure of the young Commodus, probably dating to 172 C.E. The only story Galen tells about treating the prince, it may therefore be his only significant intervention in Commodus's care.

"They say that what happened with Commodus was something very great," Galen writes modestly, "but in truth it falls short of this by a wide margin" (*Praecog.* 12, 14.661K). At about two o'clock in the afternoon, on returning from the wrestling court, the boy was suddenly struck with a hot fever. Galen took his pulse and diagnosed an inflammation. Peitholaus pointed out the boy's inflamed tonsils, and Galen identified the problem as an excessively harsh medicine of honey and sumac that the chamberlain had been applying to the boy's mouth. He ordered the medicine changed, and, when the fever had subsided after two days, Peitholaus was to feed and bathe the patient. At this point a woman of the imperial family named Annia Faustina—probably not the emperor's wife or daughter, who also went by that name, but rather his first cousin—arrived. Having heard of Commodus's fever, she had come to check on the boy and brought her entourage of Methodist physicians. In keeping with their ideology, she brashly informs Galen that he will no doubt wait until after the "suspect hour" (the hour of the attack) on the third day to feed or bathe the patient; but Peitholaus tells her that Galen's contrary instructions have already been carried out. Galen records the "joking" speech of Annia Faustina at some length—it is not clear whom he believes she is mocking, either himself or her own entourage of physicians—in which she takes one of her Methodist friends by the hand and extols Galen's superior learning before mounting her carriage again to depart. Galen mutters as he turns away that she has made him even more hated among the physicians than before, scarcely bothering to conceal his loathing of the woman.

It is not clear where the cure of Commodus occurs. Annia Faustina's arrival and departure on the same day suggest that the location was not far from Rome, if not in the city itself. There are indications that Galen was not continually absent from Rome in the period during which he treated Commodus, nor were these years entirely tranquil and unperturbed by conflict, as he implies. The story of Galen's patient Sextus Quintilius Condianus, which falls between Marcus's departure and Galen's cure of Commodus, clearly takes place in the city (the action involving visits and messengers to the houses of the main characters).

Sextus belonged to an illustrious and powerful family very close to that of the emperor. When he fell ill with fever, Galen discussed the case with Peitholaus, who asked for his prognosis. Galen predicted that the disease would come to a crisis on the sixth or seventh day, and if on the sixth day, that the feverish paroxysm would recur. Another friend of both Galen and Sextus, Claudius Severus, also became involved, quizzing Galen closely on the case. In the meantime the patient—who had indeed suffered a sweating crisis on the sixth day—stubbornly did all he could to foil Galen by avoiding a recurrence. Galen's prediction had become widely known—no doubt also, as Severus pointed out, to the emperor, through Peitholaus—and Galen's rivals publicly prayed for his failure. When it looked at first as though the prognosis would be proved wrong, they exulted; only to be humiliated again, for just as Galen had predicted, the paroxysms returned.[34] We see Galen in the thick of Rome's ever competitive culture in this story, hounded by the very "malice" he claims to have escaped while Marcus was away: "You, O Epigenes [his addressee], know the malice of almost all the doctors; they prayed openly that I would fail, and sent people every day to find out and report to them on what would happen" (*Praecog.* 10, 14.656K).

It is likely that Galen continued his medical practice as usual during such intervals. He does not seem to have lived in the palace when he was in the city (see the story of his cure of Marcus, below), staying instead in his own house, to which his clinic was attached. Thus, it is likely that many of his innumerable stories of treating patients, men and women of all walks of life, date to this period. He also clearly continued his anatomical experiments, for he writes that after the publication of *On the Usefulness of the Parts* he made certain discoveries which he then included in *On Anatomical Procedures*, "once I had persuaded myself and the others to whom I demonstrated it that I

---

34   *Praecog.* 9–10 (14.650–57K). For the identity of the patient and his full name, Nutton (1979, 213–14).

had discovered this [certain muscles of the upper eyelid] also" (*Libr. Propr.* 2, 19.20K). Nor should we imagine that the act of writing books was a private function removed from the pressure-cooker of professional competition: far from it.

Returning to Rome, Galen relived his experience at Pergamum, if on a larger scale: books that he had written for friends and had never intended for a wider audience had circulated without his knowledge, sometimes under the names of other people, and including, to his horror, the treatise *On Venesection against Erasistratus* that he had produced for Teuthras, now dead. Friends brought him copies of the works they had, which he updated and corrected and to which he affixed proper titles. Many of these he designated "for beginners," as he began to develop the idea of a curriculum for his friends and students—*On the Sects for Beginners*, *On the Bones for Beginners*, *On the Pulse for Beginners*, and *Outline of Empiricism*—all of these, apparently, took their current form at this time (*Libr. Propr.* 1, 19.10–13K).

But this aggravating flurry of editorial activity was only the beginning. Demands for Galen's services as author had not abated. As always, friends about to set out on journeys requested works to take with them: Glaucon, for example, the philosopher-friend whom Galen had so impressed with the cure of the Sicilian doctor (see chapter 4), received *On the Method of Healing to Glaucon* (*Meth. Med. Glauc.* 2.13, 11.145–46K). Other works produced for friends setting out on journeys in the years 169–176 include *On the Anatomy of the Muscles* ("My friends [*hetairoi*] compelled me, so that they might have my memoranda when they departed," *Anat. Admin.* 1.3, 2.227K); and the first books of his massive treatise *On the Method of Healing* ("which I took up writing long ago to please Hiero, when he was suddenly forced to make a long journey, not long after which it was announced that he was dead, and I left off my writing," *Meth. Med.* 7.1, 10.456K).

Indeed, Galen insists that it is only at the urgent demand of his friends that he writes the vast majority of his treatises. Of *On the Method of Healing*, in another passage: "[I wrote it when] my friends (*hetairoi*) were asking for it" (*Meth. Med. Glauc.* 2.13, 11.145–46K). Of *On Anatomical Procedures*: "I had no copies of the memoranda [originally written for Boethus and lost on his death] to give to my friends, for the ones I had at Rome were destroyed, and … for this reason they [the friends] were calling on me [to write a replacement]" (*Anat. Admin.* 1.1, 2.215K). Of the first books of *On the Mixtures and Powers of Simple Drugs*: "my friends … called on me to recall, as much as possible, the things written incorrectly about the powers of simple drugs" (*Simp. Med.* 3.1, 11.540–41K). Of *On the Differences in Pulses*: "I have discussed [these subjects, the contents of *Diff. Puls.*] because of the inane loquacity of recent physicians, convinced by the prayers of my friends, whom I resisted very much" (*Diff. Puls.* 4.1, 8.696K).

The demands of Galen's friends were, as this last quotation suggests, sometimes aimed at the outrages of his enemies. Galen was, as he claims, drawn into writing *On the Differences of Pulses* as a response to the wrongheaded claims of other physicians that were apparently being bruited around the city. A similar, if more extreme, situation is the uproar that greeted Galen's publication of *On the Usefulness of the Parts*, which seems to have coincided with the arrival in Rome of the anatomical works of Lycus of Macedonia—a student of Quintus (see chapter 2), whom Galen had never met personally. Lycus himself was dead; but he published an exhaustive work on anatomy in nineteen books, nearly as long as that of Marinus, and clearly a rival to Galen's new comprehensive work. Lycus's writings became, for a short time and to Galen's intense annoyance, the toast of the Roman medical community (*Anat. Admin.* 4.10, 2.469–70K). *On the Usefulness of the Parts*, as Galen writes, was received enthusiastically by all the better trained doctors and by Aristotelian philosophers; but his enemies—"certain slanderers motivated by jealousy"—spread the rumor all over the city that Galen described in his anatomical works things that could not, in fact, be seen. Galen's friends insisted that he stage a public dissection to prove them wrong—"in one of the large auditoria," that is, before a great crowd. Galen refused. His enemies upped the ante: "they would not cease going to the Temple of Peace every day to mock me; for before the fire, it was customary for all those who practiced the rational arts to gather there."

Galen relented and staged a series of demonstrations over several days. The method he chose was to gather all the anatomical works of his predecessors and array them before him—in itself an impressive display of erudition, for not only did Galen possess this immense heap of scrolls himself; his performance would require him to locate passages among them at a moment's notice. Before Galen, also, must have lain the corpse of the animal on which he proposed to demonstrate his claims; at his side, a number of slave assistants would have been standing ready to fetch instruments and scrolls at his direction. He invited the audience to name a part for dissection, his plan being to show systematically the difference between what his predecessors had written and the observable facts, and also the accuracy of his own published descriptions of those facts. The first part to be named was the chest. Galen intended to begin his commentary with the most ancient of the previous works, but his audience quickly demurred: "Some of the noteworthy doctors in the front row" insisted that he compare his writings only to the work of Lycus of Macedon, student of Quintus, "the greatest anatomist" (literally "most anatomical man"), and who, as they claimed, summed up all the knowledge of the previous centuries. Galen must have gritted his teeth hearing Lycus, and not one of his own teachers, identified as Quintus's star disciple, and Lycus's work praised above his own. He was, however, equal to the challenge, proceeding to demolish his rival's fashionable treatise step by step.

The entire series of demonstrations he later published in a lost treatise called *On Lycus' Ignorance of Anatomy*. Galen would also publish a summary of Lycus's anatomy in two volumes (*Libr. Propr.* 4, 147, 153 Boudon-Millot); and *On the Anatomy of the Muscles*, in response, apparently, to the circulation of a shorter work of Lycus in Rome: "The compilation of Lycus had just been brought to us, running to about 5,000 lines, in almost every one of which he makes a mistake" (*Anat. Admin.* 1.3, 2.227K).[35]

---

35   For the story of the demonstrations, see *Libr. Propr.* 2 (19.20–23K); the treatise is also mentioned in *Libr. Propr.* 4 (154 Boudon-Millot), in a passage only recently restored to the text; and see the editor's note on p. 201. See also *Anat. Admin.* 14.1 (232 Simon). The extant *Against Lycus* (18A.198–245K) is a different work, namely the one mentioned in *Plac. Hipp. Plat.* 8.7 (5.704–5K). On the date of publication of *Musc. Dissect.*, see Garofalo and Debru (2005, 96–97).

In 176 Marcus returned to Rome for a year before departing again, this time taking the young Commodus with him.[36] Galen met the emperor at least once while he was in the city (and probably more than that, if it is true that Galen endured Marcus's continued questioning about theriac: see below). And, whereas Galen humbly describes his earlier cure of Commodus as overrated, "what happened with the emperor himself was truly amazing" (*Praecog.* 11, 14.657K). Among other things, the story illustrates Galen's mastery of the pulse, and he concludes it with a rumination on the errors of other physicians too insensitive to be able to discover the subtle signs of the onset of a feverish paroxysm.

Marcus is surrounded by "the doctors who had travelled with him" on campaign, the responsibility Galen himself had dodged. They feared the onset of a paroxysm of fever; any kind of feverish illness brought with it the dread of death, and the anxiety of those around the patient in this story is palpable, as it is also in the story about Commodus. Galen describes the onset of the trouble in detail: The previous day Marcus took a medicine of bitter aloe in the morning, and then theriac at noon "as was his custom every day;" in the evening he bathed and ate a little. All night he was racked by colic and diarrhea. The "physicians around him"—three in number, as we learn later in the story—examined the emperor, took his pulse, ordered rest, and fed him porridge the following afternoon. At this point, Galen writes, he was sent for to sleep in the palace (our evidence that he did not normally live there). "As the lamps were being lit, a messenger from the emperor arrived, summoning me" (*Praecog.* 11, 14.658K).

Hearing the diagnosis of the emperor's three physicians, Galen remained conspicuously silent. When pressed, he refused to take Marcus's pulse or offer a diagnosis, citing his lack of familiarity with the emperor: surely those who had attended him for so many years and knew the characteristics of the patient's normal pulse were more competent to pronounce on his condition. The emperor, of course, insisted; whereupon Galen made his best guess based on the pulse typical for one of Marcus's age and nature, saying

---

36 Birley (1987, 195–206).

that his problem was not the onset of fever but indigestion; "his stomach was oppressed by the food he had eaten" (this perhaps a barb aimed at the physicians who had prescribed porridge before Galen's arrival).

This was a tense moment in which the stakes were very high. It was Galen's first and, perhaps, only opportunity to cure the emperor, and he took a great risk in diagnosing a trivial illness where the other doctors suspected something dire, enough to fetch Galen to the palace at nightfall. But his guess proved correct. Obviously relieved, Marcus praised Galen's diagnosis enthusiastically, exclaiming three times in succession: "That's it! Exactly what you said!" (*Praecog.* 11, 14.659K). Galen now prescribed an application of wool soaked in warm nard ointment, adding that for an ordinary citizen he would advise the riskier (and much cheaper, for nard was an expensive imported substance) therapy of wine with pepper.[37] Marcus conspicuously used both the ointment and the peppered wine, and Galen precisely records the words with which he praised him to Peitholaus: "We have *one* physician only [emphasizing Galen's superiority over the three other doctors on the scene], and he is entirely noble" [*eleutheros*, literally "free;" he is validating Galen's claim to elite status based on his professional skill]. "As you know," Galen adds, "he was always saying about me that I was the *first* of physicians." "First and only" is a phrase common on agonistic inscriptions honoring victors in contests; and what more qualified judge of an excellent physician than Marcus, the philosopher-emperor?[38]

Marcus's habit of taking theriac every day, which Galen mentions above, was well-known enough to be recorded in the history of Cassius Dio, writing in the third century:

He took very little food, and always at night; for he never ate anything during the day except the medicine called theriac. He took this medicine not so much because he was afraid of something [sc. a poison plot], as because he was ill in his stomach and chest. And they say that

---

37   On nard, see Nutton (1985, 143).

38   Agonistic inscriptions: Moretti (1953, 38, 152) and Mattern (2008a, 234 n. 33).

because of it [the medicine] he was able to endure both this [illness] and other things. (72[71].6.3)

The word *theriake* in Greek is derived from *ther*, meaning a wild animal; it denoted, above all, an antidote against venomous bites; but theriac recipes claimed effectiveness against many venoms or poisons or all of them, and against a range of other ailments. Galen is our most abundant source for the history of theriac in antiquity. His treatise *On Antidotes* collects recipes and describes their provenance. Two treatises of doubtful authenticity *On Theriac* have also come down to us under Galen's name; of these, *On Theriac to Piso* was believed authentic as early as the sixth century C.E. and is today widely accepted as genuine; *On Theriac to Pamphilianus* is probably spurious.[39]

A drug for royalty and other exalted figures who had reason to fear deadly conspiracies, theriac had an undeniably romantic aura about it. Many recipes were written in verse; complex and often secret, they contained dozens of ingredients. Some authors, Galen complains, falsified their recipes when they wrote them down; and even when they didn't, quantities in theriac recipes were easily corrupted, the signs for numerals being especially susceptible to copyist error.[40] Rome's most charismatic enemy, Mithradates VI (see chapter 1), famously developed an antidote that protected him against all known poisons, experimenting on condemned criminals, much as Attalus III of Pergamum did (*Antid.* 1.1, 14.2K). Legend held that among the other booty Pompey seized from the defeated king in 63 B.C.E. and brought back to Rome were Mithradates' notebooks, full of the knowledge he had assembled from his medical experiments and from correspondence with subjects throughout his kingdom (Pliny *Naturalis historia* 25.3.6–7). Galen transmits several

---

39   On Galen and the preparation of the emperor's theriac, Schlange-Schöningen (2003, 187–204). On theriac in antiquity, see Mayor (2010, 239–46), who argues that Mithradates' original recipe must have perished and provides up-to-date references. Totelin (2004) traces the development of theriac in Roman times. See also Gilbert Watson (1966). On the authenticity of *Ther. Pis.*, see Nutton (1997); Swain (1996, appendix D).

40   "Some people lie on purpose when they give out recipes [*graphai*] to those who ask for them, and some alter the writings they have received from others. As for the books shelved in the libraries, the ones that use signs [i.e. numerals] for numbers are easily distorted" (*Antid.* 1.5, 14.31K).

recipes for "Mithridatium" in the second book of *On Antidotes*, but it seems that Mithradates' authentic recipe had long vanished.[41]

Many Roman emperors used theriac—Galen names Augustus, Tiberius, Nero, Trajan, Hadrian, and Antoninus Pius, and also transmits the recipe developed by Nero's physician, Andromachus, who supposedly used Mithradates' antidote as a starting-point. Galen thought very highly of Andromachus's remedy, which was called, coincidentally, *galene*, or "tranquility." He also considered it a cure for a huge range of ailments of the eyes, stomach, liver, kidneys, joints, reproductive organs, and psyche, as well as for fever, convulsions, rabies, and (as mentioned above) the great plague (*Ther. Pis.* 15–16, 14.270–84K). The recipe that Galen eventually mixed for Marcus differed only slightly from Andromachus's prescription.

Marcus's official preparer of theriac, until he died sometime during the northern campaigns of 169–174, was named Demetrius. Because the recipe required rare ingredients obtainable only at Rome—some of them only in the imperial warehouses—Demetrius remained in the city while Marcus was on campaign and sent the medicine from there (*Antid.* 1.1, 14.4K). When Demetrius died, Marcus asked his supervisor of accounts, Euphrates, to name a successor from among those on the imperial payroll. Euphrates replied that Galen had always been present when Demetrius prepared the theriac, whereupon Marcus ordered Galen to assume that duty.[42] We learn here incidentally that Galen was receiving an imperial salary, starting in 168, when he was summoned to Aquileia, or 169, when Marcus placed him on call in case Commodus became ill; and probably considered himself, as he would have been considered by others, an *archiatros* or imperial physician, a word Galen himself applies to his predecessor Demetrius.[43]

Marcus, ever curious about the drug's composition, questioned Galen repeatedly about it when he came to Rome. Finally Galen replied with

---

41   On Mithradates' antidote, see Mayor (2010, 239–47); Totelin (2004); Touwaide (1994, 1941–43).

42   *Antid.* 1.1 (14.4K); Schlange-Schöningen (2003, 189). It is possible that Demetrius's gravestone survives, dating to 170, in Ostia (ibid. n. 73).

43   Schlange-Schöningen (2003, 190).

some embarrassment that he had not altered the recipes of previous imperial physicians by an iota (*Antid.* 1.1, 14.4K). Theriac, Galen writes, was much in fashion among the rich in Marcus's reign, as they emulated the emperor's habit (*Antid.* 1.4, 14.24–25K), and Galen himself prepared theriac for some aristocrats who requested it (*Antid.* 1.14, 14.71K).[44] Commodus would not use theriac; but its popularity revived under Severus (*Antid.* 1.13, 14.65–66), from whose reign the treatises *On Antidotes* and *On Theriac to Piso* date.

Theriac as Galen prepared it contained sixty-four ingredients, the quality and type of which was, he believed, critical to the drug's efficacy, and he discusses at length the correct provenance of the wine, herbs, honey, and other substances comprising it.[45] Among the most important of these, ever since Nero's physician Andromachus added it, was the flesh of vipers (*echidnai*, in Greek). This made current theriacs more efficacious against snakebite, in Galen's view, than the recipe of Mithradates, which had used only lizards.[46] The palace employed at least one snake-hunter, most likely for the purpose of supplying this commodity, rather than simply ridding the imperial grounds of reptilian pests. "One of the imperial servants, whose job was to hunt vipers, was bitten; and for a while he drank the usual medicines," Galen writes. "But when his whole color changed and he turned leek green, he came to me and told me the whole story [of his illness]" (*Loc. Affect.* 5.8, 8.355K). Galen treated him successfully with theriac.

Viper's flesh was obtainable, too, from a rather shadowy caste of professionals known as the Marsi, to which this individual may have belonged.[47] The Marsi were, strictly speaking, an ethnic group of the central Apennines,

---

44 Cf. ibid., 197).

45 Galen also prepared an "antidote of one hundred ingredients, which I use, and which I provided to the Emperor [as a remedy or prophylactic] for all things, and especially for deadly things" (*Antid.* 2.9, 14.155K); this recipe is quite different from the *galene* or theriac of Andromachus (and Galen does not call it a theriac). It is not clear which emperor he has in mind (*On Antidotes* was composed under Severus) nor, if the emperor was Marcus, that this is the theriac he took daily rather than another medicine. It seems clear that the theriac Galen prepared for Marcus was Demetrius's adaptation of Andromachus's *galene*.

46 *Antid.* 1.1 (14.2K); *Ther. Pis.* 5 (14.232K).

47 On the Marsi and snake-handling, see Dench (1995, 158–64); Nutton (1985, 138–39).

renowned as magicians and diviners, and with a related reputation for their knowledge of venomous snakes, as well as their skill in hunting and charming them. Legend held that their chants could put snakes to sleep (Silius Italicus, *Pun.* 8.495–97) or make them explode (Lucilius 575–76). They were also rumored to be impervious to snakebite (Pliny, *Naturalis historia* 7.15), and inscriptions record Marsi among the medical personnel attached to Roman military units, probably to treat soldiers for snake and scorpion bites.[48] There was a contingent living in Rome, whose advice—on the differences among poisonous snakes, and specifically, on whether there was a viper whose bite caused insatiable thirst—Galen sought out at least once (*Simp. Med.* 11.1, 12.316K). In his treatise addressed to Glaucon, Galen notes that his friend has no doubt seen the Marsi in the city preparing viper's flesh for consumption: First they cut off four finger-widths' worth from the tails and heads (considered the viper's most poisonous parts); then they gut what remains of the carcasses, skin them, and wash them (*Meth. Med. Glauc.* 2.12, 11.143–44K). Galen also mentions a patient whose profession was "capturing vipers alive" (*Simp. Med.* 11.1.1, 12.315K), and one theriac recipe required roasting live vipers (*Ther. Pis.* 19, 14.291K); perhaps this patient was one of the Marsi, but snake-handling is well-attested in other sources, and the Marsi probably did not monopolize the art. Besides being a critical ingredient in theriac, viper's flesh was also considered a remedy for elephantiasis (leprosy), and Galen tells many stories about this, some distinctly folksy in character; he endorsed this popular belief and used the remedy on elephantiasis patients with self-reported success.[49]

Imperial theriac also contained opium ("juice of poppy-heads," *opos mekonos*). Opium, originally native to the western Mediterranean and probably first domesticated there, was grown in some parts of the Mediterranean basin and in Europe even in Neolithic times, and seems to have been commonly available in Galen's world. It was used in salves or plasters for earaches,

---

48   Davies (1989, 212).
49   Viper's flesh and elephantiasis: *Subfig. Emp.* 10 (75–78 Deichgräber); *Simp. Med.* 11.1.1 (12.312–15K, mostly a transcription of the same stories recorded in *Subfig. Emp.*); *Meth. Med. Glauc.* 2.12 (11.143–44K).

eye infections, headaches, erysipelas, and gout, and internally for diarrhea, cough, insomnia, and other complaints. These remedies are attested in innumerable sources including, from the Roman period, Dioscorides, Scribonius Largus (physician to the emperor Claudius), Pliny the Elder, and Galen himself, who transmits several opium-containing remedies for throat and respiratory problems including one of his own invention.[50]

Marcus, finding that he was falling asleep while trying to conduct his daily business, asked Demetrius to remove the opium from the theriac; with the result that he suffered from insomnia at night, and the missing ingredient had to be restored. As Galen writes, Marcus had become used to it (*Antid.* 1.1, 14.4K). Was Marcus then addicted to opium, as some scholars have argued?[51] The theriac recipe that Galen probably used—that of Andromachus, slightly modified by Demetrius—contained about 3.4 percent opium. At the time that Galen began preparing theriac, Marcus took a dose "the size of an Egyptian bean" every day (*Antid.* 1.1, 14.3K). Each dose should have contained about 33 milligrams of opium.[52] For raw opium this is a small dose, probably enough to have an effect (though one should not rule out the possibility that Marcus was a placebo responder; opium was known to have soporific properties), but Marcus cannot on this basis be described as an addict. The famous early nineteenth-century opium-eater Thomas de Quincey, for instance, at the height of his addiction, ingested opium in quantities as large as 10,000 or 20,000 milligrams per day; a regimen of renunciation for him was a daily dose of 800 to 2,600 milligrams, enough in itself to kill a casual user.[53] Had Marcus gradually increased his intake of theriac (a possibility that Galen's language leaves open), he still could not have been in the same league, and Galen makes no comment on

---

50   On the domestication of opium in the Neolithic, see recently Zohary (2012, 109–11) and Bogaard, Krause, and Strien (2011). Dioscorides: 4.64. Beck (2011) is a good translation of his *De materia medica*. Galen's list of remedies: *Comp. Med. Loc.* 7.2 (13.38–45K), and he mentions opium many other times. On opium in ancient medicine, see Scarborough (1995).

51   For recent discussion and references, see Schlange-Schöningen (2003, 198–204).

52   Schlange-Schöningen (2003, 202); the original calculation was made by Africa (1961,102).

53   de Quincey (2003, 61, 87).

any effect that the drug might have had on Marcus's behavior or character besides sleepiness.[54]

One of the more exotic ingredients in theriac, and the one which receives the most comment in Galen, was cinnamon, imported from India. Galen procured his supply from the imperial storehouses and, apparently, had no other source: "When I was preparing the theriac for Antoninus [sc. Marcus] I observed many wooden vessels containing cinnamon, some placed in storage under Trajan, some under Hadrian, and some under Antoninus who reigned after Hadrian" (*Antid.* 1.13, 14.64K). The strength of the cinnamon's taste and odor, he remarks, diminished with age. The best cinnamon, he goes on to write, came from a tree brought whole to Marcus "from barbarian lands"—perhaps as a gift—in a case seven feet long. So powerful was this cinnamon that Marcus was able to drink the theriac prepared with it right away, instead of waiting the normal two-month period for it to cure. The tree was sold together with all the more recent cinnamon by Commodus, who did not use theriac; Galen saved bits of it for himself and kept them among his most precious possessions in storage near the Temple of Peace, where they were destroyed in the fire of 192. Thus, when Severus ordered Galen to begin preparing theriac again, he had to use the much weaker samples from the reigns of Trajan and Hadrian, some of which must have been fifty years old, and which were (as he notes) much diminished in strength from the time he had last used them, some three decades previously (*Antid.* 1.13, 14.65–66K; *Ind.* 6).

Galen's face-to-face interaction with Marcus and his family seems limited, and he never suggests otherwise.[55] They play only a minor role in his stories and most likely they are more prominent there than they were in actual experience; Galen would have boasted about any contact with the imperial

---

54 Africa's suggestion (1961, 97) that Marcus placed a "wall of narcotics" between himself and the stresses of empire and an unhappy marriage to a faithless wife is thus implausible. Africa's argument is based mainly on the grim and unhappy tone of the *Meditations* which, while depressing indeed, is not more so than other Stoic tracts of the same genre. For a useful commentary and discussion of its themes, see Rutherford (1989).

55 See Schlange-Schöningen (2003, 185–86).

family, yet he tells just one story of a cure of Commodus and one of a cure of Marcus, relating them as though they were extraordinary events. The care of the imperial household was not his sole preoccupation, then, and even in the period from 169 to 176, Galen cannot accurately be described as a court physician. True, he spent a fair amount of time in the palace. He was "always present" when Demetrius prepared theriac; he rummaged through the emperor's storerooms; he followed the young Commodus around Italy; and his relationship with Peitholaus, the imperial chamberlain, seems to have been close. Later, he complained about the time he was forced to waste in the emperor's court. But he did not live at the palace, and it is unclear how much time he actually spent outside of Rome with Commodus. Moreover, he continued to treat other patients including plague victims, and even to engage in his old rivalries, to which he returned his attention during or soon after Marcus's sojourn in Rome in 176.

Later Galen recalled the days of Marcus's absence, when he was receiving an imperial salary for a job that was, in fact, little more than a sinecure, as a period of relative peace and freedom in which he produced a huge quantity of writing; but he was hardly detached from public life, from his incessant rivalries, or from his regular medical practice. Indeed, what Galen remembered as a time of relative leisure was, by some standards, intensely stressful. He was anything, then, but a sheltered flower in the greenhouse of the imperial palace. Nor is it clear that that lifestyle was open to him, or to anyone.

Like other ethnic Greeks of the Roman period, Galen was ambivalent about his relationship to the emperor, the very center of power in his world. He was proud to have been called upon by Marcus, clear proof of his preeminence in his profession. Still he resented the compulsions laid upon him—his near-drafting to the German front, his recall from his home in Pergamum, his enforced service at the imperial palace. Later in life, as a sexagenarian, Galen prided himself on his Stoic indifference to "the time wasted in the imperial court, which I not only did not want, but even when fate was dragging me forcefully toward it, I resisted not once or twice, but many times" (*Ind.* 49). Here, in the same breath, Galen boasts of his relationship to the palace and insists on his resistance to the emperor's demands.

Greeks like Galen formed the ruling class of the ancient Hellenic cities that, pre-dating Roman rule by centuries, were the soul of Greco-Roman learning and culture, and they were very conscious of this. Like Aelius Aristides and others, Galen was of the establishment, then, but occupied that position uneasily, trying vaguely to distance himself from Roman culture and authority.[56] The tense mixture of arrogance and servility evident in Galen's story about treating Marcus typifies the attitudes of his class toward Rome.

Galen's decision not to accompany Marcus on campaign had consequences that he may not have anticipated or thought through. In the first place, he never achieved the power that might have been his had he ever ranked as one of the emperor's "companions." Although he may have been called *archiatros*, Galen received none of the honors or elevations in status attested for certain other imperial physicians.[57] C. Stertilius Xenophon, for example, was one of Claudius's doctors and accompanied the latter on campaign in Britain. He held the prestigious position of "secretary of Greek letters" and obtained tax immunity for his native town of Cos, where his name appears in numerous honorific inscriptions and his face on Coan coins. Likewise, Trajan's doctor Crito went with him on campaign in Dacia and also wrote a history of the Dacian wars. The emperor later elevated him to equestrian rank and called him "friend," and his home town of Heraclea declared him an honorary "founder" in return for the benefits he had obtained for them. Galen certainly would have recorded receiving any such honors; but the only imperial recognition for his services that he mentions besides a salary is the emperor's praise, and on one occasion only. Had he chosen to accompany Marcus to the German war—had he, that is, been in constant attendance on the emperor during those years 169–176, instead of in Italy writing books—he might well have achieved honors similar to Xenophon's or Crito's. And it is entirely possible that Galen consciously and deliberately chose freedom and scholarship, as he claims, over power and status. The legacy of the works that he produced

---

56   On the Second Sophistic and its relationship to Roman authority, see chapter 1, n. 11.
57   For the following examples, see Mattern (1999a).

in relative quietude has far outlasted the effect of any honors he might have received, had he been more conventionally ambitious.

But there was a more unexpected consequence of his decision, one more directly related to the scientific work Galen valued above all else: for, while human dissection was generally taboo in Roman society, the physicians who accompanied Marcus Aurelius to the German war were permitted to dissect one or more slain "barbarians." It is clear from Galen's work that he never dissected a human. The anatomy of his philosophical-medical masterpiece *On the Usefulness of the Parts* is based mainly on his exhaustive dissections of animals (see chapter 5).

Strive though he might, then, to describe human anatomy, Galen had very limited access to information on the interior of the human body beyond what he could see from treating wounds. I have mentioned his recommendations to study human skeletons where they were available at Alexandria, or the exposed bones of unburied bandits, and so forth (*Anat. Admin.* 1.2, 2.220K). But such opportunities were paltry compared with those enjoyed by the physicians who had accompanied Marcus on his campaign, and about this he was embittered. Regarding his standing in the Roman aristocracy and with the emperor, Galen was conflicted: but regarding medical research his passion was intense and unambiguous. There can be no doubt that if he had known he would be allowed to dissect a human, he would have braved the perils and discomforts of the campaign and endured the importunities of the emperor. Unsurprisingly, he heaps scorn on his undeservedly lucky colleagues for their ignorance, writing that they made little of their extraordinary opportunity because of their lack of expertise in animal dissection:

> Therefore if you see frequently in monkeys the position and size of each tendon and nerve, you will remember them accurately, and if sometime you have a way of dissecting a human body, you will discover each thing as you have observed it; but if you are entirely without practice you will profit not at all from such an opportunity, as those doctors who, in the German war, having the opportunity to dissect barbarian bodies, *did not learn more than butchers know.*
>
> (*Comp. Med. Gen.* 3.2, 13.604K; cf. *Anat. Admin.* 2.384K)

Surely Galen would have done much better. And so it is likely that he looked back at his decision to remain home from the war, in relative quiet and retirement, with ambivalence, if not regret.

Galen represents the pinnacle of the ancient anatomical tradition—an extensive tradition that depended on rigorous and painstaking transmission by text and demonstration, from teacher to student, over centuries, and formed the springboard for Renaissance discoveries once human dissection became common practice. It is an impressive legacy to say the least, but the fact remains that it was based almost entirely on animal dissection. Had Galen—the ancient world's greatest and most skilled anatomist—turned his critical eye to the human body, one can only imagine the insights he might have contributed; as it was, these would have to wait thirteen centuries.

Chapter Seven

GALEN AND HIS PATIENTS

t this point we lose the narrative thread of Galen's life. We know—from one vague reference—that he suffered in the reign of Marcus's son and successor, the unstable and narcissistic emperor Commodus, fearing for his home and property if he should be arbitrarily exiled (*Ind.* 54–55). Galen's writings, which contain many internal and cross-references, can be more or less organized in relative chronological order, but they contain few references to dateable events in his own life or in the world around him. There is a major exception—the fire of 192 C.E., which changed his life and which will be described in the next chapter. His treatise *On Theriac to Piso*, long considered spurious but now accepted as genuine by many scholars, addresses the emperors Severus and Caracalla and must date to after 204 C.E. because it refers to an event from the Secular Games of that year. If he did write this treatise, it proves that Galen was still to be found in Rome forty years from the date that Marcus Aurelius recalled him to Italy.[1] He seems to have visited Pergamum, where he still owned property, at least

---

1   On the year of Galen's death: Nutton (1995a); Strohmeier (2007); and see further discussion in chapter 8. On the authenticity of *Ther. Pis.*, Swain (1996, Appendix D); Nutton (1997). Strohmeier (2007) doubts the authenticity of the treatise but considers the abundant evidence of Arab commentators decisive for a late date of Galen's death.

once; he stopped at Lemnos for the second time on the way, as mentioned in previous chapters. But there is no obvious evidence in his writings of a long stay outside of Italy. He implies that he served each successive emperor after Marcus Aurelius in turn in some capacity, in his discussion of cinnamon from *On Antidotes* (see chapter 6), and probably remained on the imperial payroll. He continued to anatomize—this is very likely, because he continued work on the exhaustive treatise *On Anatomical Procedures* and rewrote the final books when they were lost in the fire of 192 (*Anat. Admin.* 11.11, 135 Simon). He continued to write very prolifically; his lengthy pharmacological treatises and the second half of his great therapeutic tract *On the Method of Healing*, among many other works, date to after the fire and the last decades of his life. But most importantly, he treated patients.

Galen describes hundreds of individual cases, anecdotally, in his surviving works. Visits to patients were a normal part of his daily life, and he performed these so diligently that it is difficult to understand how he also had the time to anatomize and to write, as he clearly did, or even to mix the emperor's theriac. He visited his sick patients every day, sometimes more than once. He might respond to a summons in the middle of the night and might begin his round of examinations before dawn; he mentions visiting patients in the morning, afternoon, evening, and late at night. Into the room of one patient, suffering from a wasting illness, Galen brought a lactating donkey so that he could suckle its milk directly. Another patient, a steward (probably a slave or freedman) suffering from an eye inflammation, lived in a suburb too far for Galen to visit, so Galen brought him home to live in his house, where he bled him twice and treated him several times per day with eye salve.[2]

While this seems to be an exceptional case—most of Galen's patients did not live with him—it is clear that he operated a clinic in his own house, as for example in the story of the patient with chalkstones from the preface to this book: this old man was carried to Galen's doorstep, and the wording of several other stories suggest that patients came to Galen rather than the other

---

2   On Galen's case histories, see Mattern (2008a). On visiting patients, ibid. 140–41. Middle of the night: *Meth. Med.* 9.4 (10.611K); *Praecog.* 7 (14.636K). Before dawn: *Meth. Med.* 11.16 (10.792K). Donkey: *Meth. Med.* 7.6 (10.474K). Steward: *Cur. Ven. Sect.* 17 (11.299–302K).

way around. Just as other craftsmen in antiquity lived in or adjacent to their shops, so physicians like Galen worked from their homes, where they not only treated patients but also, for example, mixed drugs. One patient, arriving at Galen's door with a knee injury exacerbated by a cold winter, asked him for a heating drug to relieve the pain and then departed for the baths. Galen did not have the drug he requested but prepared a concoction of euphorbia, oil, and melted wax, and handed it over when the patient sent for it (no doubt via slave messenger).[3]

Galen's diagnostic techniques were extraordinarily subtle. He had trained himself since childhood to notice minute changes in a patient's pulse and published several treatises on the subject. Galen built on an ancient tradition of pulse lore, tracing back through Herophilus, that had already developed an evocative and controversial terminology; he did not invent the "worm pulse," the "ant pulse," and so on, although he sometimes used these terms. The highly specialized and esoteric nature of pulse knowledge and of its vocabulary gave it pride of place in Galen's diagnostic repertoire: few could perceive the minute distinctions of size, speed, strength, frequency, fullness, hardness, regularity, and rhythm that he claimed to feel, and still fewer could grasp the definitions over which he and his colleagues argued so strenuously.[4]

The pulse, as he believed, could reveal changes in internal organs, internal growths, mental conditions (especially anxiety), and fever, of which it

---

3   *Comp. Med. Gen.* 3.2 (13.574–75K). On treating patients at his own house, see Mattern (2008a, 56–57) with notes 31–32 for further references and discussion of physicians' houses in Pompeii. Knee injury: *Comp. Med. Gen.* 3.2 (13.574–75K). On the vocabulary of mixing drugs, see Gourevitch (2003).

4   On Galen's diagnostic techniques, see Mattern (2008a, 149–52) for discussion and further references. Trained since childhood: *Dign. Puls.* 1.1 (8.770–71K). Extant pulse treatises are *On the Pulse for Beginners*; *On the Differences in Pulses* (four books); *On Diagnosis of Pulses* (four books); *On the Causes of Pulses* (four books); *On Prognosis from Pulses* (four books); and *Synopsis of the Books on Pulses* (8.453–9.549K). Notable ancient contributors to pulse lore include Herophilus; see von Staden (1989, 267–88 and testimonia 144–88b) for full discussion. Galen wrote a lost treatise specifically discussing Herophilus's pulse lore (von Staden 1989, 287 and testimonium 162 = *Dign. Puls.* 4.3, 8.161K). On the vocabulary of touch in ancient medicine, including a discussion of Galen on the pulse (p. 235), see Boehm (2003). On Galen's pulse lore, including social and cultural aspects, see Kuriyama (1998, 23–37, 63–70); Tamsyn S. Barton (1994, 152–163).

was, in Galen's view, the most accurate diagnostic indicator. In the case of Boethus's son Cyrillus and in the case of the emperor Marcus Aurelius, discussed in previous chapters, Galen pronounced his patients free of fever based on a reading of their pulses; and Antipater's fever, discussed below, will be detected from his pulse. In one patient Galen diagnosed an internal tumor from the pulse alone, before palpating the patient although the growth could be easily felt:

> When I felt his pulse, I diagnosed a large visceral tumor, which had reached such a stage that it was apparent to the sight and touch, (even) to non-medical men. Those in attendance were amazed that I diagnosed a visceral tumor from the patient's pulse.
>
> (*Opt. Med. Cogn.* 5, 80 Iskandar, tr. Iskandar)

On the pulse as on other points Galen insisted on individual variation; ideally the physician had intimate knowledge of a patient's normal, baseline pulse, which would also change as the patient moved through the stages of life from childhood to old age. The same for temperature; Galen could measure small changes in heat by touch, and a patient's normal temperature would vary according to age, individual temperament, and other factors. Long before laboratory testing, he examined urine and feces, sweat, sputum, and other substances coughed up by the patient, vomit, pus, and blood for color, texture, viscosity, and sediment. He scrutinized his patients' faces for signs such as a change in skin color or the sunken eyes of wasting or extreme dehydration. He boasted that he could take in many of these features at a glance and sometimes this allowed him to show off with a flashy diagnosis.[5]

It is not clear that Galen had a routine procedure for examining patients; he seems to have drawn on the techniques described above as circumstances

---

5   Trained sensitivity to differences in heat: *Temp.* 2.2 (1.594–99K). Familiarity with pulse: e.g., *Syn . Puls.* 7 (9.451K); *Praecog.* 11 (14.659K); *Cris.* 2.4 (9.638K). Bodily fluids: Diamandopoulos and Goudas (2003, 2005); Mattern (2008a, 150).

suggested. He could, however, be very thorough, as in the story of a youth with fever:

> Finding that his fever was rather hot, but that his pulse was regular, very large, swift, frequent and vigorous; that the heat was not of the type that is biting to the touch, and that his urine was not much different from its usual state in density and color; and learning that the man had neglected his habit of exercise for around thirty days, and that on the day before he had exercised vigorously, but not too much; and that he had nevertheless taken his accustomed food, and had managed to digest it, but slowly and with difficulty … and since the man appeared ruddy and plump, and even said that he perceived a sense of fullness …
>
> (*Meth. Med.* 9.4, 10.610K)

Here Galen comments on several characteristics of the patient's temperature, pulse, and urine, as well as on his physical appearance (ruddy, plump). This passage also illustrates another feature of Galen's clinical procedure: he talks to his patients, here eliciting information about history (the patient's neglected exercise routine) and perceptions ("[he] said that he perceived a sense of fullness"); these are indicators, in Galen's view, that the patient requires bloodletting.

Galen considered patient history critical to clinical practice and often comments on events that happened prior to the illness and may have caused it. For example, one patient's dangerous fever is related to a host of subtle causes that have heated and dried his body, including travel, temperament, character, and a fight at the gymnasium (this is one of Galen's most fascinating cases but it is little-known today, and so I will quote it at length):

> The youth, who was now seized with fever, was twenty-five years old, slender and muscular in body like a dog, and of a markedly dry and warm temperament. He enjoyed gymnastic exercises and was otherwise a serious and industrious type. While out of town, this man received some bad news, and was vexed; exerting himself, he hurried to the city.

Throughout the previous day he had exerted himself moderately and bathed and dined, and rested at an inn, but for the most part without sleeping. On the next day, he hurried still more and completed the journey, which was entirely sandy and dusty, under a hot sun; and he arrived at about the seventh hour and a half in the city. Learning better news about the matters on account of which he had hurried, he went to the gymnasium intending to bathe; when he had been oiled, he had a massage together with one of the youths there. And when asked by [the other youth] to move a little, a quarrel arose between them, the kind which gymnastic types are often accustomed to fall into, and he exerted himself more than usual; and he was already unusually dried out. As he was leaving the gymnasium, he encountered some of his friends fighting; he separated them, without realizing that he was again undertaking no small additional exercise as he dragged them apart, and shoved some of them, and seized others around the waist, and objected to some of them that they were doing wrong, and became angry on behalf of the wronged, so that he returned home extremely dry, and became aware of his own fatigue and that something was abnormal. Therefore he drank water as he was accustomed to, but he became no better; rather, the abnormal feeling increased, and he vomited.

(*Meth. Med.* 10.3, 10.671–73K)

This is a complex and subtly sympathetic portrait of a patient of the urban leisure class, male, in the prime of life, susceptible to vexation (note his stress response to the "bad news") and righteous indignation (over his place on the massage table at the gymnasium and in the fight among his friends outside, in which he enthusiastically intervenes; but the youth avoids actual violence, which would be distasteful to Galen). He is also vulnerable to the stresses of intellectual life, being "serious and industrious"—the first of these words, *phrontistes*, being one that Galen here and elsewhere associates with the health hazards of intellectual work and worry. In this case Galen has formed a compelling image of the patient, of his lifestyle among other competitive youths at the gymnasium, and of the events leading to his illness—all of which could only have come from a careful questioning of the patient or his entourage, for Galen himself does not arrive on the scene until several days into the illness.

This patient is one of Galen's best-developed characters, and he does not go into such detail in all of his stories. But many of them describe or hint at or suggest—in offhand, and therefore illuminating, ways—Galen's discussions with, and interrogations of, his patients. Little comments show that he took note of their exact words: "his fingers were difficult to move and numb and, as it were, making a crackling noise, as he himself called it" (*San. Tuend.* 6.11, 4.434K); "someone bitten by a scorpion said that he seemed to be struck by hailstones" (*Loc. Affect.* 3.11, 8.195K); "I asked if he felt bitten at the wound by the medicine. And he said that he was not 'bitten,' but had a sort of itching sensation" (*Comp. Med. Gen.* 3.2, 13.585K). Here Galen is questioning patients not about history but about current symptoms, including perceptions of pain, which can only be elicited by such questioning:

> In cases of pain around the head I am accustomed to ask the patients, what kind of quality [of pain] they have. Some perceive a sense as though their body is worn away with pain, while others [feel] as though they are being stretched or crushed, or pounded, or that violent heat or cold alone predominates.
>
> (*Comp. Med. Loc.* 2.1, 12.545K)

Galen gave thought to the question of how to distinguish the different types of pain that patients might experience and describe. He rejected the formal terminology of pain developed by Archigenes, a physician of his grandfather's generation (who had also developed a new and specialized vocabulary of the pulse of which Galen is equally critical); but Galen clearly paid attention to his patients' sometimes very striking analogies and word choices. He could also become frustrated when some patients lacked the vocabulary and intellectual sophistication to describe their pain (*Loc. Affect.* 2.6–9, 8.86–120K).

Most of the stories Galen tells are about successful diagnosis and treatment, and it is rare that a patient in his stories dies despite Galen's best efforts.

An exception is a case well known at the time: "Everybody knows," Galen writes, "what happened to Antipater the physician." This patient was "less than sixty but more than fifty years old," younger than Galen himself, if the case happened recently before its publication in *On the Affected Parts*. It is an example of subtle diagnosis from the pulse. Antipater's pulse had developed an irregularity ("anomaly") after a brief fever. Unsure what to make of it, one day when he met Galen by chance he laughingly asked for his colleague's advice. Galen was shocked when he felt the pulse and surprised that Antipater was still alive. Hedgingly, he asked whether the patient suffered any difficulty breathing; Antipater said no. Galen continued to monitor his patient's condition for six months, and when Antipater asked for his diagnosis, told him that he had an inflammation of the pulmonary vein, which had become clogged with viscous substances; and that his fever, caused by the inflammation, had in fact never resolved. In consultation with his patient, Galen prescribed the same regimen as for asthma. But over the next six months Antipater developed breathing difficulties, as Galen had predicted, along with heart palpitations. These attacks became more frequent until they were occurring fifteen times per day; then Antipater died. Today's physicians would disagree with Galen's diagnosis of the cause of Antipater's problem in the pulmonary vein; but not only did Galen predict the disease's course despite misidentification of its cause, he also provides enough detail to pose an intriguing puzzle. Modern diagnostic guesses might be atrial fibrillation and/or aortic insufficiency following an infection of the heart muscle or of the endocardium or pericardium. His heart unable to pump strongly enough to clear fluid from the lungs, the patient developed pulmonary edema and died, either of suffocation or ventricular fibrillation.[6]

A sick person coming to Galen for treatment would, then, find him- or herself the central focus of the intense, penetrating intellect that has emerged so clearly in our investigation of all other aspects of his life. Galen brought this focus not only to his anatomical researches, his studies, and his debates

---

6   *Loc. Affect.* 4.11 (8.293–96K). Modern diagnosis: I am grateful for the opinions of Drs. Joseph M. Garland and Philip G. Haines in private correspondence.

with rivals; he brought no less of it to his clinical practice, to which he devoted unlimited energy both mentally and physically. Even when patients needed extensive hands-on therapy, Galen seems to have performed many these tasks himself. It is clear that he also delegated work to the patient's servants or to his own slave assistants (these last are shadowy figures, but it is likely that they followed him everywhere—he calls them "my [people]"). But in his world of abundant servile labor, there is, perhaps surprisingly, no clear division between the functions of a physician and those of an assistant or domestic servant. In the case of the "ruddy and plump" patient mentioned above: Galen bled the patient in the middle of the night (taking so much blood that the patient fainted, then broke out in diarrhea, vomiting, and a cold sweat; 10.612K). Galen gave the patient food and orders to rest; on a later visit, he writes, he gave the patient gruel broth, suggesting that he fed the patient himself and perhaps even cooked the food himself. Elsewhere Galen writes of bathing, massaging and feeding patients, applying plasters, and mixing drugs. While it is possible or likely that "I did *x*" or "we did *x*" in the first person sometimes means "my slaves did *x*," this is probably not true of all examples; especially when Galen could, and does, describe delegating tasks to servants in some passages.[7]

Regarding his female patients, Galen sometimes mentions midwives—as in the case of Boethus's wife, discussed in chapter 5—and acknowledges issues of modesty. He seems to avoid touching women's genitals, but otherwise does not treat them noticeably differently than his male patients. Galen interrogated midwives and laywomen on obstetrical matters (accumulating folk wisdom about conception and pregnancy; he accepted the notion, attested also in the Hippocratic corpus but apparently common among the women of his era, that women could feel conception taking place as the uterus contracted around the semen). He mentions speaking with many women who described themselves as "hysterical," that is, having an illness caused, as they believed, by a condition of the uterus (*hystera* in Greek) whose symptoms varied from muscle contractions to lethargy to nearly complete asphyxia

---

7   See Mattern (2008a, 138–145) for further discussion.

(*Loc. Affect.* 6.5, 8.414K). Galen, very aware of Herophilus's discovery of the broad ligaments anchoring the uterus to the pelvis, denied that the uterus wandered around the body like an animal wreaking havoc (the Hippocratics imagined a very actively mobile womb). But the uterus could, in his view, become withdrawn in some direction or inflamed; and in one passage he recommends the ancient practice of fumigating the vagina with sweet-smelling odors to attract the uterus, endowed in this view with senses and desires of its own, to its proper place; this technique is described in the Hippocratic Corpus but also evokes folk or shamanistic medicine. Galen attributed "hysterical" conditions to the noxious accumulation of female seed or menstrual fluid and was inclined to explain a wide variety of women's disorders by disruption of the menstrual cycle.[8]

Galen accepted and expanded the ancient Hippocratic theory of humors, as I have described in chapter 2, and a humoral view of the body pervades his ideas about disease and his approach to medicine. Still, in practice, he does not apply a rigorous doctrine of humors but takes a more general approach, often emphasizing the elemental qualities of hot, cold, wet, and dry rather than the humors *per se*. To see this we need look no further than his youthful patient with fever, described above. The patient's innate temperament, which is warm and dry, his stage of life, his lifestyle, habits, and state of mind (worried, anxious, angry), and his history of travel in hot, dry weather, all contribute to the hot, dry imbalance that causes the anomaly, or disease. Galen never invokes a humor here—if he did, it would certainly be the hot, dry humor of yellow bile—but a sense of the delicate balance of qualities,

---

8   Talking to women about conception: see *Sem.* 1.2 (4.514K) (and cf. *Nat. Fac.* 3.3, 2.149K). On hysterical conditions: *Loc. Affect.* 6.5 (8.417–19K, 426–34K); *Uter. Dissect.* 4 (2.893K); *Comp. Med. Loc.* 9.10 (13.319–20K); *Hipp. 1 Prorrhet.* 3.121 (16.773K); *Hipp. Aph.* 5.35 (17B.823–24K). Fumigation: *Meth. Med. Glauc.* 1.15 (11.54K). On the wandering womb in the Hippocratic Corpus and fumigation, see Dean-Jones (1994, 69–77). For a recent collection and analysis of the evidence for hysterical conditions in antiquity, see Faraone (2011). Interrogation: *Hipp. 6 Epid.* 3.29 (17B.95K); *Sem.* 1.2 (4.514K). Modesty (of both men and women, regarding different parts): *Hipp. Off.* 1.13 (18B.687–88K). Observing women's conditions and illnesses: e.g., *Hipp. 6 Epid.* 1.2 (17A.811K, prolapsed uterus?); *Meth. Med. Glauc.* 2.12 (11.140–41K, breast cancer). Galen on menstruation: see especially *Ven. Sect. Eras.* 5 (11.164–66K); on women's diseases in Galen, see Flemming (2000, 331–42); on fumigation, see ibid. 347.

and of the intricate relationship between internal and external, individual and environment, body and soul, reflect the subtle, ancient and Hippocratic "humoral" view of disease.

The humors yellow bile, black bile, or phlegm might cause fever, if they accumulated in excess and putrefied; excess blood might cause fever if it changed into some other humor. Tumors, inflammations, ulcers, cancers, and rashes were noxious accumulations of undigested, unevacuated humors, or of rotten and putrefied humors. Accumulations of humors in the brain could cause apoplexy, epilepsy, melancholy, and other conditions. Diet could rebalance the humors or elemental qualities, if foods of the right sort were eaten. Medicinal ingredients, too—herbs, minerals, parts of animals—had their own qualities and could be used to restore balance, as Galen explains in *On the Mixtures and Powers of Simple Drugs*, in which he assigns qualities and sometimes degrees of strength to the ingredients he describes. Exercise, bathing, and massage, as well as purgative and emetic drugs could evacuate noxious substances. So could bloodletting, especially in patients with certain signs indicating that an excess of blood, or *plethos*, was the problem; but Galen interpreted these indications liberally, and considered venesection a good treatment for virtually any serious illness.[9] He sometimes took pints of blood from a patient, in a procedure that could be so drastic that one observer jokingly compared him to a butcher:

> I carefully drew enough [blood] from him [the patient] that he fainted, having learned from reason and experience that this is the best remedy for continual fevers when [the patient's] strength is vigorous. At first his body moved rapidly to the opposite state, chilled by the loss of

9   Fevers: see especially *Diff. Febr.*, book 2 (7.333–405K). Brain: *Anim. Mor. Corp.* 3 (4.776–77K); *Loc. Affect.* 3.9 (8.173–79K). Diet: see Galen's *Aliment. Fac.* and the discussion of Powell (2003, 10–13). Drugs: see especially *On Mixtures* (English translation available in Singer 1997), book 3 (1.646–94K) and *On the Mixtures and Powers of Simple Drugs*, books 1–5, with the discussion of Vogt (2008). On bloodletting generally and for what follows, see Galen's treatises *On Venesection Against Erasistratus*, *On Treatment by Venesection*, and *On Venesection Against the Erasistrateans at Rome*, with translation and discussion by Brain (1986). See also Galen's treatise *On Plenitude*, available with German translation in Otte (2001).

consciousness. It would be impossible to discover anything more pleasant or useful than this.... In bodies of this kind an evacuation of the stomach necessarily follows, and sometimes also a vomiting of bile, and immediately following these things a dampness over the whole body, or sweats. When all of these things in turn happened to him [the patient] too, they immediately extinguished the fever, so that some of those who were present said, "man, you have slaughtered the fever," whereupon we all laughed.

(*Meth. Med.* 9.4, 10.612K)

Galen was well aware that taking a lot of blood from a patient would cause a severe reaction, which he describes accurately in this passage; in this case of fever with *plethos* he deliberately provoked the reaction by bleeding the patient until he fainted, which also, as he believed, cured the disease. Venesection was a dangerous treatment when used aggressively, as here, with a narrow margin for error between perceived efficacy and lethality. Galen knew that patients could die of being bled. One must monitor their pulse carefully to prevent this, as he wrote, and he knew doctors who had killed their patients by taking too much blood. Other patients might recover but their constitutions were permanently cooled; they became pale and weak and susceptible to other diseases, which more easily claimed their lives.[10]

Bloodletting plays a minor role in the Hippocratic Corpus, but was an established therapy by Galen's time, and would go on to have a very long history in European, Islamic, and Jewish medicine, partly as a result of his influence, and also in some other cultures. Today bloodletting retains a very limited place in western biomedicine, but it is so pervasive in history that scholars still sometimes search for observable positive effects that would explain its popularity. This is probably futile, as it is hard to avoid concluding that the damage done by bloodletting outweighed any placebo effect or the occasional clinical benefit for some conditions. It is best to see

---

10   Dead patients: *Meth. Med.* 9.10 (10.637K); *Cur. Ven. Sect.* 12 (11.288–89K). Debility: *Meth. Med.* 9.10 (10.367–68K).

bloodletting in the context of ancient ideas of disease—Galen attributed most diseases to the buildup of toxins in the body, and this view seems to have remained deeply embedded in western culture.[11] Thus, it was not only physicians who foisted the procedure on their patients; Galen writes that it was a custom of "the people among us" (that is, the area around Pergamum) to be bled every spring and tells of a peasant youth who asked for a routine venesection only to have an inexperienced doctor slice into an artery (*Meth. Med.* 5.7, 10.334K).

Nevertheless, we must acknowledge that, by enthusiastically endorsing the practice of bloodletting, Galen contributed to the suffering and death of many patients in the future. While it is perhaps wrong to blame him for failing to break from a tradition that his followers, including the great physicians of the Islamic Middle East and of the European Renaissance and Enlightenment, also mostly did not question, one wishes that he had turned his scorn on this therapy, rather than on the Methodists' three-day fasting cure. For while Galen did not invent bloodletting, he had the power to consign it to oblivion.

Bloodletting was contraindicated if the patient was weak, too young (under age fourteen), or too old, if the patient was pregnant, if the weather was hot and dry (because excesses could then be evacuated by sweat and breathing), and in certain other circumstances. However, Galen did not shrink from using venesection on a woman—she was "not obscure," and the case won him many similar patients—who was so wasted with anorexia that she had not menstruated in eight months. (Galen does not name the cause of this patient's failure of appetite, but it could have been psychological; *anorexia nervosa* is not a condition limited to the western world or the modern era, and many historical and cross-cultural cases are known.) In Galen's view suppressed menstruation was an ominous condition; residues were being retained, and venesection was the cure. From this patient he

---

11   On the history of bloodletting and for a modern evaluation of the practice, see Schneeberg (2002, 157–85). On bloodletting in western and Chinese culture (where its role is much more circumscribed), see Kuriyama (1999, chapter 5; 1995). On bloodletting in medieval Islamic medicine, see Pormann and Savage-Smith (2007, 121).

took over a pint of blood on the first day and as much again over the next two days.[12]

Galen opposed narrow specializations in medicine, and his position on the status of the professional surgeon (the Greek *cheirourgos*, one who "works with the hand") is not clear. Nevertheless, he rarely mentions performing surgery himself—his operation on the slave of Maryllus is the major exception to this—and in general he wrote little about it.[13] He may often have left these procedures to surgical specialists, or patients sought out the specialists on their own. He avoided cranial trepanation (cutting a hole in a patient's skull with a chisel or circular saw), a common procedure that he gratefully relegated to the specialists in Rome; if he had stayed at Pergamum, he might have had to become more proficient at the skill himself, as he writes (*Meth. Med.* 6.6, 10.454–55K). However, Galen clearly performed some trepanations, discussing his preferred methods in one passage from *On the Method of Healing* (6.6, 10.446–55K). The main condition he mentions treating this way is skull fracture, as in a case when he removed part of one patient's frontal bone (Galen's comment that "even now [the patient] has lived many years" suggests that this was unusual). He emphasizes the need to protect the *dura mater* from perforation and describes the effects of pressing on it too hard during the procedure.[14] In general, however, Galen considered surgery a last resort and thought those doctors most worthy of praise who could treat conditions such

---

12   Anorexic patient: *Hipp. 6 Epid.* 3.29 (17B.81–82). *Anorexia nervosa*: Keel and Klump (2003). Contraindications: Brain (1986, 131–33).

13   Galen on specialization: see especially *On the Parts of Medicine*, which survives in Arabic; and *To Thrasybulus on Whether Health belongs to Medicine or Gymnastics* (5.806–98K). English translations are available of both: Lyons (1969); Singer (1997, 53–99). Galen's longest discussion of surgery appears in his *Hipp. Off.* 1.17–25 (18B.694–718K).

14   *Plac. Hipp. Plat.* 1.6 (5.186K); *Loc. Affect.* 2.10 (8.128K). Quotation: *Meth. Med.* 6.6 (10.452–53K); see also the case that follows (10.453–54K). On trepanation, see further Rocca (2003, 181–84). On the skeletal evidence for trepanation in Roman Italy, see Mariani-Costatini et al. (2000, 305–7). Only three skeletons are known; one is that of a five-year-old child treated as a last resort for an "intracranial expanding lesion" that probably was the cause of death. The skeleton comes from Fidenae, near Rome, and dates to the first or second century C.E. It is conceivable that the patient, who was well-fed and otherwise healthy despite modest means, and whose parents clearly sought out the most expert care, was one of Galen's, though it seems more likely that the child saw one of the specialists in trepanation that Galen mentions.

as abscesses, tumors, or kidney stones with diet and drugs (*Opt. Med. Cogn.* 10, 116 Iskandar).

A passage from his commentary on the sixth book of the Hippocratic *Epidemics* describes the attention to many factors demanded in therapy (and also suggests that Galen's typical patient was an urban resident with servants):

> Thus in medicine it is not the same thing to learn the art and to make appropriate use of what one has learned, knowing to ask and to speak at the right time, and to listen at the right time to the patient or to his household [*oikeioi*] and to talk with them [about] how they might be most useful for service, and to pay attention to the external things, which have been overlooked by the doctors and the household of the patient. Among which the most useful things pertain to sleep, or to either the whole house or the rooms in which the patients are lying, if they are squalid because of a foul odor or air that is very hot or cold or full of mold. And, regarding disturbances from neighbors or from those in the public streets, it is necessary for the doctor to pay attention, and to talk about all of these things with the household and the friends of the patient.
>
> (*Hipp. 6 Epid.* 2.47, 17A.1000K)

This passage also evokes the social aspects of illness in Galen's world: the hypothetical patient is surrounded by friends, household, servants, neighbors on the other side of a dividing wall, multiple physicians, people in the street just outside the courtyard. It could be impossible to clear a room of busybodies even for surgery, where the modesty of the patient required privacy and the physician could do no more than promise to try his best to hide genitals or buttocks from prying eyes (*Hipp. Off.* 1.13, 18B.687–88K). (Male) friends of (male) patients in particular played a key role in illness: they seem to be present day and night, to help with the patient's care (applying cold compresses, assisting in procedures such as bloodletting), and they argue with physicians about the best treatment. Illness was not a private experience but a social event that rallied one's connections and created both cohesion and rivalries, as one group might support one physician's advice against another's.[15]

The patient's bedside could be a scene of dramatic conflict, rivalry, victory, and humiliation. Sickroom contests were similar to the public debates and demonstrations typical of Galen's life in Rome that I have discussed in earlier chapters, and Galen makes no clear distinction between them. I mentioned in chapter 4 one of his early conflicts with Erasistrateans, including Martianus who would become his bitter enemy, over the treatment of a young woman desperately in need (in Galen's view) of bloodletting. The debate moves from the bedside to the street when Galen's friend Teuthras produces and reads publicly from Erasistratus's own case histories as proof of the necessity of bloodletting (these patients, whom the famous physician had not bled, died); and the question of the usefulness of bloodletting was also posed in what had become a daily public debate on medical (or philosophical?) points. Galen himself responded, and Teuthras had his friend's comments transcribed by a slave so that he could bring the resulting treatise on a projected return home to Pergamum, "so that he might say the same things [that I said] against Martialius [sc. Martianus] in his examinations of patients."[16] Thus, a prodigious contest between the upstart Galen and Rome's most illustrious physicians begins at the patient's bedside, is dragged out into the street, and then back to the sickroom in the form of Galen's treatise, ammunition in the hands of his friends against their enemies.

Galen's case histories often feature rivalries with other doctors or, more commonly, groups of physicians (sometimes labeled Methodists, Erasistrateans, or something else), with much bitter polemic, dramatic proof of Galen's superiority, and affirmation from the astounded witnesses. A good example is the story of the twenty-five-year-old youth who enjoyed gymnastic exercises, whose history is quoted earlier in this chapter (*Meth. Med.* 10.3, 10.671–78K). In this story Galen's rivals are "doctors of the *diatritos*"

---

15   On the role of friends in the sickroom, see Mattern (2008a, 84–87).
16   *Libr. Propr.* 1 (19.14K) and *Ven. Sect. Eras.* 1 (11.190–94K), two similar but not entirely harmonious accounts of the same events.

(that is, proponents of a trendy three-day fasting treatment popularized by Methodists).

The patient had become feverish—he was "seized by fever"—as a result of the circumstances described in the history, namely travel, vexation, physical exertion in more than one fight, hot and dry weather. "He returned home extremely dry and became aware of his own fatigue and that something was abnormal" (Galen uses the ominous word *anomalia*, *Meth. Med.* 103. 10.672K). The patient drank water but only became more ill ("the anomaly increased") and vomited. At the eleventh hour of the day—about 4 P.M.; this will become the "suspect hour" of the story, the hour of the paroxysm's onset every two days—he lay down. He spent a sleepless night. The next day some Methodist "physicians of the *diatritos*" came to call on him, and prescribed their trademark three-day fast; they returned that evening, saw that the fever was in decline, and stood by their advice, although at this point another physician (Galen does not say who) argued strenuously that the patient ought to be fed. They returned on the morning of the third day and repeated their advice.

Galen now visited the patient for the first time, on the third day of the illness, in the afternoon, after the Methodist doctors had left. (He does not say whether he was summoned or was simply paying a call on a friend.) A glance showed him the ominous "sharp nose, concave eyes" of Hippocrates' *Prognostic*, which Galen quotes here (ibid. 10.674K); this is still known today as the *facies Hippocratica* or "Hippocratic face" of impending death. The patient was dangerously ill and was, in Galen's view, on the verge of lapsing into a combined hectic and wasting fever, which would be fatal and incurable.[17] "The suspect hour," as he writes, "was the eleventh of that day" (ibid. 10.673K); Galen anticipated a serious paroxysm, and was alarmed at the thought that the patient would endure it without food. Seizing control of the situation, "I prepared a porridge of groats as quickly as possible and I gave it to him to eat" (ibid. 10.674K; note that Galen writes as though he did this with his own hands).

---

17   Incurable: *Diff. Febr.* 1.10 (7.314K); *Meth. Med.* 10.10 (10.720K).

At the eleventh hour, the paroxysm struck. The patient's extremities went cold; his pulse nearly vanished ("his pulse became small and extremely weak"). The next day Galen fed the patient twice, in the morning and the evening—not only, as he writes, to strengthen the patient, but to rehydrate him, "for his skin was dry, like a hide" (ibid. 10.674K). On the fifth day, anticipating another paroxysm, Galen mixed pomegranate seeds in with the groats, hoping to correct for the hot and dry imbalance of the patient's stomach. Again the paroxysm struck, "about the same" as before (ibid. 10.675K). Galen returned on the sixth, seventh, and eighth days; "we fed him … in the same way."

With Galen in firm control of the patient, the Methodists had, nevertheless, not entirely left the scene. They continued to advocate fasting. It was apparent to Galen and, as he claims, to everyone else that the patient would never have survived his second paroxysm—the third night of the illness—if Galen had not intervened and insisted on feeding him. For a while Galen ignored their "madness" and "contentiousness," not daring to try to refute them with a demonstration while the patient's health was so delicate. But the paroxysm of the ninth day was a little less severe; the patient's pulse was a little stronger. At this point Galen gave way to his aggravation and the weakness he calls "love of contention" (*philoneikia*): "I could no longer bear the jabbering of the doctors" (ibid. 10.676K). He announced to the patient's friends that he would prove unequivocally that his treatment had saved the patient, and, without feeding the patient, he allowed the paroxysm to attack. The result was one of the most theatrical events of his long career.

"Complete asphyxia occurred … and an extreme chilling of the whole body, so that he could not utter a sound nor scarcely feel things pressing on him" (ibid. 10.676K). Galen called together all the doctors who had been treating the patient. Also present were the patient's *oikeioi*, a word Galen uses of the household or intimate friends: these, he writes, might be angry enough almost to tear him and the other doctors apart, for the doctors' ignorance and for his own risky move that endangered the patient's life to prove a point. The Methodists, sensing a trap, "became paler and colder than the patient himself, and were considering a means of escape." Galen ordered the entryway door to be locked and gave the key to one of his (or the patient's) friends. "Standing in the middle," Galen now berated the other doctors for their stupidity. In order to refute them and to convince those whom they had swayed to their views (Galen probably means the patient's friends, companions, and household here) he had allowed his treatment to lapse, based on his considered judgment that the patient would survive the paroxysm. Now Galen would further prove his point by reviving the comatose patient. "I opened his jaws and poured in three cyanthes' worth of barley broth through a funnel" (ibid. 10.677K). The patient miraculously sat up "and began to hear and speak and recognize those present, when before he had been stretched out dry and insensible and speechless."

Somewhat unusually, Galen omits to record his large audience's response to this Lazarus-like demonstration. Perhaps this seemed unnecessary: the astonishment and wonder and spontaneous expressions of praise that he so often attributes to those who witness his superior skills can be assumed here and need not be described.[18] Galen ends the story with a summary of how he treated the patient over the following week, resulting in a complete recovery.

The story of the "gymnastic" youth, as it builds toward Galen's head-to-head confrontation with his rivals, is an excellent example of the agonistic theme in Galen's case histories. His rivals may be an individual physician (even the patient himself, as in the story of Glaucon's friend, chapter 4) or—and this is more common—an anonymous group of physicians (like the physicians treating Boethus's wife in chapter 5 or those treating Marcus Aurelius in chapter 6). Galen's deed might be a dramatic cure or a preternaturally accurate prediction. His audience might be the patient; or the patient's friends; or the other physicians, who may admit defeat or convert to his views; or sometimes an authority figure (the head of household, as in the stories about Boethus's family; the owner of a slave; the emperor Marcus Aurelius), whose judgment and expressions of admiration carry special weight.[19]

---

18   On astonishment etc., see Mattern (2008a, 80–83) and cf. the case of Glaucon's friend, chapter 4.

19   On agonistic themes in Galen's stories, see Mattern (2008a, chapter 3).

The same story also illustrates other important themes, however. I have remarked how Galen's detailed history of this patient reflects the intimate knowledge gleaned from close questioning—his dialogue with the patient and/or with those around him. This is also one of the stories in which Galen's clinical practices are best described, and we see him visiting the patient twice daily over a two-week period, preparing his meals and overseeing his care.

I also emphasize that Galen's stories about patients usually had a scientific purpose—they are not only literary creations, although they are not documentary "records" either. This particular story, for example, may have happened early in Galen's career (he opens by saying that this was the patient "on whom I first dared, led by reason, to disregard the *diatritos*") and is thus being told long after the fact, sometime in the 190s when he composed the second half of *On the Method of Healing*. Galen probably wrote this story from memory after having repeated it orally many times. It aggrandizes Galen, and it creates a sympathetic portrait of the patient and of the social class to which both he and Galen belonged. When Galen locks the door on his rivals to prevent their escape from his verbal assault he recalls a famous scene from the *Odyssey*, the hero's slaughter of the suitors, and this embellishment, along with others, may have crept into the story as it was told and retold. But Galen introduces the case with reference to none of these things (though he is not above making his own triumphs the overt message of a story, as in the case of Glaucon's friend or most of the stories in *On Prognosis*) but with a subtle epistemological point: this is the *first* case in which he dared to ignore the *diatritos*, the dominant prescription for fever in his day. It describes an initial experiment which Galen afterwards confirmed by many repetitions, a classically Empiricist method. But Galen also writes that he was inspired by "indication"—*endeixis*, a type of logical inference specifically banned in Empiricist doctrine.[20] The story, then, is not simply an entertaining or self-aggrandizing anecdote; it offers a kind of proof.

In his introductory sentence, Galen calls the patient an *arrhostos*—"I shall tell you about an *arrhostos* of this type on whom I first dared, led by reason,

---

20 See *Meth. Med.* 2.7 (10.126–27K) with the commentary of Hankinson (1991a, 202–5).

to disregard the *diatritos*" (*Meth. Med.* 10.3, 10.671K). Galen normally calls his patients *kamnon* ("sick one") or *anthropos* ("person") or by any number of other words; *arrhostos* (meaning literally "the weak one") had a special significance. It is the word for the patients in the case histories of the Hippocratic *Epidemics*; Galen and others used it to mean, substantively, the Hippocratic stories themselves. One could read an *arrhostos* or write an *arrhostos*. Thus, it was a technical word approximating our term "case history." Significantly, the other context in which Galen often uses *arrhostos* is when he appeals to clinical experience as evidence, which he does often: "I have observed this among the *arrhostoi*."[21]

Galen thought the story of the gymnastic youth and most of his stories served a purpose similar to that of the Hippocratic case histories and, perhaps, also was influenced by his Empiricist background, as I have argued in chapter 2. Galen cited case histories in oral debates with his teachers, and they played a role in at least one of his bedside disputes and discussions with rivals and colleagues. Discussing the famous case of Pausanias, cured of nerve damage to his fingers, with the other physicians in attendance, Galen queries them to make a point concerning the distinction between motor and sensory nerves:

> I said, "and so have you never observed the opposite, that movement is lost but sensation preserved?" Almost all the others said they had never seen this, but one claimed that he had, and he gave the name of the patient and he promised to provide witnesses.
>
> (*Loc. affect.* 1.6, 8.58–59K)

(Both sensation without motion and motion without sensation can happen in Galen's view, although the distinction he traces between motor and sensory nerves is complex.)[22] Thus, case histories could teach and transmit

---

21   On the role of case histories in Galen's work, see Mattern (2008a, 40–43); on words for patient, also 101–2. On "among the *arrhostoi*," see ibid. 42 n. 142 for references.

22   Regarding cranial nerves, Galen distinguishes between hard nerves of motion and soft nerves of sensation arising from harder and softer parts of the brain and brainstem in *Usu Part.* 9.11

medical knowledge, as they still do today, even though in antiquity they were mostly told orally and we have no evidence for systematic patient records.

Galen offers no diagnosis for the patient in the story of the gymnastic youth, but it is likely he would have called the disease tertian fever. A possible modern diagnosis, given the patient's neurological symptoms, is falciparian malaria, the most dangerous form of malaria (also sometimes called by its old-fashioned name "malignant tertian fever"). The life-cycle of the *P. falciparum* protozoon is forty-eight hours, and especially in established infections this can cause a cyclical pattern of paroxysmal symptoms. But intermittent fever is at best only a coarse indicator of malaria.[23] Symptoms of dehydration in the story are very striking (sunken eyes, leathery skin). Dehydration can be a symptom of malaria, but this patient also had a history of physical exertion and travel in hot, dry weather, which Galen and the patient himself considered highly relevant. Heatstroke and/or severe dehydration, either of which can cause low blood pressure, weak pulse, and neurological symptoms, could be primary or complicating factors.

Fever had pride of place in Galen's practice. As I have mentioned in chapter 5, he devoted several treatises to describing and classifying fevers, with much attention to their periodicity, which could reach dizzying levels of mathematical complication: *On Critical Days*, *On Crises*, and *On the Differences in Fevers*. In this he reflected an environment rife with infectious, febrile diseases, and a medical tradition, many centuries old, that sought to predict the course of fevers by mapping their waxing and waning over days. The story of the gymnastic youth is a good example of Galen's view of fever as a series of paroxysmal attacks. Among other diseases that he treated I have mentioned tuberculosis and leprosy (in chapter 4) and "the great plague" (in chapter 6). Most poignantly, he treated children for kidney stones, although he does not mention performing the dangerous surgery that is described in book 7 of

---

(3.274–75K); but as the limbs had only hard nerves originating in the spinal column, his theory becomes more complicated in this context (*Sympt. Caus.* 1.5, 7.111–115K). On Galenic neurology, see Rocca (2003).

23   Pearson (2009).

Celsus's first-century treatise *On Medicine* (and may have left this procedure to Rome's surgical specialists); Galen picked up the children and shook them to dislodge the stone. When blood clots develop in the urinary tract as a result of stones or other causes, Galen writes, one can try to break up the clot with medicines, and in one case he succeeded in removing the clot with a catheter; but almost all of these patients die (*Loc. Affect.* 6.4, 8.408–9). He treated women for breast cancer, which he believed to be the most common type of cancer, and his treatise *On the Method of Healing to Glaucon* preserves a striking description of an advanced case:

> We have often seen in the breasts a tumor exactly similar to that animal, the crab [*cancer*, in Latin; *karkinos*, in Greek]. For just as in the crab the feet are on either side of the body, so also in this disease the veins, extending from the unnatural tumor, make a shape similar to a crab. This disease we have cured often in its beginning, but when it has progressed to a substantial size no one can cure it without surgery.
>
> (*Meth. Med. Glauc.* 2.12, 11.140–41K)[24]

Galen believed the condition was caused by the accumulation of black bile, if it was not adequately cleared through menstruation, and that he could cure it in early stages with purgative drugs. He purged one woman every year in the spring, "and if ever the purgation was neglected, the pain arose from the depths, and she herself would call me."[25] Galen recognized that some cancers were incurable by any method available to him, and that some, including those on the roof of the mouth, would only be made worse by cutting or cauterizing, and should not be treated. Intervention in such cases might shorten the patient's life or cause unnecessary suffering.[26]

---

24   Breast cancer most common: *Meth. Med. Glauc.* 2.12 (11.139K). I translate Galen's terms *karkinoma* and *karkinodes onkos* as "cancer." For a brief review of the medical references to breast cancer in antiquity, see Retief and Cilliers (2011, 513–15).

25   *Hipp. Aph.* 6.47 (18A.80K); the same patient also mentioned in *Purg. Med. Fac.* 1 (11.344–45K).

26   *Hipp. Aph.* 4.24 (17B.688K), 6.38 (18A.60K).

Galen was especially proud of his prowess in healing patients with nerve damage and of his knowledge of the anatomy of the nervous system. One case was especially well-known because of the patient's celebrity; he was a renowned sophist, whose name, Pausanias, Galen reveals in one version of the story. (Very likely he is Pausanias of Caesarea in Cappadocia, who studied in Athens with the great Herodes Atticus. The biographer Philostratus grants this Pausanias a perfunctory paragraph in his *Lives of the Sophists*, telling us that he spoke his brilliant declamations with a vulgar, heavy Cappadocian accent, and that he was therefore called, in a reference to Plato's *Phaedrus*, "a cook who prepares expensive delicacies badly." This Pausanias held the chair of rhetoric at Athens and also at Rome, where he spent much of his life and where he died approaching old age.)[27]

The cure of Pausanias happened some time before the mid-170s, when Galen composed the earliest of his four surviving versions of the story, and went something like this (the four versions are all slightly different and contradictory but agree on enough detail to safely identify the patient): Pausanias fell out of a vehicle, perhaps on the way from Syria to Rome. (In *On the Examinations by which the Best Physicians are Recognized*, which survives only in Arabic, he falls off an animal he is riding rather than from a carriage.) He landed on his upper back, which hit a rock. For six days he suffered intense pain, which resolved; but beginning on the fifteenth day, he began to lose sensation in the two little fingers and half of the middle finger of his left hand. This gradually became worse, and he consulted either a single physician, or two or more physicians, whom Galen labels Methodists in one version of the story. They applied plasters to the affected fingers, but with no result. After some time—a month; three or four months—Pausanias consulted with Galen, who first summoned and interrogated the patient's other doctor(s) about the drugs. But the treatment seemed appropriate. Galen then questioned the patient: Had he been beaten or chilled? Had there been any inflammation? Hearing no, he pressed on: Had Pausanias not suffered some blow to the spine? Of course! The patient recalled his fall from

---

27   Philostratus, *Vitae Sophistarum* 13.

the carriage and told Galen all about it. Galen now knew and explained exactly what had happened: the nerve below the seventh cervical vertebra had been damaged in the fall. Galen's diagnosis of what would now be called a textbook case of cervical radiculopathy at the C8 nerve was certainly correct, although his treatment would probably be considered ineffective today (modern remedies, which include physical therapy and sometimes surgery, are of contested effectiveness but most patients improve on their own over time).[28] In any case Galen applied an external medicine (he does not say what it was) to the area of the nerve root. Pausanias, as he writes, recovered immediately, much to the surprise of those who witnessed the events: "it seemed amazing and surprising to those who saw it [sc. the rival physicians, implied later in this passage], that the fingers of the hand were cured when medicine was applied to the spine" (*Loc. Affect.* 1.6, 8.58K). Galen lectures his rivals patiently on the nature of nerve injuries at the end of one version of the story.[29]

Epilepsy was an illness of some mystique in antiquity and, indeed, throughout western history, which may explain its prominence in Galen's work. In popular belief it was vaguely supernatural and contaminating; people spat to ward it off, and epileptics felt the shame and disgrace of public revulsion. A popular and particularly gruesome folk remedy, according to Pliny, was drinking the blood of gladiators (*Naturalis historia* 28.4). Beginning with the treatise called *The Sacred Disease* in the Hippocratic corpus, ancient medicine had directly and deliberately challenged the common, superstitious view of epilepsy. The term *epileipsia* has its root in the Greek word "to seize," and it signified an attack, or recurrent series of attacks, that struck the patient down unconscious, with or without full-body convulsions of classical grand mal type. A number of causes were postulated, but for Galen, loosely following Hippocratic tradition, its origin was a blockage in the brain: specifically,

---

28   Coincidentally, I have suffered from almost exactly the same condition as Pausanias myself and am well familiar with the causes and symptoms.

29   The Pausanias story: *Anat. Admin.* 3.1 (2.343–45K); *Loc. Affect.* 1.6 (8.56–59K), 3.14 (8.213–14K; this is the version that names the patient); *Opt. Med. Cogn.* 9 (106–8 Iskandar). The versions in *Anat. Admin.* and *Opt. Med. Cogn.* were composed earliest and are roughly contemporary.

a thick humor, either phlegm or black bile, blocked the outlet of cerebral *pneuma* from the ventricles. This blockage could be either primary or secondary to something else; that is, in some patients, a problem arising elsewhere (especially in the cardia, between the stomach and esophagus) could affect the brain and cause epileptic seizures and other neurological problems, if vaporous exhalations carried the suspect humors upward.[30]

Galen seems to have treated many patients for epilepsy, including some that I have already mentioned: two boys he saw with his teachers as an adolescent, in Smyrna (chapter 2); the boy who was protected by his amulet of peony root (chapter 5). Galen wrote a special treatise on the disease for a Roman father, one Caecilianus (many identifications are possible), about to depart for Athens with his physician and his epileptic son; Galen had never examined the boy, but agreed to offer advice nevertheless. This was under Severus, after the fire.[31]

Galen's most illustrious patient with epilepsy was Diodorus the Grammarian, whom he mentions several times, although only once by name. Diodorus is a "youth" in the story; that is, a man in the prime of life, probably between about twenty-five and forty. "He was seized by the epileptic disorder if he taught very forcefully, or worried [*ephrontisen*], or fasted for a long time, or became angry [*ethumothe*]." Galen diagnosed the problem as arising from the cardia, and he prescribed a special diet and thrice-yearly purgations with aloe. The patient did well on this regimen, but would occasionally suffer an attack if a busy schedule caused him to skip meals.[32]

The case of Diodorus calls attention to the prominent role of emotions and psychology in Galen's practice. Galen makes no special distinction between physical causes of epileptic seizures and psychic ones; in particular, the emotions of anger or worry might precipitate them. The emotions Galen most

---

30   On epilepsy in ancient medicine, see Temkin (1971, part 1). Galen's primary discussion of the etiology of epilepsy and other brain disorders is in *Loc. Affect.* 3.8–4.5 (8.168–237K).

31   Treatise on epilepsy: *Puer. Epil.* (11.357–78K); cf. *Libr. Propr.* 7 (19.31K). On the date of the treatise, see Ilberg (1896, 183, 195); for possible identifications of Caecilianus, see *Prosopographia Imperii Romani* (1933–66), C13.

32   *Loc. Affect.* 5.6 (8.340–41K); also *San. Tuend.* 6.14 (6.448–49K) and *Ven. Sect. Eras. Rom.* 9 (11.241–42K).

often implicates in disease are anger, fear, grief (called *lupe*), and anxiety (also called *lupe* but linked to words for worry, for example, about a guilty secret, an upcoming contest, or a future contingency—rational or irrational—rather than loss).

The full proof of my last statement is subtle and will have to wait for another venue, but it evokes discussion of one of Galen's most famous cases, the case of the wife of Justus, whom he also calls "the woman in love." This happened early in his career, during his first visit to Rome, and (as he implies in *On Prognosis*) shortly after his anatomical demonstration for Boethus and other intellectuals. Galen mentions it several times, always comparing it to the legend or folktale of Erasistratus, who discovered that prince Antiochus of Syria, son of the Hellenistic King Seleucus I, was in love with his stepmother (or, in the version of the story that Galen knew, with his father's concubine).[33] Some scholars have doubted the truth of Galen's story, based on (I think) an unnecessarily stringent interpretation of the language in one of Galen's versions of it. I have no doubt that Galen's memory tailored the story to enhance its resemblance to the legend of Erasistratus, which clearly delighted him, but I do not think he invented it from whole cloth—also because he writes as though it were a well-known event.[34]

Galen is very specific, here and elsewhere, that what he detected and diagnosed in his patient was not, strictly speaking, love; nor did Erasistratus do this. There is no "erotic pulse," he explains, and no way that his famous predecessor could have identified the emotion of love through the pulse, as legend seemed to imply. What Erasistratus had felt was a change in the pulse (it became "anomalous and irregular") when the concubine entered the room, and a change back to normal when she left (*Hipp. Prog.* 1.8, 18B.40K). In the case of Justus's wife, Galen was called because she was

---

33   References to the story: *Praecog.* 5–6, 7, 13 (14.625–26, 630–33, 634, 640, 669K); *Hipp. 2 Epid.* (207–8 Wenkebach and Pfaff); *Hipp. Prog.* 1.8 (18B.40K). Concubine: *Praecog.* 6 (14.630–31K).

34   For the argument, see Mattern (2008a, 38–39 with n. 128). That the event was well-known is implied in *Praecog.* 5 (14.625–26K), where he places it in the context of other predictions and cures that enhanced his reputation.

suffering from insomnia, an ominous symptom in his view. He questioned her, but she was mostly unresponsive, and finally, when she wrapped herself in her veil and turned away in her bed, Galen gave up and left. Since he found no sign of fever, he determined that she was either suffering from depressed mood (*dysthymia*) caused by black bile, or she was distressed by something that she was unwilling to reveal. Galen returned the next day and the next, but was sent away by the chambermaid. On the fourth day he had better luck with the maid: he managed to engage her in casual conversation, in which she revealed that her mistress was worn down with *lupe*, an anxiety or grief.

At this point someone happened to walk in, coming from the theater, and say that Pylades was dancing that day. Galen noticed a change of gaze and color in the patient's face, and her pulse became suddenly irregular, indicating, as Galen writes, that her soul was disturbed. "The same thing," he says, "happens to those who are about to compete [*agonizein*]." Galen formed the hypothesis that the woman was in love with Pylades. A secret crush on a low-class entertainer, probably a slave, was a plausible cause of mental anguish in a married lady of the leisure class. Galen proceeded to test his theory: the following day (he seems to have visited this patient daily for some time) he told one of his servants to come in as he was examining the patient and say that Morpheus was dancing. No change in the patient's pulse. Galen tried the same ploy every day using the name of a different dancer, and although it is hard to believe that the patient did not become suspicious after the second or third try, she was unable to control her reaction on the fourth day, when Pylades' name was mentioned; her pulse became "disturbed in many ways" (*Praecog.* 6, 14.630–33K). Galen does not say what advice he gave the patient, or her husband.

He mentions this distinct pulse of anxiety in other places: recall that he found out the funny secret of Cyrillus, Boethus's little son who was hiding food, by feeling his pulse. In that story too Galen writes that he knew from the pulse that the child was not feverish but rather "disturbed," like someone about to compete in the *pankration* or plead in court (*Praecog.* 7, 14.640K). He claimed to be able to use the pulse as a lie-detector and, for example, to know whether a patient had followed his instructions or not.[35] Fear, anger, anxiety, and joy all had specific pulses and physical symptoms. Fear and, paradoxically, joy could be instantly fatal, in extreme cases.[36] Anxiety could be fatal in the long term: first it caused insomnia (as in the case of the woman in love), then fever, then the patient would waste until he or she died. As an alternative, anxiety might change to melancholy, an accumulation of black bile in the brain, which in Galen causes not just depression and a dark mood (misanthropy, suicide) but also, and especially, psychosis. The prognosis is especially bleak if the underlying worry is irrational (*Hipp. Aph.* 23,18A.35–36K).[37]

Some of Galen's most intriguing stories are about patients suffering extreme cases of anxiety. A patient of Erasistratus believed a ghost was calling him by name from the cemetery and was wasted by insomnia and fever. The famous doctor cured him by pretending that he had been the one who called the patient's name, shouting for help against bandits (*Hipp. 2 Epid.* 2, 207–8 Wenkebach and Pfaff). A man of Pergamum, Meander the augur, died of anxiety after predicting his own death. His symptoms, according to Galen, were similar to those of the woman in love when she heard the name of Pylades: "He went from the bird-flight area back to the city demolished, wretched and yellow in color, so that everyone who met him asked him whether he had some bodily illness. He told the truth to those in whom he trusted. Then he began to lie sleepless at nights while grief oppressed him all day, so that he deteriorated entirely" (*Hipp. 6 Epid.*, 485–86 Wenkebach and Pfaff). Finally he developed a fever and took to his bed; two months later he was dead, having gradually wasted away.

---

35   *Praes. Puls.* 1.1 (9.218K), 1.4 (9.250K).

36   *Sympt. Caus.* 2.5 (7.191–93K); *Puls. Tir.* 12 (8.472–74K); *Caus. Puls.* 4.2–6 (9.157–62K). Fatal: *Symp. Caus.* 2.5 (7.193–94K); *Loc. Affect.* 5.2 (8.302K).

37   Galen's most substantial discussion of melancholy is in *Loc. Affect.* 3.10 (8.190–93K), which appears to be heavily indebted to Rufus of Ephesus; see also *Sympt. Caus.* 2.7 (7.202–3K). On mental illness in Galen and in ancient medicine generally the most important author is Jackie Pigeaud, especially (1988) and (1981, chapter 1). On melancholy, which in antiquity was a psychotic illness in some ways similar to the modern diagnosis of schizophrenia, a new edition of the fragments of Rufus of Ephesus's lost treatise on the subject is especially important (see Pormann 2008).

My favorite patient—one Galen says that he saw himself[38]—believed that Atlas would grow tired of holding up the world and drop it, causing universal catastrophe.

> I know a man from Cappadocia, who had gotten a nonsensical thing into his head and because of that declined into melancholy.... His friends saw him weeping and asked him about his grief. At that he sighed deeply and answered, saying that he was worried that the whole world would collapse. He was worried that the person, of whom the poets relate that he carries the world and is called Atlas, would become tired because he had carried it for so long. Thus there was a danger that the sky would fall on the earth and smash it.
>
> (*Hipp. 6 Epid.*, 487 Wenkebach and Pfaff)

In this passage, surviving only in Arabic (and that I have used in its German translation), Galen's theory of anxiety progressing to melancholy shines through several retranslations in an especially striking example of mental illness. "When [this patient] was with us in the morning, as usual," he writes elsewhere, "he said in response to a question that he had lain awake all night considering what would happen if Atlas became sick and decided no longer to hold up the sky. And when he said this, we deduced that this was

---

38   I was startled to learn that the passage containing Galen's nonspecific reference to a hypo-thetical patient worried about Atlas in *Loc. Affect.* 3.10 is attributed to Rufus of Ephesus in an obscure ninth-century Latin commentary by Agnellus of Ravenna on Galen's *Sect. Intro.* and in another commentary on the same text, apparently derivative from this one, attributed pseudepi-graphically to John of Alexandria (Fischer 2010). If the passage is indeed from Rufus's lost treatise on melancholy (it was overlooked by Pormann 2008 in his edition of the fragments of this text), and if Galen invented his own stories about the Atlas patient based on the reference in Rufus, it is the only example known to me of Galen inventing a patient (see Mattern 2008a, 38–40). Another possibility is that Galen met a patient with this delusion and that he diagnosed melancholy based on the reference in Rufus; this may seem unlikely but it is suggested by Galen's wording in the passage from *Hipp. 1 Epid.* cited below ("and when he said this, we deduced that it was the begin-ning of a melancholic episode"). Full consideration of this complication must await a future project. I am grateful to Pauline Koetschet and Klaus-Dietrich Fischer for drawing my attention to the problem.

the beginning of a melancholic episode."[39] Galen obviously considers this patient's anxiety irrational, and thus the dangerous course of its progress is not surprising.

Galen recognized many kinds of illness affecting reason, memory, or other functions of the rational soul, and arising from a disorder in the brain, either primary or secondary; they might have positive symptoms (psychosis) or negative ones (lethargy, coma, loss of memory).[40] For psychotic symptoms, that is, delusions and hallucinations, he most frequently uses the words *paraphrosyne* and *phrenitis*; these are both often translated as "delirium" in English. Although he explains that *phrenitis* is *paraphrosyne* or psychosis with fever causing inflammation of the brain or meninges, and *mania* is psychosis without these factors (thus *paraphrosyne* is the more general term and *phrenitis* the more specific one), he does not maintain this usage rigorously, and sometimes uses *paraphrosyne* where we would expect (by this definition) *mania*. He also sometimes writes of *paraphrosyne* as psychosis secondary to causes outside the brain, whereas *phrenitis* has its primary cause in the brain and meninges, or possibly the diaphragm (*Loc. Affect.* 5.4, 8.327–29K).[41] Psychosis might arise as a complication of pleurisy or pneumonia, or might result from aggressive cauterization of the head, or an accumulation of black or yellow bile in the head, during a burning fever or as a secondary result of gastric problems. It might be caused by anything that inflames the brain or meninges, or the diaphragm, which Galen considered highly sympathetic with the brain, explaining in this way the belief of many ancient writers who located the seat of intelligence in the thorax.[42]

Psychosis affected either reason or perception or both: Galen offers the example of Theophilus the physician, who when ill retained his ability to talk reasonably, but thought he saw oboe-players in the corner of his room

---

39 *Hipp. 1 Epid.* 3.1 (17A.213–14K); relying on the emendation of Wenkebach and Pfaff. Galen also perhaps refers this patient in *Loc. Affect.* 3.10 (8.190K).

40 *Sympt. Caus.* 2.7 (7.200–4K); *Loc. Affect.* 2.10 (8.126–35K), 3.6 (8.160–62K).

41 Galen's terminology: *Sympt. Caus.* 2.7 (7.202K); *Loc. Affect.* 2.10 (8.127K), 3.7 (8.166K); *Hipp. 1 Prorrh.* 1.4 (16.517–18K); *Hipp. 3 Epid.* 3.45 (17A.698–99K). See further Pigeaud (1988, especially 161–162 on *phrenitis*).

42 *Loc. Affect.* 2.10 (8.127–28K), 3.9 (8.177–78K), 4.2 (8.225–26K); *Sympt. Caus.* 2.7, 7.202–3K.

and kept ordering them to be thrown out of the house. He remembered the oboe-players even when he had recovered (*Sympt. Diff.* 3, 760–61K). Galen himself as an adolescent, suffering from a burning fever—most likely during the illness he describes contracting in Pergamum as a result of eating fresh fruits—thought he saw pieces of straw sticking out of his mattress, and pills of wool on his clothes, and kept plucking at them. When he heard his friends comment on his erratic behavior he was able to understand them and asked them to help him since he was suffering from *phrenitis*. His friends brought him wet compresses, but he was up all night screaming with nightmares (*Loc. Affect.* 4.2, 8.226–27K). As a counterexample of a patient who perceived his environment clearly but had lost his reason, Galen offers, perhaps drawing on folktale or urban myth, the story of the glassmaker who lived on the upper story of a residence in Rome. He threw his glassware out the window, naming each item precisely; then, responding to the joking demand of the crowd that had gathered, and to their horror, he threw his roommate.[43]

Galen does not sharply distinguish physical and mental illness. He believed in the existence of a *psyche* or soul, as I have mentioned earlier (chapter 5). He expressed agnosticism, as I have also mentioned, on the question of whether the soul was immortal, and on whether it was a material substance or not; for the physician's purposes, as he believed, the soul could be treated as part of the body. The rational soul, the seat of consciousness, was housed in (and possibly identical with) the cerebrospinal fluid, the *pneuma*, contained in the ventricles of the brain; remedies that would purge the noxious humors affecting the brain and causing melancholic depression or psychosis ought to cure those disorders.

Galen's psychiatric observations strike me as unusually subtle. Although he drew on a long written tradition and not all his ideas were original to him, the medical literature on melancholy being especially voluminous by his time, it is also clear that he paid close attention to psychiatric symptoms in his patients (insomnia, delusions, anxiety). His psychiatric ideas are perhaps the most readily familiar to the modern practitioner, who might be confounded

---

43   *Loc. Affect.* 4.2 (8.226, 229, 331–32K); *Sympt. Caus.* 3 (7.61K).

by Galen's beliefs about innate heat or humors, but recognize an anxiety dis-order in the Atlas patient. Galen also wrote treatises on the soul (*psyche*) that focused on ethical problems and were similar to other philosophical tracts of his time. Two of those that survive were written after a catastrophic event in his life: the fire that ravaged Rome in 192 C.E. This event, and Galen's response, is the subject of the next chapter.

Chapter Eight

THE FIRE

Another great burden has been laid upon me. For after I had written out the books of the work 'On Anatomical Dissections', as I was very nearly at the end of them, it so happened that there broke out that great fire in which the Temple of Peace was burnt down together with many warehouses and storehouses … in which were stored those books of mine on Anatomical Dissections, together with all my other books. None of my works survived, except what I had already handed over to be transcribed.

(Anat. Admin. 11.12, 135 Simon, tr. Duckworth)

alen writes here and in several other places of a great fire that scoured Rome in 192 C.E. We know about this fire from independent sources: the historians Herodian and Cassius Dio both mention it; in the historiographic tradition, it was an omen of the death of Commodus, who died on the last day of that year. Galen tells us that it happened in late winter or early spring; he was sixty-two years old.[1]

---

1   *Ind.* 23. Other ancient references to the fire: Herodian 1.14; Cass. Dio 72.24; Galen, *Ind.* 12, 18; *Anat. Admin.* 11.11 (135 Simon); *Antid.* 1 (14.65K); *Comp. Med. Gen.* 1.1 (13.362K). For

The fire consumed the Temple of Peace and the area all around it. This was a cultural catastrophe as well as a human one because the fire spread to the Palatine and consumed the libraries and archives located there, intellectual plunder from centuries of conquest and probably the most extensive collection of books in the world, unless Alexandria's collection was larger. Furthermore, and especially important for Galen, the fire destroyed the storage rooms (*apothekai*) near the Temple of Peace and along the Sacred Way. These were supposed to be fireproof; only the doors were made of wood, and they were not near any residences, which is where fires normally broke out (and, according to Cassius Dio, where the fire of 192 actually started). They were kept safe under military guard because certain imperial archives were housed there, and they fetched extravagant rents. Galen stored all his most precious possessions in one of these storerooms, possibly located in the *Horrea piperataria*, the spice warehouse where Arabian and Egyptian imports were kept. Also, by a stroke of bad luck he was visiting his estate in Campania when the fire broke out and had moved the valuable items from his home into storage for safekeeping while he, and probably most of his household, were away.[2]

Galen had survived the deaths of his beloved father and of his best friend Boethus. He had lost his friend Teuthras and most of his own household slaves in the great plague. He had witnessed famines and epidemics and the deaths of innumerable patients, attacked by gruesome and terrifying infectious diseases rarely seen in the West today. He endured chronic, life-threatening illness and enforced separation from his homeland, not to mention the continuous and ruthless assaults on his reputation that were a normal part of life in his world. But the fire seems to have been, in his subjective experience, the worst catastrophe that he ever experienced. Certainly it is the only one to which he records his emotional reaction. He seems to have struggled with

---

important analyses of the fire, including the points that follow, see Nicholls (2011); Boudon-Millot and Jouanna (2010, xxii–xxvii); Tucci (2008, 2009); Nutton (2009); Christopher Jones (2009); Boudon-Millot (2007b, 76–80); Houston (2003, 45–51).

2   On the Palatine, see Nicholls (2011). Rents: *Ind.* 9, and for other evidence, see further Rickman (1971, 194–209). Campania: *Ind.* 8–11.

this reaction; the fire tested his ability to cope in a way that the other events, perhaps, did not.

Galen's treatise *Avoiding Distress* (*Peri Alupias* or *De Indolentia*, literally "On Non-Grief"), written directly in response to the fire and long believed lost, was recently discovered in a collection of thirteen Galenic treatises at a monastery in Thessaloniki. (Galen mentions the work in *On My Own Books*, and fragments had survived in Arabic.)[3] It takes the form of a letter addressed to an unknown and longtime friend, someone educated with Galen (*Ind.* 57), perhaps a compatriot, who has expressed surprise that he has never seen Galen distressed by anything. Galen writes from Rome to the addressee, who is living elsewhere, perhaps (but not certainly) at Pergamum.

Galen's treatise resembles other philosophical works of the Hellenistic and Roman period, many of which concerned ethics, and notably Plutarch's *On the Tranquility of the Soul.* It is related to the ancient philosophical genre of *consolatio*, consolation for a loss, although Galen himself does not seem to have placed his work in that category.[4] "Consolations" classically addressed the loss of a person, especially a child; but Galen laments, or rather resists lamenting, the loss of property. Indeed Galen may strike readers as cold in his casual references, in this very treatise, to the deaths of his household slaves and of Teuthras in the plague (*Ind.* 1, 35). But this may be misleading. Galen wrote no surviving treatise on the human catastrophe of the plague, which was mostly in the past by 192, and the ethical stance of *Avoiding Distress*, as also of his treatises on the soul discussed below, makes it clear that he would resist expressing any tender emotion he might feel. This attitude may, indeed, qualify him as cold and uncaring, but we must also remember that for all his privilege, Galen experienced suffering and witnessed horrors throughout his long life of a kind that modern readers can scarcely imagine, and it would be unsurprising if his attitudes were affected in ways that seem alien

---

3   The *editio princeps* is Boudon-Millot (2007b); more accessible is the Budé edition, Boudon-Millot and Jouanna (2010). We should soon have a new English translation by Vivian Nutton; I am using his translation of the treatise's title.

4   Boudon-Millot and Jouanna (2010, ix–x); Boudon-Millot (2007b, 75–76). Galen wrote a separate, lost treatise which he called *On Consolation: Libr. Propr.* 15 (19.45K).

today. We might also speculate that Galen found it easier to talk about the loss of material possessions than of people precisely because it was thus easier to avoid indulging in the emotions he sought to control.

Thanks to the recovery of *Avoiding Distress*, we have a good idea of what Galen lost and also new insight into how he acquired his library and published his own works. The fire destroyed gold, silver, silver plate, and IOUs for the debts that people owed him (in an era without bank drafts or credit cards, *Ind.* 4). He lost medical instruments, including the irreplaceable wax prototypes of instruments he had designed himself (*Ind.* 4–5, 10). He lost medicines, both simple and complex, and pharmaceutical ingredients, including eighty Roman pounds, by weight, of theriac, and a large quantity of cinnamon, difficult to acquire except by imperial gift.[5]

But more than any other loss by far, Galen mourned the destruction of his books. He lost two rare collections of drug recipes, some of them "most amazing" and, to his knowledge, unique in the Roman world. One of his friends, a fellow Pergamene, had amassed a large collection of recent and historic recipes at great expense, paying as much as a hundred gold pieces for some recipes. These were preserved on parchment, and when the unknown collector died his heir, spontaneously and to the recipient's surprise, gave them to Galen. Galen inherited another collection, also on parchment, from Teuthras when he died. Teuthras had himself inherited it from a Pergamene doctor, Eumenes. Galen augmented these collections himself by trading copies of individual recipes for new ones, so that his recipes all told ran to some eighty ancient books.[6] All of these perished, but much worse than that—as Galen writes—was the loss of the original text of *On the Composition of Drugs*

5   *Ind.* 5–6. In *Antid* 1 (14.64–66K), Galen writes that he acquired his cinnamon from the imperial storerooms, transferring a large quantity to his own storeroom, which was all lost in the fire. When Severus ordered him to resume making theriac, he used cinnamon stored under Hadrian and Trajan, which had survived. See chapter 6.

6   Eighty books: *Ind.* 6. First collection: *Ind.* 32–33; see Boudon-Millot and Jouanna (2010, xxxi). The heir's name was Claudianus, also a Pergamene (*Comp. Med. Loc.* 1.2, 12.421–23K). Teuthras: *Ind.* 34–35. Boudon-Millot and Jouanna (2010, 106–7) consider, but decide against, amending the text to identify this physician with the Pergamene physician named Eudemus (not Galen's patient in *On Prognosis*) mentioned in a few other passages. Trading copies: *Ind.* 36.

by Type, of unknown length, one of three major and massive pharmacological works that he composed.[7] Galen was certain that some one among his friends must have a copy of the first two books, which he had circulated, but he was unable to find anyone who admitted possessing them and had to rewrite the whole treatise. He thought the first two books might still turn up, and felt obliged to explain why two different versions of these books might be in circulation.[8]

Galen writes that only a few of his recipes survived, those he had given to his students (*Ind.* 37). Either he is failing to mention some other collection in his possession or his rewritten treatise *On the Composition of Drugs by Type* and its sequel, *On the Composition of Drugs by Part*, represent the great labor of his declining years. As I have mentioned, Galen had already written one version of *On the Composition of Drugs by Type*, which was entirely lost; at least part of that earlier work had been completed by the early 170s, when he mentions it to Glaucon in his treatise *On the Method of Healing to Glaucon*. To this earlier era also belong the first eight books of *On the Mixtures and Powers of Simple Drugs*, Galen's long work on medical ingredients and pharmacological theory, which survives. The surviving versions of the two later works on compound drugs were both written after the fire, as were the last two books of *On the Mixtures and Powers of Simple Drugs*.[9]

Together, they run to seventeen books. The recipes Galen records— like the ones he lost—were the products of long tradition and have much

---

7   Galen's language, read carefully, confirms that he had completed the treatise before it was destroyed, and not only the first two books, as many scholars have assumed. "I had already written the treatise (*pragmateia*), and the first two books of it had been given out, but they [sc. his copies of the first two books] were left in the storeroom on the Sacred Way together with the other [books], at the time when the entire Temple of Peace was burned along with the great libraries of the Palatine. At that time many books of others were lost and those of my own that lay in that storeroom, and none of my friends in Rome has admitted to having copies of the first two [books]." *Comp. Med. Gen.* 1.1 (13.362–63K).

8   *Ind.* 37; *Comp. Med. Gen.* 1.1 (13.632–33K).

9   On the chronology of these works, see Peterson (1977, 489–91); Ilberg (1889, 226–228). On the chronology of *Simp. Med.*, see *Simp. Med.* 9.3.21 (12.227K). Glaucon: *Meth. Med. Glauc.* 2.9 (11.124K). The most important study of the structure and method of composition of Galen's pharmacological works is still Fabricius (1972).

of the character of folk medicine. The pharmacological works are vast, nearly impenetrable collections of hundreds of remedies culled from previous authors, organized by form (for *On the Composition of Drugs by Type*, that is, plasters, laxatives, and so forth), or part treated (for *On the Composition of Drugs by Part*, which begins at the top of the head with remedies for hair loss). Galen annotates the recipes with much commentary reflecting his own experience, sometimes including stories of patients healed, and occasionally the results of deliberate experiment. It is in *On the Composition of Drugs by Type* that he transmits recipes for the plasters he used on wounded gladiators, describing his own experience, mentioning the low number of gladiators that died of their wounds in his care, and also that he had given out his recipes to the other doctors of Pergamum and other cities "so that their efficacy could be confirmed by use" (*Comp. Med. Gen.* 3.2, 13.599–603K). This was, as he would have us understand, an unselfish gesture in a time when medicine was competitive and much knowledge was kept secret. In another work, *On the Organ of Smelling*, he describes an experiment with a nasal drug: a person, perhaps a patient of Galen's, had tried inhaling a concoction containing black caraway (*melanthion*, probably the modern *Nigella sativa*) up through his nose to cure a chronic sinus problem; the remedy worked but gave him a terrible headache on the fourth day, from which Galen concluded that the drug was affecting the ventricles of the brain. The headache resolved, and Galen decided to test the promising remedy on his household servants. "Some perceived no pain and some a slight one, and some a grave one deep in the head" (*Instr. Oder.* 4, 2.868–69K).

Whatever we may think of Galen's human-subjects ethics, the point is that his pharmacological works were intended to reflect his own experience and also that of others: "I gave some of my writings also to my friends, when they asked for drugs like these; the drugs, tested by these very people, seem to have lived up to their promise" (*Comp. Med. Gen.* 1.18, 13.453K). He describes the first version of *On the Composition of Drugs by Type,* incinerated in the fire, as "a handbook [*pragmateia*] that I composed with great accuracy about the composition of drugs, in which I recalled how I myself prepared the most famous of my drugs" (*Ind.* 37).

In his practice, Galen missed the medicines and recipes destroyed in the fire every day (*Ind.* 12). He also lost a large number of the rare books he had collected and edited himself. In his decades at Rome he had pored over the libraries there and had found genuine texts not listed in the official catalogues of ancient works and thus unknown to the world, and texts whose authors had been misidentified, including, perhaps, a genuine work of Aristotle misattributed to his pupil Theophrastus.[10] The fire destroyed this precious discovery and Galen's only copy of it on the same day. Further, Galen was a diligent editor and textual critic and kept his own editions of many ancient works in the storeroom—he names the philosophers Theophrastus, Aristotle, Eudemus [of Rhodes], Cleitus, Phainias [of Eresus], Chrysippus, "and all the ancient doctors" (*Ind.* 15).

Galen also lost much of his own work, which devastated him, although we should not exaggerate the extent of what was destroyed. He lost the original text of *On the Composition of Drugs by Type*, as I have mentioned (*Comp. Med. Gen.* 1.1, 13.362–63K); and books twelve through fifteen of *On Anatomical Procedures* (*Anat. Admin.* 11.12, 135 Simon). He also lost the second half of his massive dictionary of words in classical Athenian authors. The half that survived, on prose writers, ran to an astounding forty-eight books. The lost half, on comic writers, was perhaps the more precious to Galen, who admired the comedians for their command of common idiom.[11]

This may exhaust the list of major original works that perished in the fire, although Galen does not offer a full accounting. He seems to have believed that *On Prognosis*, his autobiographical treatise on his rise to prominence in Rome, was lost, because he does not list it in his catalogs *On My Own Books* and *On the Order of My Own Books*, although he mentions it a few times in earlier works.[12] Much of Galen's writing—more than half of all known treatises,

---

10   *Ind.* 16–17. This is my own interpretation of the very difficult passage. On the catalogue or catalogues, see Nicholls (2011, 135–37).

11   *Libr. Propr.* 19 (19.47K) and *Ind.* 20, 23–24, 28 with the notes of Boudon-Millot (2007a) and Boudon-Millot and Jouanna (2010, ad loc).

12   See Nutton (1979, 48–51). Galen also lost an epitome of Didymos's work on Attic vocabulary, a large number of his synopses of the works of others, and a couple of short treatises; for a fuller analysis, see Boudon-Millot and Jouanna (2010, xxxi–xxxviii).

including the very substantial philosophical treatise *On Demonstration* in fifteen books, which had already partly disappeared in Greek by the ninth century, as well as the forty-eight books of his Attic dictionary that had survived the fire, and dozens of other treatises listed in *On My Own Books*—has since disappeared for other reasons.[13] But a great deal survived the fire, because Galen circulated most of his works. He addressed them to friends and gave copies of them away; sometimes he expresses horror that works circulated beyond his intended, private audience, but there is no sharp distinction between these and works that he produced for broader publication. The procedure was the same: he had copies made for friends, students, followers, or anyone who asked for them, and copies in turn might be made from those copies. Some probably ended up in Rome's public libraries, although he does not say this. Some books circulated in more than one edition; an early version, intended for a friend or student, might acquire its own life even after a newer version, corrected by Galen, had also been released. Draft copies of a work, with marginal corrections, might also circulate without Galen's knowledge.[14]

Plagiarism and forgery were also problems. Books might be stolen and published under someone else's name. Or books might be forged and falsely attributed to famous authors, to increase their value. In a well-known story I have mentioned already, Galen was in the Sandaliarion, the district where "most of the booksellers in Rome" could be found, when he overheard an argument that had broken out about the authorship of a book that someone had just bought, called *The Physician*. The buyer thought it was by Galen, whose name was on the volume; but a bystander, not recognizing the title and inquiring about the subject, pronounced it a forgery after hearing only the first two lines. Galen was no doubt delighted by this stranger's intimate

---

13 A catalog of all known Galenic and Pseudo-Galenic works, surviving and lost, is supplied by Fichtner (2004). He lists 441 titles.
14 On Galen's publications, the study of Hanson (1998a) is especially helpful; also Johnson (2010, 85–91). Copies retrieved and corrected: *Libr. Propr.* 1 (19.11–12K), 2 (19.16–17K); copies circulating unintentionally, ibid. and *Libr. Propr.* 1 (19.15K), 6 (19.33K), 11 (19.41–43K); *Anat. Admin.* 5.6 (2.504K), 8.2 (2.659–60K); *Plac. Hipp. Plat.* 8.2 (5.663–64K); and many other references. See Hanson (1998a, 28–35) and Johnson (2010, 86–87). Multiple editions, cf. *Comp. Med. Gen.* 1.1 (13.362–63K), discussed above. Marginalia: *Hipp. 1 Epid.* 1.36 (17A.80K).

knowledge of his work, and at this point launches into a moralizing disquisition on the benefits of the old-fashioned Greek education possessed, as he imagined, by this gentleman but not, unfortunately, by most of those pretending to study medicine or philosophy in his time. This particular forgery may survive today as the treatise commonly called *Introductio seu Medicus* ("Introduction, or The Physician"), transmitted under Galen's name through the Renaissance, but not by Galen.[15]

One could retrieve lost copies of books from friends, if they had copies (*Libr. Propr.* 14, 19.41K); thus Galen's irritation with the friends who lost the first two books of *On the Composition of Drugs by Type*. Boethus, too, had died in possession of the original, short version of *On Anatomical Procedures*; Galen's copy had perished in a mishap of unknown date (not the fire of 192, which came later). Boethus's copy may have survived, but since he had died in Palestine, Galen was unable to lay hands on it and had to rewrite the work (*Anat. Admin.* 1.1, 2.215K). Galen also did his best to keep copies of his works in multiple locations (this is analogous to today's "remote back-up storage"). He regularly had two copies of his works made, and stocked his house in Campania with one set, while he donated the other to a public library at Pergamum, at the request of friends there. In fact, as he writes, had the fire struck two months later, copies of all his works would have been safely stored in Campania and in Pergamum. The most recent batch of copies was in the storeroom awaiting transport when it burned (*Ind.* 20–22). We should not, by the way, imagine Galen making all these copies himself, although it is one of the tragedies of the fire that it destroyed "works of the ancients, [copied] by my own hand" (*Ind.* 6). He employed a staff of slave stenographers, trained at great expense in shorthand, as well as fine bookhand, and criticized as materialistic those who preferred to spend their money on other things (*Anim. Affect. Dign.* 9, 5.48–49K). Twice he mentions that friends, Teuthras and Boethus, sent stenographers, probably slaves from their

---

15 *Libr. Propr.* 1 (19.8–9K); see Petit (2009, xlv–xlix). Books plagiarized: *Libr. Propr.* 2 (19.17K); cf. ibid. 14 (19.41–42K). On the bookshops in Rome, their location, and their role in intellectual life, see Peter White (2009, 268–87).

households, to transcribe lectures he had delivered.[16] Galen also apparently used hired scribes, because he complains that his copies of the rare works he had acquired from Rome's libraries, that perished together with the originals in the fire, had been expensive to obtain (*Ind.* 19).

The tools available to Galen for managing his grief were the ethical principles of Hellenistic philosophy, a discipline to which he devoted himself all his life. Galen had written pointedly and at length on the soul in his youth, in *On the Doctrines of Hippocrates and Plato*; he returned to the subject later in life with a somewhat different emphasis, in a number of short works including the curious treatise *That the Soul Follows the Mixtures of the Body*, as well as *On Diagnosing and Curing the Affections and Errors of the Soul*; and the treatise *Avoiding Distress*, which I have mentioned. The other works that Galen lists, in a passage from *On My Own Books*, as his contributions to ethical philosophy have all disappeared, including some that one wishes especially had survived: his work *On Characters* (or *On Ethics*) in four books, of which only a summary comes down to us, in Arabic translation; and "*On Slander*, in which [there is] also [material about] my own life" (*Libr. Propr.* 15, 19.46K). [17] *Avoiding Distress* was written directly in response to the fire of 192, as I have described, and *On Diagnosing and Curing the Affections and Errors of the Soul* seems closely related and may have been written at about the same time. That the treatise *On Characters* seems to date to the same period is a further indication that the subject of ethics preoccupied Galen in the wake of the fire.[18]

In both *Avoiding Distress* and in the corresponding section of *On Diagnosing and Curing the Affections and Errors of the Soul*, Galen responds to an interlocutor who asks him how it is possible that he has never seen Galen express the emotion of *lupe*, grief or distress. The two interlocutors

---

16   *Ven. Sect. Eras. Rom.* 1 (11.194–95K); *Praecog.* 5 (14.630K); *Libr. Propr.* 1 (19.14K).

17   On the summary of *On Characters* surviving in Arabic, see Mattock (1972).

18   Boudon-Millot and Jouanna (2010, lix–lxi) argue that *Anim. Affect. Dign.*, since it does not mention the fire, must precede it. But, as they also explain, it refers to Galen's lost treatise *On Characters*, which itself referred to a historical incident from the reign of Commodus that probably could not have been mentioned while the emperor was alive. This would place *Anim. Affect. Dign.* after the death of Commodus and after the fire.

are different people. The addressee of the *Avoiding Distress* is a compatriot living abroad who posed his question in a letter (*Ind.* 1), but Galen's interlocutor in *On Diagnosing and Curing the Affections and Errors of the Soul*, although also apparently a Pergamene (*Anim. Morb. Dign.* 7, 1.46K) is someone nearby:

> One of the youths among my intimate acquaintance, who denied that he became upset over small things, later became aware of it; he visited me at daybreak, and said that he had been sleepless the whole night because of this matter; and meanwhile somehow he arrived at the recollection that I did not become as upset over great matters, as he did over small ones.
>
> (*Anim. Affect. Dign.* 7, 5.37K)

That is, unless one or both of these interlocutors is imaginary (which is quite possible), more than one of Galen's friends noticed his extraordinary resilience and asked him about it. Galen seems especially proud of his response to the fire, a great catastrophe. He knew more than one person who perished of grief in its wake. In his commentary on the sixth book of Hippocrates' *Epidemics* he mentions the example of Callistus, the grammarian, "whose books were destroyed in the great fire in Rome in which the ... Temple of Peace burned." Callistus developed insomnia, and then fever, and then wasted away until he died, like other cases of anxiety or despair that Galen describes in that passage.[19] This Callistus may or may not be the same grammarian he mentions in *Avoiding Distress*, here called Philides, who died "consumed by depression [*dysthymia*] and grief" (*Ind.* 7). In *On the Composition of Drugs by Type*, which he had to rewrite after the fire, Galen comments that he knows one doctor who died of distress after losing his remedies in the same way, and another who, in despair, stopped practicing medicine (*Comp. Med. Gen.* 2.1, 13.458–59K). More even than the plague that claimed almost his entire household, Galen considered the fire a nearly unendurable disaster (*Ind.* 1–2).

---

19   *Hipp. 6 Epid.* (486 Wenkebach and Pfaff).

Not everyone, according to Galen, is by nature capable of great virtue. This he considered abundantly clear from his observation of personality differences in children. Some are temperate and generous; others are greedy, violent, and selfish. While our rational souls may share a universal preference for the good and beautiful, we differ greatly from one another in the strength or weakness of this soul, relative to the passions and appetites—anger, fear, and grief; lust, greed, and gluttony—that compete for influence over us. Galen had good cause to wonder, in childhood and perhaps in adolescence, about the nature of the soul he had inherited; for the contrast in his parents' characters was very great, as I have described (see chapter 1). But he had always, as he writes, naturally preferred the qualities of his father and strove to imitate them.[20]

Some characters are, then, hopeless from birth; but some respond to training. Education, in philosophy and in sciences such as geometry and astronomy, strengthens the rational soul. One must also diligently work to maintain a sense of perspective. The purpose of the appetites, and of the "vegetative" soul in the liver (so called because it shares its nature with both animals and plants), is to keep the body alive and to reproduce; beyond that, if our basic needs for food and shelter are met, the appetites can only cause grief and despair when we fail to satisfy them or when we lose something we have acquired. Galen advises constantly reminding oneself that what is adequate for one's basic needs is enough: "Always have in mind the idea of self-sufficiency." The philosopher Artisippus of Cyrene, when he had lost one of the four estates he owned in his homeland, and one of his fellow citizens expressed sympathy for him, laughed and asked why his friend should feel pity when Aristippus still owned much more property than he did? "Perhaps," said Aristippus to his interlocutor, "I should feel sorry for you." Following the hero's advice in Euripides' lost tragedy *Theseus* (a passage famous in his time and preserved in other authors), Galen

---

20   Children: *Anim. Affect Dign.* 7 (5.37–39K); *Anim. Mor. Corp.* 2 (4.768, 816–18K); *Mor.* 1 (29–30 Kraus). Natural preference for the beautiful: *Anim. Mor. Corp.* 11 (815–16K); *Mor.* 1 (33 Kraus), 2 (36 Kraus). Father and mother: *Anim. Affect. Dign.* 8 (5.40–41K); father: *Ind.* 58–62.

meditated every day on the worst possible calamities, physical torment, exile, and premature death:

> I bring calamities to mind always,
> I set before myself exile from my country, and premature deaths, and
> other ways of evil,
> so that, if one day I should suffer one of the things I have imagined,
> it will not sting my soul the more for being new.[21]

Galen recommends recruiting a brutally honest friend, perhaps someone older of Galen's own generation, to correct one's moral faults constantly, and to point out failures to control the passions and appetites until good habits are internalized. We cannot see our own faults, writes Galen, but only those of others, correctly identifying what modern psychologists would call self-serving bias. Whether he practiced this method himself we do not know (he nowhere mentions having such a mentor), but this friend is only a more efficient substitute for the self-monitoring of one's own reactions that he also recommends. He advises beginning every day with the thought of how much better it is to maintain self-control than to be a slave of the passions, constantly keeping the ugliness of anger in mind, constantly taking note of mistakes of overindulgence in food, wine, and sex. With this kind of practice one may see slow improvement over years and must not become discouraged if change does not occur right away. Finally, in his unusual treatise *That the Soul Follows the Mixtures of the Body*, he explains that because the character of the soul depends on the elemental qualities (hot, cold, wet, and dry) of the body it inhabits, some faults in character can be corrected with the proper diet. There is a question, in this view, whether those of evil character are truly

---

21 Hopeless: *Anim. Affect. Dign.* 7 (5.38–39K). Education: *Mor.* 3 (52–53 Kraus). Appetites and grief: *Anim. Affect. Dign.* 9 (5.49–51K); *Mor.* 1 (27 Kraus), 2 (41 Kraus). Aristippus: *Ind.* 39–42. Self-sufficiency: *Anim. Affect. Dign.* 8 (5.43–44K), 9 (5.48–52K); *Ind.* 39–76. Theseus and Commodus: *Ind.* 52–54, 77. The quotation is also known from Cicero and seems to have been commonly cited when discussing the theme of enduring grief; see Boudon-Millot and Jouanna (2010, 137–38).

responsible for their faults, since some people are by natural temperament incapable of virtue. But for Galen it does not follow that we should not be punished for our vices, even with death.[22]

Galen's ethical ideas were not original to him, and he borrowed freely from the Stoics, the Epicureans, Plato, Aristotle, and their followers (even as he criticizes, especially, certain Stoic doctrines). He drew, that is, on the common wisdom of his culture regarding the regulation of emotion and behavior. This advice on moral improvement was quite sound. Psychologists tell us that the daily practice of self-control can increase willpower over time, that the monitoring of one's own emotions and reactions is an important part of this process, and that an "attitude of gratitude" is a helpful safeguard against depression. Galen's therapies were both cognitive (avoiding certain thoughts, cultivating other thoughts) and behavioral (monitoring and modifying certain behaviors, especially angry reactions, until the desired behavior becomes routine). Scientists today often acknowledge modern cognitive behavioral therapy's debt, or at least resemblance, to ancient ethical philosophy, usually singling out Stoicism, though similar principles are found in the other traditions from which Galen also draws. Even Galen's dietetic approach to ethics in *That the Soul Follows the Mixtures of the Body* is not alien to modern ideas of nutrition or of mental disease as chemical imbalance, although he offers no specific advice in this treatise and I would not make extravagant claims for his insights.[23]

While grief has a special place in Galen's work because of the fire of 192, the main focus of much Hellenistic and Roman-era ethical thought was anger and the control of violence, and this theme is also prominent in Galen.

---

22   Friend: *Anim. Affect. Dign.* 3 (5.8–14K), 5 (5.24K), 6 (5.30–31K), 7 (5.36K), 10 (5.55K). Blind to one's own faults: *Anim. Affect. Dign.* 2 (5.5K); *Mor.* 4 (47 Kraus). Self-monitoring: *Anim. Affect. Dign.* 4 (5.15–16, 20–21, 25–26K), 6 (5.30–31K), 7 (36K). Slow improvement: *Anim. Affect. Dign.* 4 (5.20–21K), 6 (5.33K), 10 (5.54K). Food, responsibility: *Anim. Mor. Corp.* 9 (4.807–8K), 11 (815–21K).

23   Gratitude: Watkins (2004). On self-control perhaps the most frequently cited article is the ethically oriented essay of Baumeister and Exline (1999; see esp. 1176–1179). See also, more recently, Baumeister and Tierney (2011). On Galenic psychotherapy, see Gill (2010, chapter 5); Hankinson (1993, 199–204). On psychotherapy in Greco-Roman and early Christian philosophy generally, see Sorabji (2000); chapter 15 reviews the evidence for psychotherapeutic exercises.

Examples often involved anger against slaves, perhaps reflecting a pervasive ethical challenge for the aristocratic class who studied and wrote philosophy. Galen's memorable story about the Cretan who almost murdered two of his slaves in a rage over lost luggage, which impressed itself on his memory and which he repeated often, is an example of this theme. Galen was a slave owner himself; his anecdotes mention domestic servants and stenographers, and the presence of slaves can be inferred in many stories where they are not specifically mentioned. He often calls them "mine" ("my [people]"), using a single substantive pronoun. He tested a nasal drug on his household, as I have mentioned, and lost a large number of household slaves to the great plague.[24]

As I have mentioned before in chapter 1, Galen argues that one should never hit slaves with one's own hands and especially not in the heat of anger; rather, he suggests delaying punishment until good judgment has returned and substituting lectures for blows where it is possible to do so. A similar argument is made by Seneca in his treatise *On Anger*, and this idea that slaves should not be punished in the heat of anger or hit with one's own hands was a philosophic commonplace. Galen tells us that this is how Plato treated his own slaves. Although Galen claims never to have hit a slave himself, arguments like this, and other references, like the story of the Cretan, are discomfiting and even shocking in the level of everyday, casual violence they imply. Galen condemns friends of his father's who bruised their hands hitting slaves in the teeth, wounds that often became infected later. Galen's notorious passage about his own mother, quoted in chapter 1, describes how she would fly into rages and bite her slaves. In another treatise, Galen treats a master who wounded his finger while hitting a slave. Galen claims to have seen a man poke a slave in the eye with a reed-pen, something the emperor Hadrian is also supposed to have done. While Galen himself condemns

---

24   On anger in ancient philosophy and culture, see the magisterial study of Harris (2001), including a discussion of anger in Galen (120–23). On slavery and violence, see, e.g., Harris (2001, chapter 13); Fitzgerald (2000, chapter 2); Saller (1991); Bradley (1987, chapter 4). On slavery in Galen, including the evidence for Galen's own slaves, see Schlange-Schöningen (2003, chapter 9). The Cretan: *Anim. Affect. Dign.* 4 (18–20K) and chapter 6 above.

these brutal acts, he does not oppose the corporal punishment of slaves per se, and elsewhere he accepts violence against slaves as routine and commonplace, as virtually all ancient writers do. A passage from *On the Doctrines of Hippocrates and Plato* refers, in a general way, to the grisly punishments such as burning or beating meted out to slaves "even now"; they are inflicted upon the offending limb (for example, legs, for runaways), and Galen does not seem to find this offensive but to appreciate the poetic justice of the system.[25]

Galen treated slaves in his practice, often (but not always) at the request of their masters. He also treated peasants, as I have mentioned, and spent his formative years as a physician treating gladiators, men of ambiguous, but certainly not high, social status. It is in his relationship to slave patients, and not in his ethics as slaveholder, that we find some challenge to, or discrepancy with, the normal role of slaves in ancient culture. It is difficult to show that Galen treated his enslaved patients differently from his free ones and easier to show that he treated them the same; that is, he talked to them, visited several times a day if necessary, and generally gave them his best—sometimes heroic—efforts, as in the case of Maryllus's slave, saved by thoracic surgery that exposed his heart. Galen most often does not mention a patient's social status, because his self-image as a professional rested on other factors; the difficulty of the case, the humiliation of his rivals, the skills deployed, and the success achieved.[26]

These factors, rather than a humanistic view of medical ethics, may account for Galen's otherwise surprising lack of condescension for his low-status patients, although evidence for such humanism is not completely

25   *Plac. Hipp. Plat.* 6.8 (5.579K). Lectures instead of blows: *Anim. Affect. Dign.* 4 (5.17K), 5 (5.21–22K). Galen never hit a slave with his hand: *Anim. Affect. Dign.* 4 (5.17K). Philosophic commonplace: Seneca, *De Ira* 3.32.1–3; Harris (2001, chapter 13); Fitzgerald (2000, 34–36); Manning (1989, 1525–26); Bradley (1986, 169). Seneca: *De Ira* 3.12.5–7. Plato: *Anim. Affect. Dign.* 5 (5.21K). Hitting slaves in the teeth: *Anim. Affect. Dign.* 4 (5.17K). Wounded finger: *Syn. Puls.* 21 (9.495–96K); the patient suffers a deterioration of his condition through his own fault, when he neglects Galen's advice. Hadrian: *Anim. Affect. Dign.* 4 (5.17K). Galen's mother: *Anim. Affect. Dign.* 8 (5.40–41K).

26   On enslaved patients, see Mattern (2008a, 116–19).

lacking: Did not Hippocrates himself, as Galen writes, treat the poor? Galen did not accept fees and would sometimes provide patients with necessities that they lacked, whether food, or medicine, or servants. The only patient for whom he openly expresses disdain is a wealthy "medicine-loving" (*philophar-makos*) fool who enjoys treating his own slaves but only exacerbates their injuries in his incompetence, demands drugs with expensive, smelly ingredients, and lies about taking remedies that Galen has forbidden.[27]

Galen acknowledges that his character has never been tested by the greatest imaginable disaster: for him, this would be the loss of all his possessions, so that he no longer had enough left to survive, or the total loss of status that might come from public condemnation or exile; or, perhaps, the destruction of his homeland, or a friend coerced by a tyrant (he appears to consider this much more terrible than the loss of a friend to natural causes). He prays for health too, preferring to imagine horrific injury rather than actually to experience it for the sake of strengthening his spirit. He gave specific thought, in this later period of his life, to the precise limits of his fortitude: "I am indifferent to all loss of money as long as enough remains in my possession to avoid hunger, cold, and thirst ... and I am indifferent to pain as long as it remains possible for me to converse with a friend or follow the words of someone who is reading me a book." With uncharacteristic humility, then, Galen doubts his ability to endure all the contingencies that might come his way, and perhaps he looked forward with apprehension to the inevitable trials of declining health and death. He prays to Zeus not, as the Stoic Musonius Rufus did, to send him whatevever circumstances the god wished; rather, Galen asks Zeus to send him no circumstance that he cannot endure.[28] He may have planned suicide if his sufferings surpassed his capacity to bear them, but we do not know what actually happened.

---

27 Hippocrates: *Opt. Med. Philosoph.* 3 (1.58K), referring to the *Epidemics* ("the poor of Cranon, Thasos, and other cities"). *Philanthropia* as characteristic of medicine: ibid. 2 (1.56K) and *Plac. Hipp. Plat.* 9.5 (5.751–52K). For scholarship on this issue, see Pigeaud (1997); Temkin (1991, 28–33, 220–33); Gourevitch (1984, 276–78, 281–88). On fees, see Meyerhof (1929, 84). Charity: ibid. and *Anim. Affect. Dign.* 9 (1.48K). Wealthy patient: *Praesag. Puls.* 1.1 (9.218–20K); *Comp. Med. Gen.* 3.8 (13.636–38K).

28 *Anim. Affect. Dign.* 8 (43–44K); *Ind.* 71–78. Quotation: *Ind.* 78.

Old age cast a long shadow.[29] It is true that Galen mentions no emperors by name after Septimius Severus, who ruled from 193 to 211, and no specific events after the fire of 192, except for the Secular Games of 204 (if the treatise *On Theriac to Piso* is genuine). The *Suda*, an encyclopedia in Greek of the tenth century C.E, records in its entry on Galen that he lived to age seventy. Western scholars long believed this, while finding it difficult to understand how he could have composed, in just six years, the lengthy list of his works that must postdate the fire. These include not only the two long works on compound drugs, but his diagnostic masterpiece *On the Affected Parts* in eight books; lost dictionaries on Attic usage in certain comic writers (though he never rewrote the comprehensive work that was destroyed); the last four books of *On Anatomical Procedures*; the last three books of *On the Mixtures and Powers of Simple Drugs*; the second half, in seven books, of *On the Method of Healing*; *On Antidotes* in two books; the three treatises on ethics that I have described above; the treatise *The Art of Medicine*; the two bibliographic treatises; the treatise *On My Own Opinions*; and other minor works.

Many testimonies to Galen's longevity far beyond age seventy survive. His old enemy, Alexander of Aphrodisias, is supposed to have quipped about *On My Own Opinions* that it took Galen eighty years to figure out that he knew nothing. Byzantine historians record that he was still alive in the reign of Caracalla, which began in 209; and sources in Arabic are unanimous in the view that he died at age eighty-seven (except for two that place his death a year or two later, in the reign of Elagabalus). The authors of the *Suda* misunderstood a tradition that his *career* lasted seventy years, after seventeen years of childhood and early education. If the Arabic tradition is accurate, Galen lived a further twenty-three years after the great fire and died in 216 or 217.

We do not know where he died. Only sources in Arabic (and one in Persian) comment on the location of his tomb, and their testimony sounds

---

29 For what follows on Galen's age at death and his tomb, see Strohmeier (2007); Nutton (1995a). On the quotation of Alexander of Aphrodisias, see additionally Nutton (1999, 37–38).

more like legend than fact. According to one version of the story, Galen went to the city of Lycopolis (Asyut) in Upper Egypt to study the properties of opium; there he decided to return to Pergamum, his homeland, but on the way he died. His place of death was Pelusium on the eastern Nile delta, where his tomb, according to these sources, could be found. Another story, impossible to reconcile with historical fact, tells that Galen heard of the miracles of Jesus, and set out from Rome for Palestine to meet Jesus' disciples. But he died on the journey, in Palermo, Sicily, which also claimed his tomb.

As he advanced in years he gave thought to the fate of his literary legacy. In *On My Own Opinions*, perhaps his last work—impossible to date precisely, but later than *On My Own Books,* and no other work of Galen's refers to it—he summarizes his views on innate heat and the heart, nutrition and the liver, the humors, the temperaments and stages of life, the efficacy of drugs, the nervous system, the embryo, creation, and (especially) the soul, condensing all of this to a single book. His purpose was to confirm and authenticate the ideas expressed over a lifetime. Like *On My Own Books*, which begins with Galen's story about overhearing an argument on a falsified work attributed to himself, *On My Own Opinions* also opens with an anecdote about authenticity: the poet Parthenius of Nicaea, who lived in the first century B.C.E., while travelling happened upon two schoolteachers (*grammatici*) debating the meaning of his poems. When Parthenius tried to intervene in the argument, claiming at first to have heard himself, the poet, expounding the correct meaning, his opponent refused to believe him; Parthenius, lamenting his failure at argumentation, could only win his point by calling on witnesses from his entourage to prove that he was the author of the poems in dispute (*Plac. Propr.* 1, 172 Boudon-Millot and Pietrobelli).[30]

It is this problem that Galen sought to forestall, looking forward, no doubt, to the time after his death when he would no longer be able to authenticate his own works or prove the fraudulence of forgeries. *On My Own Opinions* and *On My Own Books*, also written late in life—after the fire of 192 but before *On My Own Opinions,* and thus possibly as late as 210 or so,

---

30   On the manuscript transmission of *Plac. Propr.*, see above, chapter 5, n. 60.

although the most recent historical event it mentions is the reign of Pertinax in 193[31]—suggest anxiety on this point. In another treatise he remarks:

> Some do not have successors for their teaching, and some do not publish books while they are alive, and then when they are dead, the one or two surviving copies are lost. For it can happen that they [the authors] are disdained, and their works are neglected and, in time, completely destroyed. And sometimes certain jealous people hide them, or even erase the books of older writers. Others do the same thing by saying that what is written in them is their own.... To set aside all other causes, I will mention only two of those that recently happened in Rome. Often temples have burned, and often they have fallen down in earthquakes, or for some other reason, and they [these causes] seem to be responsible for the loss of many books.
>
> (*Hipp. Nat. Hom.* 1.1, 15.23–24K)

In the background was Galen's own long and painstaking labor on the Hippocratic Corpus, identifying those works he deemed orignial to the legendary physician based on style, language, manuscript tradition, and also dogma, and correcting the mistakes of generations of venal or incompetent scribes and commentators.[32] But in the passage quoted above he also seems to recall his own intellectual ancestors. Quintus published little; Pelops and Heraclianus suppressed the writings of Numisianus, Pelops's teacher and Heraclianus's father; Pelops's and Numisianus's works were eventually destroyed by fire. When Galen writes that "often temples have burned," he may well be thinking of the event of 192, which would date this passage and the work it comes from to that year or later. Thus the fire, as well as advancing age, caused Galen to ruminate on the fragility of his legacy.

Galen could not control the text of his works, which were doomed to be transmitted imperfectly. Even during his lifetime, to his frustration, multiple

---

31   Boudon-Millot (2007a, 8–9), on the date of *Libr. Propr.*
32   Cf. Hanson (1998a) and Nutton (1999, 127).

versions of some works circulated, some uncorrected, some altered by authors who passed them off as their own. But he did his best to help future generations distinguish his genuine treatises. *On My Own Books* is a catalog of Galen's genuine works, by title; it has helped modern scholars greatly in understanding his contribution and in identifying some inauthentic works. *On My Own Opinions*, on the other hand, is a guide to Galen's genuine views on a variety of medical subjects including, as I have mentioned, the creator and the substance of the soul. He represents these ideas as perfectly consistent and unchanging with only one exception (for he describes, not entirely accurately, a development over time in his views on the order in which the parts of the embryo are formed).[33] Finally, *On the Order of My Own Books*, written at about the same time as *On My Own Books*, describes the proper sequence in which the diligent student or amateur ought to read his works. A similar, but shorter, list of recommended reading appears at the end of the roughly contemporary treatise *The Art of Medicine*. *On My Own Books*, *On the Order of My Own Books*, and *On My Own Opinions* are unique works; it occurred to no other ancient writer to attempt to guarantee his legacy in this way. But it is just the sort of thing that Galen would do.[34]

Galen was aware that, by his time, much writing of great value had already been lost—"even among the Athenians there are found some famous comic and tragic poets whose plays no longer survive" (*Hipp. Nat. Hom.* 1.2, 15.24K)—and he felt keenly the losses that occurred in his own lifetime, as I have described. His own works were not immune to the wreckage of time, but a relatively large proportion has nevertheless survived. This is in some ways surprising, as Galen's fears seem to have been reasonable: we are well-informed about his enemies, but we know the name of no devoted student who carried on his teachings.

---

33   *Propr. Plac.* 11 (182 Boudon-Millot and Pietrobelli), with the commentary of Nutton (1999, 176–79).
34   On the relationship among these works, see Boudon-Millot (2007a, 3–8). On the authenticity of *Ars Medica*, see Boudon-Millot (2000, 157–64); on the catalog, ibid. 192–93. An invaluable catalog of all known Galenic and Pseudo-Galenic works, surviving and lost, is supplied by Fichtner (2004).

In fact, we know little about the Greco-Roman medical tradition after Galen at all. Later medical writers—Oribasius, Caelius Aurelianus, Paul of Aegina—published excerpts and translations of older authors, Galen and his predecessors and contemporaries. It is as though, after Galen, nothing noteworthy was written. We do not know why. Surely one factor was the political crisis of the mid-third century c.e., which rocked the Roman Empire to its foundation and coincides with a steep drop in surviving intellectual product. In the fourth and fifth centuries the rise of Christianity, ambivalent at best in its attitude toward science, made its own contribution to the decline of medicine. Although medicine continued to be valued, taught, and practiced in the Byzantine period, there were virtually no new theories or anatomical discoveries, no sectarian rivalries or bitter public feuds—no Galen. In his time, medicine was still very much alive. After Galen it became more antiquarian in focus, preserving his works as though in a refrigerator, but without the vibrant context of debate, rivalry, and performance that produced them, and without which their meaning is so much impoverished.[35]

35　On intellectual decline in the third century, see MacMullen (1976, chapter 1; 1990, 1–15). The later antique period was not entirely devoid of innovation and experimentation, notably the therapeutics of the brash Jacob Psychrestus of Constantinople and possibly some advances in the anatomy of the tongue at Alexandria, but there is a very sharp contrast with the productivity of Galen's century. See Nutton (1984a; also for the refrigerator metaphor); Temkin (1962).

EAST AND WEST; OR, GALEN AND TWO DISCIPLES

G alen became a figure of legend, like Hippocrates before him. Stories that he was Hippocrates' student, that he was a contemporary of Jesus, that he was the teacher or nephew of the apostle Luke, that he learned secrets of gynecology from Cleopatra, the last queen of Egypt, and other chronologically absurd fictions rose up around him. His own surviving works showed that they could not be true, but it did not matter. Galen became a hero of medicine, in Greek, Syriac, Arabic, and, later, in Latin literature and in the art of Western Europe. He was not so much its founding figure—Asclepius and Hippocrates had better claims to that role—as he was its greatest exemplar. John of Alexandria, writing late in the sixth century C.E. only a few decades before the fall of the city, which was still the Mediterranean world's premier center of medical education, to the Arabs, called Galen the "Seal of the Physicians"—a metaphor that saw the history of medicine as finished, with Galen as its capstone. John's scheme of a sequence of eight great physicians, beginning with Asclepius and ending with Galen, passed into Arabic tradition. Filling in yawning gaps in what is known about Galen's personal life, early Arab legends credited him variously with a sister (supposed to be the mother of the apostle Paul) and a sex manual, but not, apparently, a wife, lover, or children.[1]

The story of what happened to Galen's works, which is much of the story of Byzantine, Western European, and Islamic medicine for many centuries, is too long to recount here in full. Oswei Temkin's classic *Galenism: Rise and Decline of a Medical Philosophy*, first published in 1973, is still the most lucid and captivating version of this tale.[2] I will mention only three episodes here.

Among the many thousands of scraps of papyrus recovered from the garbage dumps of Roman Egypt and painstakingly transcribed and published, eight are fragments of Galen's works. Two of them come from the same manuscript copy of *On the Doctrines of Hippocrates and Plato*, Galen's most important surviving philosophical work, and date to the early third century, almost to Galen's own lifetime. That is, shortly after his death, Galen's work was being copied in Egypt, often enough to have left a trace for us to find. Another early papyrus, from the third or fourth century, preserves a fragment of Galen's lost commentary on the Hippocratic treatise *On Aliment*. From the fourth or fifth centuries comes a fragment of *On the Natural Faculties*; and later papyri mostly preserve excerpts from Galen's books on drugs. The papyri come from Hermopolis Magna, Antinoopolis, and the Fayyum—sites in Middle Egypt, and the Fayyum is on Lake Moeris west of the Nile, the ancient site of Crocodilopolis, also called Arsinoe. The papyri, like those of the Hippocratic Corpus and a few other medical writers (some anonymous) that have also survived, probably trace back to the modest libraries and collections of practicing physicians who treasured them and may have gone to great lengths to acquire them.[3] Very few papyri at all have been recovered near Alexandria, because the climate there is more humid and because it has remained densely populated since ancient times. Galen's works were, however, certainly being read by those who came to the legendary city to study medicine, as Galen had once done; we know this from Arab sources.

---

1   Swain (2006, p. 402 for the "Seal"); Nutton (2008).

2   For a more recent discussion, see "Histoire du texte," Boudon-Millot (2007a, xci–ccxxxviii).

3   On Galenic papyri, see Boudon-Millot (2007a, cvii–cxii); Hanson (1998b, 1985); Andorlini Marcone (1993, nos. 4–8; 2001, no. 3).

Galen had many great translators in the centuries after his death, but perhaps the greatest and most infuential was the Nestorian Christian of Baghdad, Hunain ibn Ishaq, whose life spanned most of the ninth century C.E.[4] (In Europe, when Latin translations of his Arabic editions were later produced, he was known as Johannitius.) As an adolescent Hunain came to Baghdad eager to study medicine with the great Yuhanna ibn Masawahi, but quickly annoyed his master with his incessant questions. Rejected and distraught, he left Baghdad, traveled to the Byzantine Empire and learned Greek in Alexandria (he also acquired Persian besides his native Syriac and Arabic). He then returned to the Abbasid capital, where he completed his medical studies and where he spent most of the rest of his life. Hunain was responsible for bringing much of Greek science to the Arab world, first as a young man under the caliph al-Mamun, a passionate admirer of Greek philosophy and collector of manuscripts, who once disputed with Aristotle in a dream. According to legend, al-Mamun paid for translations with their weight in gold. Later Hunain served the caliph al-Mutawakkil and was twice imprisoned when he refused to concoct a deadly poison at the caliph's request. Hunain insisted that he learned and practiced medicine only to help, not to harm humanity.

From Istanbul, two copies survive of the document called "Missive from Hunain ibn Ishaq to 'Ali ibn Yahya on all the books of Galen which, as far as he [Hunain] knows, have been translated, and on some of them which have not been translated." It was written in 855–56, when Hunain was forty-eight, and updated in 863–64 by the original author; the document was updated again after its author's death, perhaps by its recipient, 'Ali ibn Yahya, secretary and friend of the caliph al-Mutawakkil and commander of his army against the Byzantine Empire. An intellectual, lover of science, and perhaps the most powerful of Hunain's patrons, 'Ali is a sort of parallel to Galen's friend and patron Boethus. But Hunain, like Galen, had many friends and patrons for whom he produced his works, including prominent Muslim officials, as well

---

4   On Hunain and for what follows, see Meyerhof (1926); Gabrieli (1924); Pormann and Savage-Smith (2007, 24–37). Hunain's letter is published in Arabic with a German translation by Bergsträsser (1925) and with corrections, after the discovery of a second manuscript, in id. (1932).

as Christian colleagues and friends. Hunain produced his Syriac translations for the Christians, and Arabic versions for his Muslim patrons.

Hunain knew one hundred and twenty-nine works of Galen and produced new translations of nearly all of them, into Arabic, Syriac, or both. He made his first translations of Galen's work as a teenager, when he rendered *On the Differences in Fevers* and *On the Natural Faculties* into Syriac. A painstaking edition of Galen's *magnum opus* on therapeutics, *On the Method of Healing*, was lost in a fire while being shipped to Baghdad. Hunain later obtained a second, better Greek manuscript and retranslated the treatise.

Hunain was an ardent collector of Galen's works, which he sought out in all the great cities of the Middle East. He complains that he could not find a complete Greek manuscript of *On Demonstration*, although he searched the libraries of "(Mesopotamia), Syria, Palestine and Egypt," including Alexandria, but he found about half of it in Damascus.[5] He was an exceptionally rigorous scholar who not only produced meticulous translations but also critical editions of the original Greek texts, based on all available Greek manuscripts. He was obliged to invent Arabic words for many of Galen's anatomical and other technical terms, and his language became canonical. Although Hunain's work was seriously interrupted when his entire library of "all the books which I had gradually collected during the course of my whole adult life in all the lands which I had travelled" was lost, probably confiscated during one of Hunain's conflicts with al-Mutawakkil,[6] he produced no fewer than ninety-five Syriac translations of Galen's works, and thirty-five in Arabic, as well as a huge number of translations of other Greek philosophers and scientists (Plato, Aristotle, Euclid, and Hippocrates among many others) and more than one hundred original works. Of the works that Hunain knew about, but did not translate himself, many were translated by his pupils and especially by his nephew and most illustrious student, Hubaish ibn al-Hasan. Many projects were collaborations among Hunain and his students.

---

5   Meyerhof (1926, 690).
6   Meyerhof (1926, 689, tr. Meyerhof).

.

Hunain was not the first translator of most of Galen's works; by his time previous translations, which he catalogues, into Syriac or Arabic existed of almost all the items known to him. The earliest of these date all the way back to the mid-sixth century C.E. and were inspired by the privileged position of Galen's works at the medical school of Alexandria. Hunain lists twenty titles supposedly read by medical students there. This tradition of an Alexandrian core curriculum of "sixteen books"—twenty-four separate titles by modern count, mostly the same as the twenty titles identified by Hunain—is well-attested in later Arab writers. Modern scholars debate whether the list may be properly called a canon and whether any such formal institution as "the medical school of Alexandria" (in Hunain's words)[7] existed, but most do not dispute that these titles were favored and widely read at Alexandria. The texts Hunain names are *On My Own Books, On the Order of My Own Books, On the Sects, The Art of Medicine, On the Pulse for Beginners, On the Method of Healing to Glaucon, On the Bones for Beginners, On the Anatomy of the Muscles, On the Anatomy of the Nerves, On the Elements According to Hippocrates, On Mixtures, On the Natural Faculties, On the Causes of Symptoms* and Galen's five other books on the causes and symptoms of disease, here joined together as one work; *On the Affected Parts*; Galen's four treatises on the pulse, here collected into a single work on the pulse; *On Types [of Fevers]; On Crises; On Critical Days*; the monumental *On the Method of Healing*; and, as Hunain adds later, *On Healthfulness*.

At Baghdad, intellectual center of the Muslim world and home of the "House of Wisdom," which perhaps imitated Alexandria's famous Museum, medical education was modeled on the Alexandrian curriculum and included works of Hippocrates and the "sixteen books" of Galen. This remained the foundational canon of Greco-Arabic medicine for a thousand years and profoundly influenced the later development of medieval Islamic medicine, including its most brilliant representatives, al-Razi, ibn Sina, and ibn Rushd (known in in the West as Rhazes, Avicenna, and Averroes). Even today traditional medicine based on Greco-Arabic

---

7   Meyerhof (1926, 692, tr. Meyerhof).

principles is practiced widely in the Middle East and parts of India and Pakistan.[8]

In Western Europe, Galen's influence reached its peak in the Renaissance, which was also the point of its decline. "Galenism's" most critical turning point arrived in the sixteenth century, in the person of Andreas Vesalius (this is the Latinized form of his name, André van Wesele) of Brussels, the individual who did the most to undermine what had become its intellectual stranglehold on medicine.

Western European medicine had long relied on Latin translations of a few, mostly short treatises, by Galen, by Hippocrates (although the Hippocratic Corpus was known in this period mostly through Galen's commentaries), and by Islamic physicians heavily influenced by Galen.[9] A very popular handbook, the *Articella*, contained a translation of Galen's *Art of Medicine*, called the *Tegni* after its Greek title (*Techne iatrike*); also the *Isagoge* or "Introduction" to medicine of Hunain ibn Ishaq; and a few other items. The *Articella* remained popular through the sixteenth century and many printed copies survive. Other works were, however, increasingly available to the diligent; and especially from the first half of the fourteenth century, when Niccolò da Reggio translated dozens of new treatises into Latin directly from Greek, including Galen's *magnum opus*, *On the Usefulness of the Parts*. The fourteenth-century French surgeon, Guy de Chauliac, quoted from thirty-one separate works of Galen.[10]

Human dissection, which was practiced only rarely in antiquity and which Galen had never done, was part of regular university curricula in Western Europe from the early fourteenth century. The bodies were those of criminals, executed for particularly heinous offenses, as dissection was a sort of added punishment. Dissections were infrequently performed—generally only once per year, before an audience of passive students, while a professor in

---

8   On the Alexandrian "canon," see Iskandar (1976). On Yunani/Greco-Arabic medicine in the twentieth and twenty-first centuries, see Saad and Said (2011); Attawell (2007).

9   Excellent discussions of the history of the transmission of Galen's work are available in Boudon-Millot (2007a, xci–ccxxxviii) and Durling (1961).

10   Durling (1961, 236).

a lofty seat lectured from books, and a barber (for these also performed most minor surgical procedures), or a surgeon, dissected the body. This we know from, among other sources, the complaints of Andreas Vesalius himself; on which more below. Few new discoveries or corrections to Galenic anatomy were made this way, although there were exceptions.

In the fifteenth and sixteenth centuries, Renaissance humanism reinvigorated medicine with its emphasis on philology and textual criticism and the recovery of ancient works. Scholars believed that if they could only read the original works of Galen, unmediated by translations and intepreters and uncorrupted by forgeries, they would uncover troves of lost knowledge about anatomy and other subjects. New Greek texts were sought out and compared; new and more reliable editions were produced, and new translations in Latin also appeared. By 1525, a comprehensive edition of Galen's known works in Greek—the Aldine edition, from the press of Aldus Manutius in Venice—was in print. The Aldine edition contained nearly all of the Galenic treatises surviving in Greek that are known today, in five enormous folio volumes. Suddenly Galen's work was accessible, as a corpus, in a way that it had never been before, although most medical students could not afford a complete Galen and instead bought small octavo editions of his most popular treatises, which were produced in huge numbers.

Vesalius was born in 1514 in Brussels.[11] His father was a pharmacist in the retinue of the Holy Roman Emperor Maximilian and, later, Charles V. When Charles gratefully acknowledged his service by legitimizing his birth, this perhaps inspired his son, Andreas, to seek out a higher status through a medical education. This Andreas pursued first in Paris and then in Leuven. He arrived in Paris in 1533, just as humanistic Galenism was taking hold; for the curriculum at the University of Paris was relatively conservative. In 1526 its library acquired the Aldine edition of Galen, published just one year earlier, and in the following year it acquired a Hippocratic Corpus. In the years

---

11   The classic biographical work on Vesalius is still the very thorough study of O'Malley (1965). What follows is based on this work. I present a rather traditional and simplistic version of the history of Renaissance anatomy; a large scholarship offering more nuanced discussions of anatomy in Renaissance culture exists. Sawday (1995) is recommended.

that followed appeared the first Parisian editions of Galen's anatomical works in Latin translation, which is how most medical students would use them: Niccolò da Reggio's *On the Usefulness of the Parts* and Guinter of Andernach's version of the first nine books of *On Anatomical Procedures*, among other texts. Guinter of Andernach was one of Vesalius's teachers.

Another was Jacobus Sylvius, who was later known to bring the stinking, putrid body parts of hanged criminals to the lecture hall in his sleeves and dissect them before his students. This habit, so different from the traditional method of dissection in Paris and other European universities at the time, must have dated to after 1536, when Vesalius had left Paris; for it seems that in Vesalius's time he only brought in parts of dogs. But Sylvius was clearly a brazen and charismatic man who made an impression on his most famous student, who later, perhaps ungratefully, boasted of having learned anatomy without the aid of a teacher. For Sylvius remained a loyal Galenist, but Vesalius did not.[12]

Vesalius was not content to watch barbers dissect a few major organs once or twice a year, but found ways, perhaps under Sylvius, to wield the knife himself. When war broke out between France and Flanders in 1536, he was forced to relocate to Leuven for the last year of his baccalaureate in medicine. Anatomy was not taught there at all, but Vesalius received permission to perform some dissections, including one on an eighteen-year-old aristocratic female who had apparently died of pneumonia complicated by the severe compression of her organs by her corset. He continued his studies at the University of Padua in Italy, where he was appointed to the faculty as chair of surgery and anatomy before the year 1537 was out. A friend at Padua, Vitus Tritonius, was already calling him "the most skilled and diligent of all anatomists" by that time.[13]

Vesalius performed his first human dissection in Padua over the course of eighteen days in December 1537, still using Galen as his main authority. But unlike traditional instructors at Padua and elsewhere, he performed it

---

12   On body parts, see O'Malley (1965, 49); on dogs, 51.
13   Ibid., 79.

himself. In 1538 he published a series of six anatomical drawings, the *Tabulae anatomicae*, also based largely on Galenic anatomy: a completely new and stunningly original set of illustrations for medical students. But in 1540, visiting Bologna, Vesalius performed a series of dissections (on three human bodies and six dogs), in which he openly contested the views of Matteo Corti, a Galenist on the faculty at Bologna, and also of Galen himself. Before an audience of two hundred eager students on benches encircling the dissection table, he declared in response to a challenge from Corti that, whenever he said something that contradicted Galen's opinion, he would prove Galen wrong by demonstration.

Vesalius was, at this time, not only dissecting human and animal bodies and teaching anatomy but also engaged in revising Latin translations of Galen's *On Anatomical Procedures*, *On the Anatomy of the Veins and Arteries*, and *On the Anatomy of the Nerves* for a new edition of Galen's complete works, to be published by the Giunta Press in Venice. This close reading of Galen, combined with his enthusiasm for, and increasing proficiency in, human dissection, were the foundations of Vesalius's greatest work, the *Fabrica corporis humani* or *On the Structure of the Human Body*, which first appeared in print in 1543.

For all Vesalius's hostility to Galenism, there are many similarities between the two men, both superficial and psychological. Like Galen at Alexandria, Vesalius learned medicine in an era when anatomy was being revitalized; and he, like Galen, was perhaps the most important, but not the only, contributor to this change. Like Galen, he rose to the top of his profession and served the emperor, in this case the Holy Roman Emperor Charles VI. Like Galen, he was self-aggrandizing and based his reputation on the brick-by-brick demolition of the anatomical theories of his rivals and predecessors, insisting on observation as the criterion of truth. Like Galen he dissected obsessively, sometimes keeping rotting corpses in his room for weeks. Many of Vesalius's polemics are aimed not directly at Galen himself, but at the physicians of Vesalius's own time who slavishly held to his views despite the evidence before their very eyes—criticisms reminiscent of Galen's merciless diatribes against sectarianism in his own day.

The *Fabrica* is organized according to the same sequence of parts as Galen's *On Anatomical Procedures*, not on the model of medieval anatomies. That is, it is framed as an updated, corrected version of Galen's work. There can be no doubt that Vesalius was influenced on a very deep level by his close study of the work of the man he still, even in the second edition of the *Fabrica* published in 1555, called the "prince of medicine." In his preface, for example, Vesalius describes the decline of medicine from the time of Hippocrates in a way reminiscent of passages in Galen's *On Anatomical Procedures*—no longer, until recently, was dissection practiced by physicians willing to get their hands dirty; the doctors of the era preceding Vesalius had learned only from books. Indeed, who in history was more like Galen than Vesalius? And who more like Vesalius than Galen, the man who once stood before an animal's corpse with the works of all his predecessors arrayed before him, announcing that he would prove all of them wrong on any point of the audience's choice—and followed through?

Galen's most influential contribution to medicine was surely anatomy. Anatomy is a cumulative science; one cannot simply cut up a corpse and find meaning in its inner structures without knowing what to look for. Galen's exhaustive descriptions drew on many centuries of tradition before him. Virtuoso anatomist that he was, he could not have seen what he saw, nor described what he described, without that tradition; which also led him astray many times, as did the traditional views on physiology that he also espoused and elaborated. There are no perforations in the heart's septum, as Vesalius finally concluded after more than a decade of searching for them. But without Galen's *Anatomical Procedures*, Vesalius, the founder of modern anatomy, could not himself have observed nor described in such fine detail the structure of the human body.

Galen's most relevant contribution today, however, is paradoxically his clinical practice. Although his polemics, his theories of physiology, and his meticulous anatomical instructions come down to us over the centuries in large quantities, it is the voice of the healer that speaks to us most directly. Despite the energy he devoted to dissecting, writing, and showing off, Galen never lost sight of the idea that medicine is about treating patients; and he treated all kinds of patients. His anecdotes, although personal in tone, betray barely a hint of condescension toward any patient except for one silly rich man. He would root around in a farmer's yard for a suitable ingredient for a plaster. He would wheedle information from a chambermaid if it helped him make a better diagnosis. He would perform insanely risky surgery on the slim chance of saving a slave boy's life, with professional disgrace as the price of failure. Galen was egotistical, arrogant, bossy, bombastic; he was an unapologetic owner of slaves and possibly, by some definitions, a misogynist. He was not necessarily a good man. But he was a good doctor. The challenges he faced are scarcely imaginable today; paramedics, military field doctors, and physicans in very poor developing countries are in the best position to understand, but even there, the advances of the last century have obliterated much of the experience of medicine in the premodern world. Galen battled a staggering array of lethal infections day after day, year after year, and with his own hands.

The rare passages where Galen suggests his motives for practicing the profession to which he dedicated his intellect and energy so exhaustively strike modern readers as paradoxical. Through the lens of our more reserved, less openly competitive culture, Galen seems obsessed with fame and victory. But he could have achieved these as a philosopher or a sophist, or through several other professions. It was the patients that drew him to medicine.

> The aim of the physician ... is not fame or wealth, as Menodotus the Empiricist wrote; this was the aim for Menodotus, but not for Diocles, nor for Hippocrates or Empedocles or for many other of the ancients, who healed people for the love of mankind.
>
> (*Plac. Hipp. Plat.* 9.5, 5.751–52K)

Medicine was Galen's passion, one to which he devoted all his energies throughout a life that was extraordinarily long by the standards of his day and yet, as for all mortals engaged in the study of nature's secrets, all too short.

BIBLIOGRAPHY

Africa, Thomas (1961). "The Opium Addiction of Marcus Aurelius." *Journal of the History of Ideas* 22: 97–102.

Aldrete, Gregory S. (2007). *Floods of the Tiber in Ancient Rome*. Baltimore: Johns Hopkins University Press.

Allen, R. E. (1983). *The Attalid Kingdom: A Constitutional History*. Oxford: Clarendon.

Alston, Richard (2002). *The City in Roman and Byzantine Egypt*. London: Routledge.

_____ and Onno van Nijf, eds. (2008). *Feeding the Ancient Greek City*. Leuven: Peeters.

Ando, Clifford (2000). *Imperial Ideology and Provincial Loyalty in the Roman Empire*. Berkeley: University of California Press.

Andorlini Marcone, Isabella (1993). "L'apporto dei papyri alla conoscenza della scienza medica antica." *Aufstieg und Niedergang der römischen Welt* 2.37.1: 458–562.

_____ (2001). *Greek Medical Papyri 1*. Florence: Instituto Papirologico G. Vitelli.

Ascenzi, A., P. Bianco, R. Nicoletti, G. Ceccarini, M. Fornaseri, G. Graziani, M. R. Giuliani, R. Rosicarello, L. Ciuffarella, and H. Granger-Taylor (1996). "The Roman Mummy of Grottarossa." Pp. 205–18 in *Human Mummies: A Global Survey of their Status and the Techniques of Conservation*, ed. K. Spindler, Haraid Wilfing, Elisabeth Rastbichler-Zissernig, Dieter ZurNedden, and Hans Nothdurfter. Vienna: Springer.

Attawell, Guy N. A. (2007). *Refiguring Unani Tibb: Plural Healing in Late Colonial India*. New Delhi: Orient Longman.

Aufderheide, A. C., G. Rapp, L. E. Wittmers, J. E. Wallgren, R. Macchiarelli, G. Fornaciari, F. Mallegni, and R. S. Corruccini (1992). "Lead Exposure in Italy: 800 BC–700 AD." *International Journal of Anthropology* 7: 9–15.

Auget, Roland (1972). *Cruelty and Civilization: The Roman Games*. New York: Allen & Unwin (1972) and London: Routledge (1974) = *Cruauté et civilization: Les Jeux romains*. Paris: Flammarion (1970).

Ault, Bradley A., and Lisa C. Nevett, eds. (2005). *Ancient Greek Houses and Households: Chronological, Regional, and Social Diversity*. Philadelphia: University of Pennsylvania Press.

Badian, Ernst (1983). *Publicans and Sinners: Private Enterprise in the Service of the Roman Republic*. 2d ed. Ithaca, NY: Cornell University Press.

Bailey, Jillian F., Maciej Henneberg, Isabelle B. Colson, Annamaria Ciarallo, Robert E. M. Hedges, and Bryan Sykes (1999). "Monkey Business in Pompeii—Unique Find of a Juvenile Barbary Macaque Skeleton Identified Using Osteoarchaeology and Ancient DNA Techniques." *Molecular Biology and Evolution* 16: 1410–14.

Baker, Brenda J., and George J. Armelagos (1988). "The Origin and Antiquity of Syphilis: Paleopathological Diagnosis and Interpretation." *Current Anthropology* 29: 703–37.

Baker, Patricia Ann (2004). *Medical Care for the Roman Army on the Rhine, Danube, and British Frontiers in the First, Second, and Early Third Centuries A.D.* Oxford: J. and E. Hedges.

Bardong, Kurt (1942). "Beiträge zur Hippokrates- und Galenforschung." *Nachrichten von der Akademie der Wissenschaften in Göttingen: Philologisch-Historische Klasse* 7: 577–640.

Barton, Carlin A. (1993). *The Sorrows of the Ancient Romans: The Gladiator and the Monster*. Princeton, NJ: Princeton University Press.

Barton, Tamsyn S. (1994). *Power and Knowledge: Astrology, Physiognomics and Medicine under the Roman Empire*. Ann Arbor: University of Michigan Press.

Baumeister, Roy, and Julie Juola Exline (1999). "Virtue, Personality and Social Relations: Self-Control as the Moral Muscle." *Journal of Personality* 67: 1165–94.

Baumeister, Roy, and John Tierney (2011). *Willpower: Rediscovering the Greatest Human Strength*. New York: Penguin.

Beck, Lily Y. (2011). *Pedanius Dioscorides of Anazarbus: De Materia Medica*. Altertumswissenschaftliche Texte und Studien 38. 2d ed. Hildesheim: Olms.

Behr, Charles A. (1968). *Aelius Aristides and the Sacred Tales*. Amsterdam: Hakkert.

———— (1981). *P. Aelius Aristides: The Complete Works*. 2 vols. Leiden: Brill.

Bergsträsser, G. (1925). "Ḥunain ibn Isḥāq über die syrischen und arabischen Galen-übersetzungen." *Abhandlungen für die Kunde des Morgenlandes* 17.

———— (1932). "Neue Materielen zu Ḥunain ibn Isḥāq's Galen-Bibliographie." *Abhandlungen für de Kunde des Morgenlandes* 19.

Betzig, Laura (1992). "Roman Polygyny." *Ethnology and Sociobiology* 13: 309–49.

Birley, Anthony (1987). *Marcus Aurelius: A Biography.* 2d ed. New Haven, CT: Yale University Press.

Bisset, Norman G., Jan J. Bruhn, Silvio Curto, Bo Holmstedt, Ulf Nyman, and Meinhart K. Zenk (1994). "Was Opium Known in 18th Dynasty Ancient Egypt? An Examination of Materials from the Tomb of the Chief Royal Architect Kha." *Journal of Ethnopharmacology* 41: 99–114.

Bliquez, Lawrence J. (1994). *Roman Surgical Instruments and Other Minor Objects in the National Archaeological Museum of Naples.* Mainz: von Zabern.

Bodel, John (2000). "Dealing with the Dead: Undertakers, Executioners and Potter's Fields in Ancient Rome." Pp. 128–51 in *Death and Disease in the Ancient City*, ed. Valerie M. Hope and Eirann Marshall. London: Routledge.

Boehm, Isabelle (2003). "Toucher du doigt: Le Vocabulaire de toucher dans les textes médicaux grecs et latins." Pp. 229–40 in *Manus medica: Actions et gestes de l'officiant dans les textes médicaux latins. Questions de thérapeutique et de lexique*, ed. Françoise Gaide and Frédérique Biville. Aix-en-Provence: Publications de l'Université de Provence.

Bogaard, Amy, Rüdiger Krause, and Hans-Christoph Strien (2011). "Towards a Social Geography of Cultivation and Plant Use in an Early Farming Community: Vaihingen an der Enz, South-West Germany." *Antiquity* 85: 395–416.

Boudon, Véronique (1994). "Les Oeuvres de Galien pour les debutants ('De sectis,' 'De pulsibus ad tirones,' 'Ad Glauconem de methodo medendi,' et 'Ars medica'): Médecine et pédagogie au IIe siècle ap. J.-C." *Aufstieg und Niedergang der römischen Welt* 2.37.2: 1421–67.

_____ (2000). *Galien.* Vol. 2, *Exhortation à l'étude de la médecine; Art médical.* Paris: Les Belles Lettres.

Boudon-Millot, Véronique (2007a). *Galien.* Vol. 1, *Introduction générale; Sur l'ordre de ses propres livres; Sur ses propres livres; Que l'excellent médecin est aussi philosophe.* Paris: Les Belles Lettres.

_____ (2007b). "Un traité perdu de Galien miraculeusement retrouvé, le *Sur l'inutilité de se chagriner*: Texte grec et traduction française." Pp. 67–118 in *La Science médicale antique: Nouveaux regards*, ed. V. Boudon-Millot, A. Guardasole, and C. Magdelaine. Paris: Beauchesne.

Boudon-Millot, Véronique, and Jacques Jouanna (2010). *Galien.* Vol. 4, *Ne pas se chagriner.* Paris: Les Belles Lettres.

Boudon-Millot, Véronique, and A. Pietrobelli (2005). "Galien ressuscité: Édition princeps du texte grecque du *De propriis placitis.*" *Revue des Études Grecques* 118: 168–213.

Boulogne, Jacques (1996). "Plutarque et la médecine." *Aufstieg und Niedergang der römischen Welt* 2.37.3: 2762–2893.

Bowersock, Glen (1969). *Greek Sophists in the Roman Empire.* Oxford: Clarendon.

Bradley, Keith (1986). "Seneca and Slavery." *Classica et Mediaevalia* 37: 161–72.

———— (1987). *Slaves and Masters in the Roman Empire: A Study in Social Control*. Oxford: Oxford University Press.

———— (1997). "Law, Magic, and Culture in the Apologia of Apuleius." *Phoenix* 51: 203–23.

Brain, Peter (1986). *Galen on Bloodletting*. Cambridge: Cambridge University Press.

Brock, Arthur John (1916). *Galen: On the Natural Faculties*. Cambridge, MA: Harvard University Press. Reprinted (1991).

Brodersen, Kai (2001). "The Presentation of Geographical Knowledge for Travel and Transport in the Roman World." Pp. 7–21 in *Travel and Geography in the Roman Empire*, ed. Colin Adams and Ray Laurence. London: Routledge.

Cahill, Nicholas (2002). *Household and City Organization at Olynthus*. New Haven, CT: Yale University Press.

Capasso, Luigi (2000). "Indoor Pollution and Respiratory Diseases in Ancient Rome." *The Lancet* 356: 1774.

Cappelletti, Silvia (2006). *The Jewish Community of Rome from the Second Century B.C. to the Third Century C.E.* Supplements to the *Journal for the Study of Judaism* 113. Leiden: Brill.

Carter, M. J. (2006). "Gladiatorial Combat: The Rules of Engagement." *Classical Journal* 102: 97–114.

Champlin, Edward (1980). *Fronto and Antonine Rome*. Cambridge, MA: Harvard University Press.

Cohn-Haft, Louis (1956). *The Public Physicians of Ancient Greece*. Smith College Studies in History 42. Northampton, MA: Smith College Department of History.

Cruse, Audrey (2004). *Roman Medicine*. Stroud, United Kingdom: Tempus.

Curry, Andrew (2008). "The Gladiator Diet." *Archaeology* 61.6: 28–30.

Davies, Roy W. (1989). *Service in the Roman Army*. Ed. David Breeze and Valerie A. Maxfield. Edinburgh: Edinburgh University Press.

Dean-Jones, Lesley (1994). *Women's Bodies in Classical Greek Science*. Oxford: Clarendon.

Debru, Armelle (1996). "Les Demonstrations médicales à Rome au temps de Galien." Pp. 69–81 of vol. 1 in *Ancient Medicine in its Socio-Cultural Context*, ed. Ph. J. van der Eijk, H. F. J. Horstmanshoff, and P. H. Schrijvers. 2 vols. Amsterdam: Rodopi.

———— (2008). "Physiology." Pp. 263–82 in *The Cambridge Companion to Galen*, ed. R. J. Hankinson. Cambridge: Cambridge University Press.

Deichgräber, Karl (1965). *Die griechische Empirikerschule: Sammlung der Fragmente und Darstellung der Lehre*. Berlin: Weidmann.

de Lacy, Phillip (1980–84). *Galen: On the Doctrines of Hippocrates and Plato*. Corpus Medicorum Graecorum 5.4.1.2, 2 vols. 2d ed. Berlin: Akademie-Verlag.

Delson, Eric (1980). "Fossil Macaques, Phyletic Relationships and a Scenario of Deployment." Pp. 10–30 in *The Macaques: Studies in Ecology, Behavior and Evolution*, ed. Donald D. Lindburg. New York: Van Nostrand Reinhold.

Dench, Emma (1995). *From Barbarians to New Men: Greek, Roman and Modern Perceptions of Peoples of the Central Appennines*. London: Oxford University Press.

de Quincey, Thomas (2003). *Confessions of an English Opium Eater and Other Writings*. Ed. Barry Milligan. London: Penguin.

Diamandopoulos, Athanasios A., and Pavlos C. Goudas (2003). "The Late Greco-Roman and Byzantine Contribution to the Evolution of Laboratory Examinations of Bodily Excrement. Part 1: Urine, Sperm, Menses and Stools." *Clinical Chemistry and Laboratory Medicine* 41.7: 963–69.

———(2005). "The Late Greco-Roman and Byzantine Contribution towards the Evolution of Laboratory Examinations of Bodily Excrement. Part 2: Sputum, Vomit, Blood, Sweat, Autopsies." *Clinical Chemistry and Laboratory Medicine* 43.1: 90–96.

Dmitriev, Sviatoslav (2005). *City Government in Hellenistic and Roman Asia Minor*. New York: Oxford University Press.

Donini, Pierluigi (2008). "Psychology." Pp. 184–209 in *The Cambridge Companion to Galen*, ed. R. J. Hankinson. Cambridge: Cambridge University Press.

Donoghue, Helen D., Antónia Marcsik, Carney Matheson, Kim Vernon, Emilia Nuorala, Joseph E. Molto, Charles L. Greenblatt, and Mark Spigelman (2005). "Co-Infection of *Mycobacterium tuberculosis* and *Mycobacterium leprae* in Human Archaeological Samples: A Possible Explanation for the Historical Decline of Leprosy." *Proceedings of the Royal Society B: Biological Sciences* 272: 389–94.

Downie, Janet (2008). "Proper Pleasures: Bathing and Oratory in Aelius Aristides' *Hieros Logos I* and *Oration 33*." Pp. 115–130 in *Aelius Aristides between Greece, Rome, and the Gods*, ed. W. V. Harris and Brooke Holmes. Leiden: Brill.

Dubos, René Jules, and Jean Dubos (1987). *The White Plague: Tuberculosis, Man and Society*. 2d ed. New Brunswick, NJ: Rutgers University Press.

Dunbabin, Katharine M. D. (1989). "*Baiarum grata voluptas*: Pleasures and Dangers of the Baths." *Papers of the British School at Rome* 57: 6–46.

Duncan-Jones, R. A. (1996). "The Impact of the Antonine Plague." *Journal of Roman Archaeology* 9: 108–36.

Durling, Richard T. (1961). "A Chronological Census of Renaissance Editions and Translations of Galen." *Journal of the Warburg and Courtauld Institutes* 24: 230–305.

Eckstein, Arthur M. (2006). *Mediterranean Anarchy, Interstate War, and the Rise of Rome*. Berkeley: University of California Press.

Edelstein, Emma J., and Ludwig Edelstein (1945). *Asclepius: A Collection and Interpretation of the Testimonies*, 2 vols. Baltimore: Johns Hopkins University Press. (Reprinted, 1998.)

Egerbacher, Monika, Heike Weber, and Silke Hauer (2000). "Bones in the Heart Skeleton of the Otter (*Lutra lutra*)." *Journal of Anatomy* 196: 485–91.

Erdkamp, Paul (2008). "Grain Funds and Market Intervention in the Roman World." Pp. 109–26 in *Feeding the Ancient Greek City*, ed. Richard Alston and Onno van Nijf. Leuven: Peeters.

Evans, Richard (2012). *A History of Pergamum: Beyond Hellenistic Kingship.* London: Continuum.

Fabricius, Cajus (1972). *Galens Exzerpte aus älteren Pharmakologen.* Berlin: De Gruyter.

Facchini, F., E. Rastelli, and B. Brasili (2004). "*Cribra orbitalia* and *Cribra cranii* in Roman Skeletal Remains from the Ravenna Area and Rimini (I–IV Century AD)." *International Journal of Osteoarchaeology* 14: 126–36.

Fagan, Garrett (1999). *Bathing in Public in the Roman World.* Ann Arbor: University of Michigan Press.

Faraone, Christopher A. (2011). "Magical and Medical Approaches to the Wandering Womb in the Ancient Greek World." *Classical Antiquity* 30: 1–32.

Fenner, F., D. A. Henderson, I. Arita, Z. Ježek, and I. D. Ladnyi (1988). *Smallpox and Its Eradication.* Geneva: World Health Organization.

Fichtner, Gerhard (2004). *Corpus Galenicum: Verzeichnis der galenischen und pseudogalenischen Schriften.* Tübingen: Institut für Ethik und Geschichte der Medizin.

Fischer, Klaus-Dietrich (2010). "De fragmentis Herae Cappadocis atque Rufi Ephesii hactenus ignotis." *Galenos* 4: 173–83.

Fitzgerald, William (2000). *Slavery and the Roman Literary Imagination.* Cambridge: Cambridge University Press.

Flemming, Rebecca (2000). *Medicine and the Making of Roman Women: Gender, Nature and Authority from Celsus to Galen.* Oxford: Oxford University Press.

———— (2008). "Demiurge and Emperor in Galen's World of Knowledge." Pp. 59–84 in *Galen and the World of Knowledge*, ed. Christopher Gill, Thomas Whitmarsh, and John Wilkins. Cambridge: Cambridge University Press.

Fowler, Murray E., and Susan K. Mikota (2006). *Biology, Medicine, and Surgery of Elephants.* Ames, IA: Blackwell.

Frede, Michael, and Richard Walzer (1985). *Three Treatises on the Nature of Science.* Indianapolis: Hackett.

———— (2003). "Galen's Theology." Pp. 73–126 in *Galien et la philosophie*, ed. Jonathan Barnes and Jacques Jouanna. Entretiens sur l'antiquité classique 49. Geneva: Fondation Hardt.

Frend, W. H. C. (1965). *Martyrdom and Persecution in the Early Church.* Oxford: Blackwell.

Furley, David J., and J. S. Wilkie (1984). *Galen on Respiration and the Arteries.* Princeton, NJ: Princeton University Press.

Furtrell, Alison (1997). *Blood in the Arena: The Spectacle of Roman Power.* Austin: University of Texas Press.

Gabrieli, Guiseppe (1924). "Hunáyn ibn Isháq." *Isis* 6: 282–92.

Galvão-Sobrinho, Carlos (1996). "Hippocratic Ideals, Medical Ethics, and the Practice of Medicine in the Early Middle Ages: The Legacy of the Hippocratic Oath." *Journal of the History of Medicine and Allied Sciences* 51: 438–55.

Garnsey, Peter (1988). *Famine and Food Supply in the Greco-Roman World: Responses to Risk and Crisis*. Cambridge: Cambridge University Press.

_____ (1999). *Food and Society in Classical Antiquity*. Cambridge: Cambridge University Press.

Garofalo, Ivan (1988). *Erasistrati fragmenta*. Pisa: Giardini.

Garofalo, Ivan, and Armelle Debru (2005). *Galien*, vol. 5: *Les Os pour les debutants; L'Anatomie des muscles*. Paris: Les Belles Lettres.

Gill, Christopher (2010). *Naturalistic Psychology in Galen and Stoicism*. Oxford: Oxford University Press.

Gilliam, J. F. (1961). "The Plague under Marcus Aurelius." *American Journal of Philology* 82: 225–51.

Gleason, Maud W. (2009). "Shock and Awe: The Performance Dimension of Galen's Anatomy Demonstrations." Pp. 85–114 in *Galen and the World of Knowledge*, ed. Christopher Gill, Tim Whitmarsh, and John Wilkins. Cambridge: Cambridge University Press.

Golvin, Jean -Claude (1988). *L'Amphithéâtre romain: Essai sur la theorization de sa forme et de ses fonctions*. 2 vols. Publications du Centre Pierre Paris 18. Paris: Boccard.

Goudsmit, Jaap, and Douglas Brandon-Jones (1999). "Mummies of Olive Baboons and Barbary Macaques in the Baboon Catacomb of the Sacred Animal Necropolis at North Saqqara." *Journal of Egyptian Archaeology* 85: 45–53.

_____ (2000). "Evidence from the Baboon Catacomb in North Saqqara for a West Mediterranean Monkey Trade Route to Ptolemaic Alexandria." *Journal of Egyptian Archaeology* 17: 111–19.

Gourevitch, Danielle (1984). *Le Triangle Hippocratique dans le monde gréco-romain: Le Malade, sa maladie et son médecin*. Rome: École française de Rome.

_____ (2003). "Fabriquer un médicament composé, solide et compact, dur et sec: Formulaire et réalités." Pp. 49–68 in *Manus medica: Actions et gestes de l'officiant dans les textes médicaux latins. Questions de thérapeutique et de lexique*, ed. Françoise Gaide and Frédérique Biville. Aix-en-Provence: Publications de l'Université de Provence.

Green, Robert Montraville (1951). *A Translation of Galen's Hygiene*. Springfield, IL: Thomas

Grmek, Mirko (1989). *Diseases in the Ancient Greek World*. Baltimore: Johns Hopkins University Press = *Les Maladies à l'aube de la civilization occidentale: Recherches sur la réalité pathologique dans le monde grec préhistorique, archaïque, et classique*. Paris: Payot, 1983.

_____ (1997). *Le Chaudron de Médée: L'Expérimentation sur le vivant dans l'antiquité*. Le Plessis-Robinson: Institut Synthélabo.

Grmek, Mirko, and Danielle Gourevitch (1986). "Medice, cura te ipsum: Les Maladies de Galien." *Études de lettres* 1: 45–64.

_____ (1994). "Aux sources de la doctrine médicale de Galien: L'Enseignement de Marinus, Quintus, et Numisianus." *Aufstieg und Niedergang der römischen Welt* 2.37.2: 1491–1528.

Gros, Pierre (1996–2001). *L'Architecture romaine: Du début du IIIe siècle av. J.-C. à la fin du Haut-Empire*. 2 vols. Paris: Picard.

Gruen, Erich S. (2002). *Diaspora: Jews amidst Greeks and Romans*. Cambridge, MA: Harvard University Press.

Gummerus, Hermann (1932). *Der Ärztestand im römischen Reiche nach den Inschriften*. Helsinki: Societas Scientarum Fennica.

Habicht, Christian (1969). *Die Inschriften des Asklepieions*. Deutsches Archäologisches Institut, Altertümer von Pergamon VIII.3. Berlin: de Gruyter.

Hales, Shelley (2003). *The Roman House and Social Identity*. Cambridge: Cambridge University Press.

Halfmann, Helmut (1979). *Die Senatoren aus dem östlichen Teil des Imperium Romanum bis zum Ende des 2. Jahrhunderts n. Chr*. Hypomnemata: Untersuchungen zur Antike und zu ihrem Nachleben 58. Göttingen: Vandenhoeck & Ruprecht.

_____ (2004). *Éphèse et Pergame: Urbanisme et commanditaires en Asie mineure romaine*, Bordeaux: Ausonius = *Städtebau und Bauherren im römischen Kleinasien: Ein Vergleich zwischen Pergamon und Ephesos*. Beihefte der Istanbuler Mitteilungen 43. Tübingen: Wasmuth (2001).

Hall, A. J., and E. Photos-Jones (2008). "Accessing Ancient Beliefs and Practices: The Case of Lemnian Earth." *Archaeometry* 50: 1034–49.

Hankinson, R. J. (1989). "Galen and the Best of All Possible Worlds." *Classical Quarterly* 39: 206–27.

_____ (1991a). *Galen on the Therapeutic Method: Books I and II*. Oxford: Oxford University Press.

_____ (1991b). "Galen's Anatomy of the Soul." *Phronesis* 36: 197–233.

_____ (1993). "Actions and Passions: Affection, Emotion, and Moral Self-Management in Galen's Psychological Philosophy." Pp. 184–222 in *Passions and Perceptions: Studies in the Hellenistic Philosophy of Mind*, ed. Jacques Brunschwig and Martha C. Nussbaum. Cambridge: Cambridge University Press.

_____ (1994a). "Galen's Anatomical Procedures: A Second-Century Debate in Medical Epistemology." *Aufstieg und Niedergang der römischen Welt* 2.37.2: 1834–55.

_____ (1994b). "Galen's Theory of Causation." *Aufstieg und Niedergang der römischen Welt* 2.37.2: 1757–74.

_____ (2008a). "The Man and His Work." Pp. 1–33 in *The Cambridge Companion to Galen*, ed. R. J. Hankinson. Cambridge: Cambridge University Press.

_____ (2008b). "Philosophy of Nature." Pp. 225–36 in *The Cambridge Companion to Galen*, ed. R. J. Hankinson. Cambridge: Cambridge University Press.

Hanson, Ann Ellis (1985). "Papyri of Medical Content." *Yale Classical Studies* 28: 39–47.

_____ (1998a). "Galen: Author and Critic." Pp. 22–53 in *Editing Texts / Texte edieren*, ed. Glenn W. Most. Göttingen: Vandenhoeck & Ruprecht.

_____ (1998b). "In the Shadow of Galen: Two Berlin Papyri of Medical Content." Pp. 145–60 in *Text and Tradition: Studies in Ancient Medicine and its Transmission*, ed. Klaus-Dietrich Fischer, Diethard Nickel, and Paul Potter. Leiden: Brill.

Harper, Kristin N., Molly K. Zuckerman, Megan L. Harper, John D. Kingston, and George J. Armelagos (2011). "The Origin and Antiquity of Syphilis Revisited: An Appraisal of Old World Pre-Columbian Evidence for Treponemal Infection." *Yearbook of Physical Anthropology* 54: 99–133.

Harris, W. V. (2001). *Restraining Rage: The Ideology of Anger Control in Classical Antiquity*. Cambridge, MA: Harvard University Press.

_____ (2009). *Dreams and Experience in Classical Antiquity*. Cambridge, MA: Harvard University Press.

Harris, W. V., and Brooke Holmes, eds. (2008). *Aelius Aristides between Greece, Rome, and the Gods*. Leiden: Brill.

Harvey, Allison G. (2011). "Sleep and Circadian Functioning: Critical Mechanisms in the Mood Disorders?" *Annual Review of Clinical Psychology* 7: 297–319.

Hausmann, Ulrich (1948). *Kunst und Heiltum: Untersuchungen zu den griechischen Asklepiosreliefs*. Potsdam: Stichnote.

Healy, John F. (1978). *Mining and Metallurgy in the Greek and Roman World*. London: Thames and Hudson.

Hirt, Alfred Michael (2010). *Imperial Mines and Quarries in the Roman World: Organizational Aspects, 27 BC–AD 235*. Oxford: Oxford University Press.

Hoffmann, Adolf (1998). "The Roman Remodeling of the Asklepieion." Pp. 41–62 in *Pergamon: Citadel of the Gods*, ed. Helmut Koester. Harvard Theological Studies 46. Harrisburg, PA: Trinity Press International.

Holmes, Brooke (2008). "Aelius Aristides' Illegible Body." Pp. 81–114 in *Aelius Aristides between Greece, Rome, and the Gods*, ed. W. V. Harris and Brooke Holmes. Leiden: Brill.

Hong, Singmin, J.-P. Candelone, C. C. Patterson, and C. F. Boutron (1994). "Greenland Ice Evidence of Hemispheric Lead Pollution Two Millenia Ago by Greek and Roman Civilizations." *Science* 265: 1841–43.

Hopkins, Donald R. (2002). *The Greatest Killer: Smallpox in History*. Chicago: University of Chicago Press.

Hopkins, Keith (1983). "Murderous Games." Pp. 1–30 in id., *Death and Renewal. Sociological Studies in Roman History* 2. Cambridge: Cambridge University Press.

Houston, George W. (2003). "Galen, His Books and the *Horrea piperataria* in Rome." *Memoirs of the American Academy in Rome* 48: 45–51.

Hunter, Kathryn Montgomery (1991). *Doctors' Stories: The Narrative Structure of Medical Knowledge*. Princeton, NJ: Princeton University Press.

Ilberg, Johannes (1889). "Über die Schriftstellerei des Klaudios Galenos" (1). *Rheinisches Museum* n.s. 44: 207–39.

———— (1892). "Über die Schriftstellerei des Klaudios Galenos" (2). *Rheinisches Museum* n.s. 47: 489–514.

———— (1896). "Über die Schriftstellerei des Klaudios Galenos" (3). *Rheinisches Museum* n.s. 51: 165–96.

———— (1897). "Über die Schriftstellerei des Klaudios Galenos" (4). *Rheinisches Museum* n.s. 52: 591–623.

———— (1905). "Aus Galens Praxis: Ein Kulturbild aus der römischen Kaiserzeit." *Neue Jahrbücher* 15: 276–312. Reprinted in *Antike Medizin*, ed. Hellmut Flashar. Darmstadt: Wissenschaftliche Buchgesellschaft (1971), 361–416.

Isaac, Benjamin (2004). *The Invention of Racism in Classical Antiquity*. Princeton, NJ: Princeton University Press.

Iskandar, A. Z. (1976). "An Attempted Reconstruction of the Late Alexandrian Medical Curriculum." *Medical History* 20: 235–58.

Jacques, Jean-Marie (2002). *Nicandre: Oeuvres*. Vol. 3, *Les Alexipharmaques*. Paris: Les Belles Lettres.

Johnson, William A. (2010). *Readers and Reading Culture in the High Roman Empire*. Oxford: Oxford University Press.

Johnston, Ian (2006). *Galen on Diseases and Symptoms*. Cambridge: Cambridge University Press.

Johnston, Ian, and G. H. R. Horsley (2011). *Galen: Method of Medicine*. 3 vols. Cambridge, MA: Harvard University Press.

Jones, A. H. M. (1971). *The Cities of the Eastern Roman Provinces*. 2d ed. Oxford: Clarendon.

Jones, Christopher P. (1998). "Aelius Aristides and the Asklepieion." Pp. 63–76 in *Pergamon: Citadel of the Gods*, ed. Helmut Koester. Harrisburg, PA: Trinity Press International.

———— (2009). "Books and Libraries in a Newly-Discovered Treatise of Galen." *Journal of Roman Archaeology* 22: 390–97.

Jouanna, Jacques (1999). *Hippocrates*. Baltimore: Johns Hopkins University Press = *Hippocrate*. Paris: Fayard (1992).

———— (2010). "Hippocrates as Galen's Teacher." Pp. 1–21 in *Hippocrates and Medical Education*, ed. Manfred Horstmanshoff. Studies in Ancient Medicine 35. Leiden: Brill.

Junkelmann, Marcus (2000). *Das Spiel mit dem Tod: So kämpften Roms Gladiatoren*. Mainz: von Zabern.

Kanz, Fabian, and Karl Grossschmidt (2006). "Head Injuries of Roman Gladiators." *Forensic Science International* 160: 207–16.

Kayne, Donald (1968). "Antibacterial Activity of Human Urine." *Journal of Clinical Investigation* 47: 2374–90.

Keel, Pamela K., and Kelly L. Klump (2003). "Are Eating Disorders Culture-Bound Syndromes? Implications for Conceptualizing their Etiology." *Psychological Bulletin* 129: 747–69.

Keyser, Paul T. (1997). "Science and Magic in Galen's Recipes (Sympathy and Efficacy)." Pp. 175–198 in *Galen on Pharmacology: Philosophy, History and Medicine*, ed. Armelle Debru. Leiden: Brill.

Koester, Helmut, ed. (1998). *Pergamon: Citadel of the Gods.* Harvard Theological Studies 46. Harrisburg, PA: Trinity Press International.

König, Jason (2005). *Athletics and Literature in the Roman Empire.* Cambridge: Cambridge University Press.

Korpela, Jukka (1987). *Das Medizinalpersonal im antiken Rom: Eine sozialgeschichtliche Untersuchung.* Annales Academiae Scientiarum Fennicae, Dissertationes Humanarum Litterarum 45. Helsinki: Suomalainen Tiedeakatemia.

Kudlien, Fridolf (1981). "Galen's Religious Belief." Pp. 117–30 in *Galen: Problems and Prospects*, ed. Vivian Nutton. London: Wellcome Institute for the History of Medicine.

_____ (1986). *Die Stellung des Arztes in der römischen Gesellschaft.* Stuttgart: Steiner.

Künzl, Ernst (1983). *Medizinische Instrumente aus Sepulkralfunden der römischen Kaiserzeit.* Kunst und Altertum am Rhein 115. Cologne: Rheinland Verlag.

Kuriyama, Shigehisa (1995). "Interpreting the History of Bloodletting." *Journal of the History of Medicine and Allied Sciences* 50: 11–46.

_____ (1999). *The Expressiveness of the Body and the Divergence of Greek and Chinese Medicine.* New York: Zone Books.

Lane Fox, Robin (1986). *Pagans and Christians.* San Francisco: Harper & Row.

Li, Yu, Darin S. Carroll, Shea N. Gardner, Matthew C. Walsh, Elizabeth A. Vitalis, and Inger K. Damon (2007). "On the Origin of Smallpox: Correlating *Variola* Phylogenics with Historical Smallpox Records." *Proceedings of the National Academy of Sciences* 104.40: 15787–92.

LiDonnici, Lynn R. (1995). *The Epidaurian Miracle Inscriptions: Text, Translation and Commentary.* Atlanta: Scholars Press.

Littman, R. J., and M. L. Littman (1973). "Galen and the Antonine Plague." *American Journal of Philology* 94: 243–55.

Llewelyn-Jones, Lloyd (2003). *Aphrodite's Tortoise: The Veiled Woman of Ancient Greece.* Swansea: Classical Press of Wales.

Lo Cascio, Elio (2006). "Did the Population of Imperial Rome Reproduce Itself?" Pp. 52–68 in *Urbanism in the Pre-Industrial World: Cross-Cultural Examples*, ed. Glenn R. Storey. Tuscaloosa: University of Alabama Press.

Lyons, Malcolm (1969). *Galen: On the Parts of Medicine, On Cohesive Causes, On Regimen in Acute Diseases in Accordance with the Theories of Hippocrates.* Corpus Medicorum Graecorum, Supplementum Orientale 2. Berlin: Akademie-Verlag.

MacDonald, William L. (1982). *The Architecture of the Roman Empire.* 2 vols. 2d ed. New Haven, CT: Yale University Press.

MacMullen, Ramsay (1974). *Roman Social Relations, 50 BC to AD 284*. New Haven, CT: Yale University Press.

_____ (1976). *The Roman Government's Response to Crisis, A.D. 235–337*. New Haven, CT: Yale University Press.

_____ (1980a). "Roman Elite Motivation: Three Questions." *Past and Present* 88: 3–16. Reprinted in *Changes in the Roman Empire*, Princeton, NJ: Princeton University Press (1990), chapter 2.

_____ (1980b). "Women in Public in the Roman Empire." *Historia* 29 (1980): 208–18. Reprinted in *Changes in the Roman Empire*, Princeton, NJ: Princeton University Press (1990), chapter 15.

_____ (1981). *Paganism in the Roman Empire*. New Haven, CT: Yale University Press.

_____ (1990). *Corruption and the Decline of Rome*. New Haven, CT: Yale University Press.

Magie, David (1950). *Roman Rule in Asia Minor*. 2 vols. Princeton, NJ: Princeton University Press.

Manning, C. E. (1989). "Stoicism and Slavery in the Roman Empire." *Aufstieg und Niedergang der römishcen Welt* 2.36.3: 1518–43.

Mariani-Costatini, Renato, Paola Catalano, Francesco di Gennaro, Gabriella di Tota, and Luciana Rita Angeletti (2000). "New Light on Cranial Surgery in Ancient Rome." *The Lancet* 355: 305–7.

Mattern, Susan P. (1999a). "Physicians and the Roman Imperial Aristocracy: The Patronage of Therapeutics." *Bulletin of the History of Medicine* 73: 1–18.

_____ (1999b). *Rome and the Enemy: Imperial Strategy in the Principate*. Berkeley: University of California Press.

_____ (2008a). *Galen and the Rhetoric of Healing*. Baltimore: Johns Hopkins University Press.

_____ (2008b). "Galen's Ideal Patient." Pp. 116–30 in *Asklepios: Studies on Ancient Medicine*, ed. Louise Cilliers. Acta Classica Supplementum 2. Bloemfontain: Classical Association of South Africa.

Mattock, J. N. (1972). "A Translation of the Arabic Epitome of Galen's Book Περί ἤθων." Pp. 1–51 in *Islamic Philosophy and the Classical Tradition*, ed. S. M. Stern, Albert Hourani, and Vivian Brown. Festschrift for Richard Walzer. Columbia: University of South Carolina Press.

May, Margaret Tallmadge (1968). *Galen: On the Usefulness of the Parts of the Body*. 2 vols. Ithaca, NY: Cornell University Press.

Mayor, Adrienne (2010). *The Poison King: The Life and Legend of Mithradates, Rome's Deadliest Enemy*. Princeton, NJ: Princeton University Press.

McKenzie, Judith (2007). *The Architecture of Alexandria and Egypt, c. 300 BC to AD 700*. New Haven, CT: Yale University Press.

Meyerhof, Max (1926). "New Light on Ḥunain ibn Isḥāq and His Period." *Isis* 8: 685–724.

_____ (1929). "Autobiographische Bruchstücke Galens aus arabischen Quellen." *Sudhoffs Archiv* 22: 72–85.

Millar, Fergus (1992). *The Emperor in the Roman World (31 BC—AD 337)*. 2d ed. Ithaca, NY: Cornell University Press.

Miller, Stephen G. (2004). *Ancient Greek Athletics*. New Haven, CT: Yale University Press.

Minenka, Susan, David Watson, and Lee Anna Clark (1998). "Comorbidity of Anxiety and Unipolar Mood Disorders." *Annual Review of Psychology* 49: 377–412.

Mitchell, Stephen (1993). *Anatolia: Land, Men, and Gods in Asia Minor*. 2 vols. Oxford: Clarendon.

Moraux, Paul (1985). *Galien de Pergame: Souvenirs d'un médecin*. Paris: Les Belles Lettres.

Moretti, Luigi (1953). *Iscrizioni agonistiche greche*. Studi pubblicati dall'Istituto italiano per la storia antica 12. Rome: Signorelli.

Morstein-Marx, Robert (1995). *Hegemony to Empire: The Development of the Roman Imperium in the East from 148 to 62 BC*. Berkeley: University of California Press.

Müller, Helmut (1987). "Ein Heilungsbericht aus dem Asklepieion." *Chiron* 17: 193–233.

Musurillo, Herbert (1954). *Acts of the Pagan Martyrs: Acta Alexandrinorum*. Oxford: Clarendon Press.

Nevett, Lisa C. (1999). *House and Society in the Ancient Greek World*. Cambridge: Cambridge University Press.

_____ (2002). "Continuity and Change in Greek Households under Roman Rule: The Role of Women in the Domestic Context." Pp. 81–100 in *Greek Romans and Roman Greeks: Studies in Cultural Interaction*, ed. Erik Nis Ostenfeld. Aarhaus Studies in Mediterranean Antiquity 3. Copenhagen: Aarhaus.

_____ (2010). *Domestic Space in Classical Antiquity*. New York: Cambridge University Press.

Newby, Zahra (2005). *Greek Athletics in the Roman World: Victory and Virtue*. Oxford: Oxford University Press.

Nicholls, Matthew C. (2011). "Galen and Libraries in the *Peri Alupias*." *Journal of Roman Studies* 101: 123–42.

Nicolet, Claude (2000). *Censeurs et publicains: Économie et fiscalité dans la Rome antique*. Paris: Fayard.

Nriagu, J. O. (1983a). *Lead and Lead Poisoning in Antiquity*. New York: Wiley.

_____ (1983b). "Saturnine Gout among Roman Aristocrats." *New England Journal of Medicine* 308: 660–63.

Nunn, J. F. (1989). "Anaesthesia in Ancient Times—Fact and Fable." Pp. 21–26 in *The History of Anaesthesia*, ed. Richard S. Atkinson and Thomas B. Boulton. International Congress and Symposium Series 134. London: Royal Society of Medicine Services.

Nutton, Vivian (1973). "The Chronology of Galen's Early Career." *Classical Quarterly* 23: 158–71. Reprinted in *From Democedes to Harvey: Studies in the History of Medicine*. London: Variorum (1988).

———— (1977). "Archiatri and the Medical Profession in Antiquity." *Papers of the British School at Rome* 45: 191–226. Reprinted in *From Democedes to Harvey: Studies in the History of Medicine*. London: Variorum (1988).

———— (1979). *Galen: On Prognosis*. Corpus Medicorum Graecorum 5.8.1. Berlin: Akademie-Verlag.

———— (1984a). "From Galen to Alexander: Aspects of Byzantine Medical Practice in Late Antiquity." *Dumbarton Oaks Papers* 38: 1–14.

———— (1984b). "Galen in the Eyes of His Contemporaries." *Bulletin of the History of Medicine* 58: 315–24. Reprinted in *From Democedes to Harvey: Studies in the History of Medicine*. London: Variorum (1988).

———— (1985). "The Drug Trade in Antiquity." *Journal of the Royal Society of Medicine* 78: 138–45. Reprinted in *From Democedes to Harvey: Studies in the History of Medicine*. London: Variorum (1988).

———— (1993). "Galen and Egypt." Pp. 11–32 in *Galen und das hellenistische Erbe*, ed. Jutta Kollesch and Diethard Nickel. Stuttgart: Steiner.

———— (1995a). "Galen ad multos annos." *Dynamis* 15: 25–39.

———— (1995b). "Galen and the Traveller's Fare." Pp. 359–70 in *Food in Antiquity*, ed. John Wilkins, David Harvey, and Mike Dobson. Exeter: University of Exeter Press.

———— (1995c). "The Medical Meeting-Place." Pp. 3–25 of vol. 1 in *Ancient Medicine in its Socio-Cultural Context*, ed. Ph. J. van der Eijk, H. F. J. Horstmanshoff, and P. H. Schrijvers. 2 vols. Amsterdam: Rodopi.

———— (1997). "Galen on Theriac: Problems of Authenticity." Pp. 133–52 in *Galen on Pharmacology: Philosophy, History, and Medicine*, ed. Armelle Debru. Studies in Ancient Medicine 16. Leiden: Brill.

———— (1999). *Galen: On My Own Opinions*. Corpus Medicorum Graecorum 5.3.2. Berlin: Akademie-Verlag.

———— (2004). *Ancient Medicine*. London: Routledge.

———— (2008). "The Fortunes of Galen." Pp. 355–390 in *The Cambridge Companion to Galen*, ed. R. J. Hankinson. Cambridge: Cambridge University Press.

———— (2009). "Galen's Library." Pp. 19–34 in *Galen and the World of Knowledge*, ed. Christopher Gill, Tim Whitmarsh, and John Wilkins. Cambridge: Cambridge University Press.

O'Malley, C. D. (1965). *Andreas Vesalius of Brussels: 1514–1564*. Berkeley: University of California Press.

Oberhelman, Steven M. (1983). "Galen, *On Diagnosis from Dreams*." *Journal of the History of Medicine and Allied Sciences* 38: 36–47.

_____ (1993). "Dreams in Graeco-Roman Medicine." *Aufstieg und Niedergang der römischen Welt* 2.37.1: 121–56.

Oliver, James Henry (1989). *Greek Constitutions of Early Roman Emperors from Inscriptions and Papyri*. Philadelphia: American Philological Society.

_____ and R. E. A. Palmer (1955). "Minutes of an Act of the Roman Senate." *Hesperia* 24: 320–49.

Osborn, Dale J., with Jana Osbornová (1998). *The Mammals of Ancient Egypt*. Warminster, UK: Aris & Phillips.

Oser-Grote, Carolin (1997). "Einführung in das Studium der Medizin: Eisagogische Schriften des Galen in ihrem Verhältnis zum Corpus Hippocraticum." Pp. 95–117 in *Gattungen wissenschaftlicher Literatur in der Antike*, ed. Wolfgang Kullmann, Johann Althoff, and Markus Asper. Tübingen: Narr.

Otte, Christoph (2001). *Galen: De plenitudine*. Serta Graeca: Beiträge zur Erforschung griechischer Texte 9. Weisbaden: Reichert.

Papagrigorakis, M. J., C. Yapijakis, P. N. Synodinos, and E. Baziotopoulou-Valavani (2006). "DNA Examination of Ancient Dental Pulp Incriminates Typhoid Fever as a Probable Cause of the Plague of Athens." *International Journal of Infectious Disease* 10.4: 334–35.

Papavramidou, Niki, and Helen Christopoulou-Aletra (2009). "The Ancient Technique of 'Gastrorrhaphy.'" *Journal of Gastrointestinal Surgery* 13: 1334–50.

Pearson, Richard D. (2009). "Malaria." *The Merck Manual for Healthcare Professionals*. http://www.merckmanuals.com/professional/sec15/ch197/ch197g.html#v1016553, accessed August 12, 2011.

Perkins, Judith (1995). *The Suffering Self: Pain and Narrative Representation in Early Christianity*. London: Routledge.

Peterson, Donald W. (1977). "Observations on the Chronology of the Galenic Corpus." *Bulletin of the History of Medicine* 51: 484–95.

Petit, Caroline (2009). *Galien*. Vol. 3, *Le médecin. Introduction*. Paris: Les Belles Lettres.

Petsalis-Diomidis, Alexia (2008). "The Body in the Landscape: Aristides' Corpus in the Light of the *Sacred Tales*." Pp. 131–50 in *Aelius Aristides between Greece, Rome, and the Gods*, ed. W. V. Harris and Brooke Holmes. Leiden: Brill.

_____ (2010). *'Truly Beyond Wonders': Aelius Aristides and the Cult of Asclepius*. Oxford: Oxford University Press.

Pigeaud, Jackie (1981). *La Maladie de l'âme: Étude sur la relation de l'âme et du corps dans la tradition médico-philosophique antique*. Paris: Les Belles Lettres.

_____ (1988). "La Psychopathologie de Galien." Pp. 154–83 in *Le opere psicologiche de Galeno*, ed. Paola Manuli and Mario Vegetti. Naples: Bibliopolis.

_____ (1997). "Les Fondements philosophiques de l'éthique médicale: Le Cas de Rome." Pp. 255–96 in *Médecine et morale dans l'antiquité*, ed. H. Flashar and J. Jouanna. Entretiens sur l'antiquité classique 43. Geneva: Hardt.

Pormann, Peter E. (2008). *Rufus of Ephesus: On Melancholy*. Tübingen: Mohr Siebeck.

Pormann, Peter E., and Emilie Savage-Smith (2007). *Medieval Islamic Medicine*. Edinburgh: Edinburgh University Press.

Potter, David (1999). "Entertainers in the Roman Empire." Pp. 303–25 in *Life, Death and Entertainment in the Roman Empire*, ed. D. S. Potter and D. J. Mattingly. Ann Arbor: University of Michigan Press.

_____ (2012). *The Victor's Crown: A History of Ancient Sport from Homer to Byzantium*. Oxford: Oxford University Press.

Powell, Owen (2003). *Galen on the Properties of Foodstuffs*. Cambridge: Cambridge University Press.

Quass, Friedemann (1993). *Die Honoratiorenschicht in den Städten des griechischen Ostens: Untersuchung zur politischen und sozialen Entwicklung in hellenistischer und römischer Zeit*. Stuttgart: Steiner.

Radt, Wolfgang (1999). *Pergamon: Geschichte und Bauten einer antiken Metropole*. Darmstadt: Primus.

Ramesh, H. A., Mohammad Azmathulla, Malay Baidya, and Mohammed Asad (2010). "Wound Healing Activity of Human Urine in Rats." *Research Journal of Pharmaceutical, Biological and Chemical Sciences* 1: 750–58.

Ramoutsaki, Ioanna A., Helen Askitopoulou, and Eleni Konsolaki (2002). "Pain Relief and Sedation in Roman Byzantine Texts: *Mandragoras officinarum, Hyosycamos niger* and *Atropa belladonna*." *International Congress Series* 1242: 43–50.

Retief, François Pieter, and Louise Cilliers (2011). "Breast Cancer in Antiquity." *South African Medical Journal* 101: 513–15.

Richardson, L., Jr. (1992). *A New Topographical Dictionary of Ancient Rome*. Baltimore: Johns Hopkins University Press.

Rickman, Geoffrey (1971). *Roman Granaries and Store Buildings*. Cambridge: Cambridge University Press.

Rives, James B. (2003). "Magic in Roman Law: The Reconstruction of a Crime." *Classical Antiquity* 22: 313–39.

Robert, Louis (1940). *Les Gladiateurs dans l'orient grec*. Paris: Champion. Reprinted Amsterdam: Hakkert (1971).

Rocca, Julius (2003). *Galen on the Brain: Anatomical Knowledge and Physiological Speculation in the Second Century A.D.* Leiden: Brill.

_____ (2008), "Anatomy." Pp. 242–62 in *The Cambridge Companion to Galen*, ed. R. J. Hankinson. Cambridge: Cambridge University Press.

Rutherford, R. B. (1989). *The Meditations of Marcus Aurelius: A Study*. Oxford: Clarendon.

Rütten, Thomas (1996). "Receptions of the Hippocratic Oath in the Renaissance: The Prohibition of Abortion as a Case Study in Reception." Tran. Leonie von Reppert-Bismarck. *Journal of the History of Medicine and Allied Sciences* 51: 456–83.

Saad, Bashar, and Omar Said (2011). *Greco-Arab and Islamic Herbal Medicine: Traditional System, Ethics, Safety, Efficacy, and Regulatory Issues*. Hoboken, NJ: Wiley.

Sallares, Robert (1991). *The Ecology of the Ancient Greek World*. Ithaca, NY: Cornell University Press.

———— (2002). *Malaria and Rome: A History of Malaria in Italy*. Oxford: Oxford University Press.

Saller, Peter (1982). *Personal Patronage under the Early Empire*. Cambridge: Cambridge University Press.

———— (1991). "Corporal Punishment, Authority, and Obedience in the Roman Household." Pp. 151–64 in *Marriage, Divorce, and Children in Ancient Rome*, ed. Beryl Rawson. Canberra: Humanities Research Center and Oxford: Clarendon.

Sandison, A. T., and Edmund Tapp (1998). "Disease in Ancient Egypt." Pp. 38–58 in *Mummies, Disease and Ancient Cultures*, ed. Aidan Cockburn, Eve Cockburn, and Theodore A. Reyman. 2d ed. Cambridge: Cambridge University Press.

Sandys-Winsch, Lucy, director (2009). "The Giraffe." Windfall Productions, "Inside Nature's Giants," London, Channel 4.

Sapolsky, Robert (2004). *Why Zebras Don't Get Ulcers*. 3d ed. New York: Macmillan.

Sarton, George. *Galen of Pergamon*. Lawrence: University of Kansas Press.

Sawday, Jonathan (1995). *The Body Emblazoned: Dissection and the Human Body in Reniassance Culture*. London: Routledge.

Scarborough, John (1971). "Galen among the Gladiators." *Episteme: Rivista critica delle scienze mediche e biologiche* 5: 98–111.

———— (1995). "The Opium Poppy in Hellenistic and Roman Medicine." Pp. 4–23 in *Drugs and Narcotics in History*, ed. Roy Porter and Mikuláš Teich. Cambridge: Cambridge University Press.

Scheidel, Walter (1999). "Emperors, Aristocrats and the Grim Reaper: Toward a Demographic Profile of the Roman Élite." *Classical Quarterly* 49: 254–81.

———— (2001a). *Death on the Nile: Disease and the Demography of Roman Egypt*. Leiden: Brill.

———— (2001b). "Roman Age Structure: Evidence and Models." *Journal of Roman Studies* 91: 1–26.

———— (2002). "A Model of Demographic and Economic Change in Roman Egypt after the Antonine Plague." *Journal of Roman Archaeology* 15: 97–114.

———— (2003). "Germs for Rome." Pp. 158–76 in *Rome the Cosmopolis*, ed. Catharine Edwards and Greg Woods. Cambridge: Cambridge University Press.

———— (2009) "Disease and Death in the Ancient City of Rome." Version 2.0. *Princeton-Stanford Working Papers in Classics*, April. http://www.princeton.edu/~pswpc/.

———— (2010a). "Physical Wellbeing in the Roman World." Version 2.0. *Princeton-Stanford Working Papers in Classics*, September. http://www.princeton.edu/~pswpc/.

Scheidel, Walter. (2010b) "Roman Well-Being and the Economic Consequences of the 'Antonine Plague.' Version 3.0. *Princeton-Stanford Working Papers in Classics*, January. http://www.princeton.edu/~pswpc.

Schlange-Schöningen, Heinrich (2003). *Die römische Gesellschaft bei Galen: Biographie und Sozialgeschichte*. Untersuchungen zur antiken Literatur und Geschichte 65. Berlin: de Gruyter.

Schmitz, Thomas (1997). *Bildung und Macht: Zur sozialen und politischen Funktion der zweiten Sophistik in der griechischen Welt der Kaiserzeit*. Munich: Beck.

Schneeberg, Norman G. (2002). "A Twenty-First Century Perspective on the Ancient Art of Bloodletting." *Transactions and Studies of the College of Physicians of Philadelphia* 24: 157–85.

Scobie, Alex (1986). "Slums, Sanitation and Mortality in the Roman World." *Klio* 68: 399–433.

Shaw, Brent (1984). "Bandits in the Roman Empire." *Past and Present* 105: 3–52.

Shchelkunov, Sergei N. (2011). "The Emergence and Re-Emergence of Smallpox: The Need for Development of a New Vaccine." *Vaccine* 295: D49–D53.

Sherwin-White, A. N. (1977). "Roman Involvement in Anatolia, 167–88 BC." *Journal of Roman Studies* 67: 62–75.

Shuttleton, David (2007). *Smallpox and the Literary Imagination, 1660–1820*. Cambridge: Cambridge University Press.

Singer, P. N. (1997). *Galen: Selected Works*. Oxford: Oxford University Press.

Smith, Dale C. (1996). "The Hippocratic Oath and Modern Medicine." *Journal of the History of Medicine and Allied Sciences* 51: 484–500.

Smith, Wesley D. (1979). *The Hippocratic Tradition*. Ithaca, NY: Cornell University Press.

Sorabji, Richard (2000). *Emotion and Peace of Mind: From Stoic Agitation to Christian Temptation*. Oxford: Oxford University Press.

Stone, Anne C., Alicia K. Wilbur, Jane E. Buikstra, and Charlotte A. Roberts (2009). "Tuberculosis and Leprosy in Perspective." *Yearbook of Physical Anthropology* 52: 66–94.

Strohmeier, Gotthard (2007). "La Longévité de Galien et les deux places de son tombeau." Pp. 393–403 in *La Science médicale antique: Nouveaux regards*, ed. Véronique Boudon-Millot, Alessia Guardasole, and Caroline Magdelaine. Paris: Beauschesne.

Swain, Simon (1996). *Hellenism and Empire: Language, Classicism, and Power in the Greek World A.D. 50–250*. Oxford: Clarendon.

———— (2006). "Beyond the Limits of Greek Biography: Galen from Alexandria to the Arabs." Pp. 395–433 in *The Limits of Ancient Biography*, ed. Brian McGing and Judith Mossman. Swansea: Classical Press of Wales.

Tecusan, Manuela (2004). *The Fragments of the Methodists*. Leiden: Brill.

Temkin, Oswei (1962). "Byzantine Medicine: Tradition and Empiricism." *Dumbarton Oaks Papers* 16: 95–115.

_____ (1971). *The Falling Sickness: A History of Epilepsy from the Greeks to the Beginnings of Modern Neurology*. 2d ed. Baltimore: Johns Hopkins University Press.

_____ (1973). *Galenism: The Rise and Decline of a Medical Philosophy*. Ithaca, NY: Cornell University Press.

_____ (1991). *Hippocrates in a World of Pagans and Christians*. Baltimore: Johns Hopkins University Press.

Thomas, Christine M. (1998). "The Sanctuary of Demeter at Pergamon: Cultic Space for Women and Its Eclipse." Pp. 278–97 in *Pergamon: Citadel of the Gods*, ed. Helmut Koester. Harvard Theological Studies 46. Harrisburg, PA: Trinity Press International.

Tieleman, Teun (2003). "Galen's Psychology." Pp. 131–61 in *Galien et la philosophie*, ed. Jonathan Barnes and Jacques Jouanna. Vandoeuvres-Geneva: Fondation Hardt.

Todman, Donald (2007). "A History of Caesarian Section from the Ancient World to the Modern Era." *Australian and New Zealand Journal of Obstetrics and Gynecology* 47: 367–71.

Totelin, Laurence M. V. (2004). "Mithradates' Antidote: A Pharmacological Ghost." *Early Science and Medicine* 9: 1–19.

Touwaide, Alain (1994). "Galien et la toxicologie." *Aufstieg und Niedergang der römischen Welt* 2.37.2: 1887–1986.

Tsuji, L. J. S., E. Nieboer, J. D. Karagatzides, and D. R. Koslovic (1997). "Elevated Dentine Lead Levels in Adult Teeth of First Nation People from an Isolated Region of Northern Ontario, Canada." *Bulletin of Environmental Contamination and Toxicology* 59: 854–60.

Tucci, Pier Luigi (2008). "Galen's Storeroom, Galen's Libraries and the Fire of A.D. 192." *Journal of Roman Archaeology* 21: 133–49.

_____ (2009). "Antium, the Palatium and the *Domus Tiberiana* Again." *Journal of Roman Archaeology* 22: 398–401.

Vallance, J. T. (1990). *The Lost Theory of Asclepiades of Bithynia*. Oxford: Clarendon.

van Bremen, Riet (1996). *The Limits of Participation: Women and Civic Life in the Greek East in the Hellenistic and Roman Periods*. Amsterdam: Gieben.

van der Eijk, Philip J. (2001). *Diocles of Carystus: A Collection of the Fragments with Translation and Commentary*. 2 vols. Leiden: Brill.

_____ (2009). "Aristotle! What a Thing for You to Say!: Galen's Engagement with Aristotle and Aristotelians." Pp. 261–81 in *Galen and the World of Knowledge*, ed. Christopher Gill, Tim Whitmarsh, and John Wilkins. Cambridge: Cambridge University Press.

van Nijf, Onno (1999). "Athletics, Festivals and Elite Self-Fashioning in the Roman East." *Proceedings of the Cambridge Philological Society* 45: 176–200.

_____ (2000). "Local Heroes: Athletics, Festivals and Elite Self-Fashioning in the Roman East." Pp. 306–34 in *Being Greek under Rome*, ed. Simon Goldhill. Cambridge: Cambridge University Press.

_____ (2003). "Athletics, *Andreia* and *Askesis*-Culture in the Roman East." Pp. 263–86 in *Andreia: Studies in Manliness and Courage in Classical Antiquity*, ed. Ralph Rosen and Ineke Sluiter. Leiden: Brill.

van Straten, F. T. (1981). "Gifts for the Gods." Pp. 65–151 in *Faith, Hope, and Worship: Aspects of Religious Mentality in the Ancient World*, ed. H. S. Versnel. Leiden: Brill.

Veyne, Paul (1976). *Le Pain et le cirque: Sociologie historique d'un pluralisme politique*. Paris: Seuil.

Ville, Georges (1981). *La Gladiature en occident des origines à la mort de Domitien*. Rome: Ecole française de Rome.

Vogt, Sabine (2008). "Drugs and Pharmacology." Pp. 304–22 in *The Cambridge Companion to Galen*, ed. R. J. Hankinson. Cambridge: Cambridge University Press.

von Hintzenstern, Ulrich (1989). "Anaesthesia with Mandrake in the Tradition of Dioscorides and Its Role in Classical Antiquity." Pp. 38–40 in *The History of Anaesthesia*, ed. Richard S. Atkinson and Thomas B. Boulton. International Congress and Symposium Series 134. London: Royal Society of Medicine Services.

von Staden, Heinrich (1982). "*Haeresis* and Heresy: The Case of the *haireseis iatrikai*." Pp. 76–100, 199–206 in *Jewish and Christian Self-Definition*, Vol. 3, *Self-Definition in the Greek and Roman World*, ed. Ben F. Meyer and E. P. Sanders. London: SCM.

_____ (1989). *Herophilus: The Art of Medicine in Early Alexandria*. Cambridge: Cambridge University Press.

_____ (1992). "The Discovery of the Body: Human Dissection and its Cultural Contexts in Ancient Greece." *Yale Journal of Biology and Medicine* 65: 223–41.

_____ (1995). "Anatomy as Rhetoric: Galen on Dissection and Persuasion." *Journal of the History of Medicine and Allied Sciences* 50: 47–66.

_____ (1996). "'In a Pure and Holy Way': Personal and Professional Conduct in the Hippocratic Oath?" *Journal of the History of Medicine and Allied Sciences* 51: 404–37.

_____ (1997a). "Galen and the 'Second Sophistic.'" Pp. 33–54 in *Aristotle and After*, ed. Richard Sorabji. *Bulletin of the Institute of Classical Studies*, Supplement 68. London: Institute of Classical Studies, School of Advanced Study, University of London.

_____ (1997b). "Gattung und Gedächtnis: Galen über Wahrheit und Lehrdichtung." Pp. 65–96 in *Gattungen wissenschaftlicher Literatur in der Antike*, ed. Wolfgang Kullmann, Jochen Althoff, and Markus Asper. Tübingen: Gunter Narr.

_____ (2000). "Body, Soul, and Nerves: Epicurus, Herophilus, Erasistratus, the Stoics, and Galen." Pp. 79–116 in *Psyche and Soma: Physicians and Metaphysicians on the Mind–Body Problem from Antiquity to the Enlightenment*, ed. John P. Wright and Paul Potter. Oxford: Clarendon.

_____ (2003). "Galen's *daimon*: Reflections on 'Irrational' and 'Rational.'" Pp. 15–44 in *Rationnel et irrationnel dans la médecine ancienne et médiévale: Aspects historiques, scientifiques et culturels*, ed. Nicholas Palmieri. Saint-Etienne: Publications de l'Université de Saint-Etienne.

_____ (2004). "Galen's Alexandria." Pp. 179–216 in *Ancient Alexandria between Egypt and Greece*, ed. W. V. Harris and Giovanni Ruffini. Columbia Studies in the Classical Tradition 26. Leiden: Brill.

_____ (2009). "Staging the Past, Staging Oneself: Galen on Hellenistic Exegetical Traditions." Pp. 132–56 in *Galen and the World of Knowledge*, ed. Christopher Gill, Tim Whitmarsh, and John Wilkins. Cambridge: Cambridge University Press.

Waite, J. G., and M. A. Daeschel (2007). "Contribution of Wine Components to Inactivation of Food-Borne Pathogens." *Journal of Food Science* 72: 286–91.

Walker, Philip L, Rhonda R. Bathurst, Rebecca Richman, Thor Gjerdrum, and Valerie A. Andrushko (2009). "The Causes of Porotic Hyperostosis and Cribra Orbitalia: A Reappraisal of the Iron-Defiency Anemia Hypothesis." *American Journal of Physical Anthropology* 139: 109–25.

Wallace-Hadrill, Andrew (1994). *Houses and Society in Pompeii and Herculaneum*. Princeton, NJ: Princeton University Press.

Walsh, Joseph (1927). "Galen Visits the Dead Sea and the Copper Mines of Cyprus." *Bulletin of the Geographical Society of Philadelphia* 25: 93–110.

_____ (1928). "Galen Clashes with the Medical Sects at Rome." *Medical Life* 35: 408–44.

_____ (1929). "The Date of Galen's Birth." *Annals of Medical History* n.s. 1: 378–82.

_____ (1930). "Galen's Second Sojourn in Italy, and his Treatment of the Family of Marcus Aurelius." *Medical Life* 37: 473–505.

_____ (1932). "Refutation of Ilberg as to the Date of Galen's Birth." *Annals of Medical History* n.s. 4: 126–46.

_____ (1937). "Galen's Studies at the Alexandrian School." *Annals of Medical History* 9: 132–43.

Walzer, R. (1944). *Galen on Medical Experience*. London: Oxford University Press for the Wellcome Trustees.

_____ (1949). *Galen on Jews and Christians*. London: Oxford University Press.

Wankel, Hermann (1979–84). *Inschriften von Ephesos*. Inschriften von griechischer Städte aus Kleinasien 11–17. Bonn: Habelt.

Ward, R. B. (1992). "Women in Baths." *Harvard Theological Review* 85: 125–47.

Watkins, Philip (2004). "Gratitude and Subjective Well-Being." Pp. 244–85 in *The Psychology of Gratitude*, ed. Robert A. Emmons and Michael E. McCullough. New York: Oxford University Press.

Watson, David (2005). "Rethinking the Mood and Anxiety Disorders." *Journal of Abnormal Psychology* 114: 522–36.

Watson, Gilbert (1966). *Theriac and Mithridatium: A Study in Therapeutics*. Publications of the Wellcome Historical Medical Library 9. London: The Wellcome Historical Medical Library.

Wear, Andrew (2008). "Place, Health, and Disease: *The Airs, Waters, Places* Tradition in Early Modern England and North America." *Journal of Medieval and Early Modern Studies* 38: 443–65.

White, L. Michael (1998). "Counting the Costs of Nobility: The Social Economy of Roman Pergamon." Pp. 331–65 in *Pergamon: Citadel of the Gods*, ed. Helmut Koester. Harvard Theological Studies 46. Harrisburg, PA: Trinity Press International.

White, Peter (2009). "Bookshops in the Literary Culture of Rome." Pp. 268–87 in *Ancient Literacies: The Culture of Reading in Greece and Rome*, ed. William A. Johnson and Holt N. Parker. Oxford: Oxford University Press.

Whitmarsh, Tim (2001). *Greek Literature and the Roman Empire: The Politics of Imitation*. Oxford: Oxford University Press.

Wiedemann, Thomas (1992). *Emperors and Gladiators*. London: Routledge.

Wilkins, John (2003). "Foreword." Pp. ix–xxi in Owen Powell, *Galen on the Properties of Foodstuffs*. Cambridge: Cambridge University Press.

Witt, Mathias (2009). *Weichteil- und Viszeralchirurgie bei Hippocrates*. Berlin: de Gruyter.

Wrigley, E. A. (1967). "A Simple Model of London's Importance in Changing English Society and Economy 1650–1750." *Past and Present* 37: 44–70.

Wulf-Rheidt, Ulrike (1998). "The Hellenistic and Roman Houses of Pergamon." Pp. 299–330 in *Pergamon: Citadel of the Gods*, ed. Helmut Koester. Harvard Theological Studies 46. Harrisburg, PA: Trinity Press International.

Yegül, Fikret (2010). *Bathing in the Roman World*. Cambridge: Cambridge University Press.

Zaminska, Nicholas (2007). "Videos Teach China's Rural Doctors." *Wall Street Journal*, July 10.

_____ (2008). "China's Village Doctors Take Great Strides." *Bulletin of the World Health Organization* (December): 914–15.

Zohary, David (2012). *Domestication of Plants in the Old World: The Origin and Spread of Domesticated Plants in Southwest Asia, Europe, and the Mediterranean Basin*. 4th ed. New York: Oxford University Press.

Zuiderhoek, Arjan (2009). *The Politics of Munificence in the Roman Empire: Citizens, Elites and Benefactors in Asia Minor*. Cambridge: Cambridge University Press.

INDEX